The Path of the Priestess

A Guidebook for Awakening the Divine Feminine

SHARRON ROSE

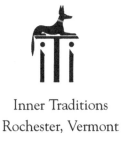

Inner Traditions

Rochester, Vermont

*This book is dedicated to my mother, Paula Bronfein Scherr,
to my guruji, Sitara Devi, and to all the wise women
and men throughout the ages whose eyes have never
strayed from the shining path of spirit.*

Inner Traditions
One Park Street
Rochester, Vermont 05767
www.InnerTraditions.com

LIBRARY OF CONGRESS CATALOGING-IN-PUBLICATION DATA

Rose, Sharron.
Path of the priestess : a guidebook for awakening the divine feminine
/ Sharron Rose.
p. cm.
Includes bibliographical references and index.
ISBN 978-0-89281-964-5
1. Women—Religious life. 2. Goddess religion. I. Title.
BL625.7 .R67 2002
291.4'4'082—dc21
2002151589

Printed and bound in the United States

10 9 8 7 6 5 4

Frontispiece: The author in the temple ruins of India.

This book was typeset in Goudy with Monsignor Elegant, Vivante, and
Avant Garde as the display typefaces
Text design by Priscilla Baker
Text layout by Virginia L. Scott Bowman

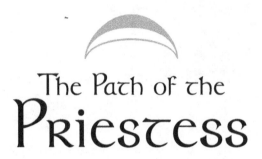

The Path of the
PRIESTESS

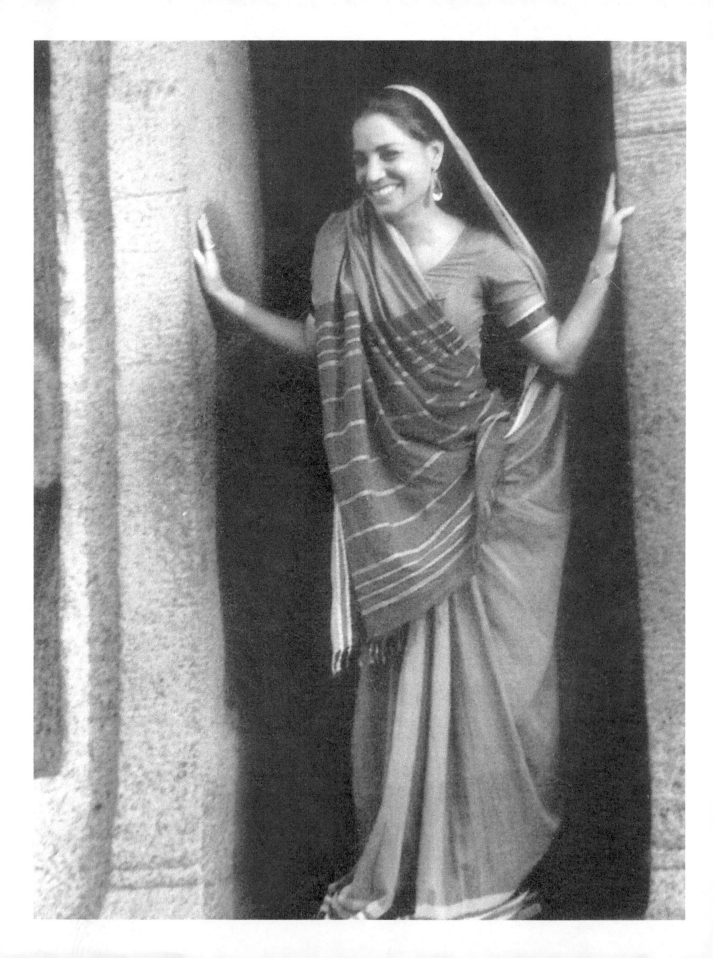

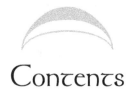

Contents

ACKNOWLEDGMENTS • vii

PREFACE • ix

Part One

Mystic Quest: A Modern-day Odyssey to Discover the Mysteries of the Goddess and Her Sacred Realms of Light • 1

1 THE CALL OF THE GODDESS • 2

2 THE DANCE OF THE DAKINI • 36

3 OPENING THE MYSTIC EYE • 67

4 THE KEEPERS OF THE LIGHT • 90

5 HISTORY AND THE FEMININE MYSTERIES:
REFLECTIONS ON THE CYCLE OF THE GREAT YUGA • 124

The Golden Age: The Age of Divinity • 128

The Silver Age: The Age of Ritual • 130

The Bronze Age: The Age of Doubt • 135

The Iron Age: The Age of Chaos • 140

The Time of Transition • 145

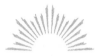

Part Two

Awakening the Divine Feminine • 149

6 LIFTING THE VEIL FROM THE FACE OF MODERNITY • 150
The Feminist Rebellion, Mind Control, and the Cult of Consumerism • 158
Our Modern Cultural Malaise • 163
Spiritual Materialism and the Birth of the New Age • 174
Reclaiming Our Sacred Heritage • 179

7 DISCOVERING STRENGTH AND POWER • 183
The Goddesses of Strength and Power • 184
The Myth of Durga • 189
The Energy Field of the Strong and Fiery Goddess • 194
The Feminine Art of Emotional Expression • 199
Expressions of Strength and Power • 201

8 EXPLORING SENSUALITY • 211
The Sensuous Goddesses • 212
The Legend of Mandarava • 220
The Energy Field of the Sensuous Goddess • 225
The Art of Sensuality • 231
Expressions of Sensuality • 232

9 EXPERIENCING LOVE AND COMPASSION • 242
The Goddesses of Love and Compassion • 243
The Story of Tara • 251
The Energy Field of the Peaceful Goddess • 255
The Art of Love and Compassion • 259
Expressions of Love and Compassion • 260

EPILOGUE • 270

NOTES • 272
BIBLIOGRAPHY • 281
INDEX • 288

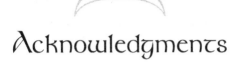

Acknowledgments

o book is written in a vacuum. There are so many factors and forces that merge to bring about a work of art, so many experiences and interactions that add to its import. How can I adequately pay tribute to the contributions of teachers, friends, family, and students who have encouraged and assisted me throughout a lifetime of learning? So many have opened their hearts and minds to me over the years, filling my life with great depth and meaning. To all of you I am grateful.

Foremost, I wish to thank my husband, Jay Weidner, whose love, devotion, and insight has sustained and assisted me through the process of writing this book. It was his belief in my capacity to transmit the wealth of my research and experience in an eloquent and meaningful way that gave me the strength and incentive to take up the task of writing this book. Our days and nights of passionate discussions concerning the essential nature of Tantra and alchemy, the history of humanity and the political milieu in which we currently abide, provided me with great fuel for *The Path of the Priestess*.

I would like to express my profound gratitude to my parents, Paula Scherr and Herbert Beckenheimer, who gave me the strength, courage, and support to pursue my dreams, even when they took me into cultures and teachings that appeared to be very different from their own. And of course to my son, Ari Ben Weiner, who has traveled so much of this path by my side.

I would also like to thank those whose knowledge and insights have contributed to the dominant themes inherent in *The Path of the Priestess*. Janet Fine, Tim and Vicki Richards, Bhanu Atthaiya, Bikram and Gina Khan, Shantilal Somaiya, Dr. Jivan Pani, Antonia Minnecola, Mark Weiner, Sister Kiran, and Roy Ulery for their insights into the art, culture, and spiritual traditions of India. Paul Leake, Shanti Shivani, and Louise Landes-Levi for their work in the field of Indian classical music and the Indo-Tibetan tradition. David Sharp, Dr. Miranda Shaw, Clark Johnson, John Reynolds, and Kyu and

Dr. Steven Goodman of the Dzogchen community for their insights into Tibetan Tantra and Dzogchen, as well as my dear friend Pat Johnson for the many hours of thought-provoking discussions concerning Tibetan Buddhism, healing, the nature of mind, and the feminine principle. Marcus Daniels, Dr. Celeste Pepe, Dr. Alberto Villoldo, and Frank Lowen for their teachings in the realm of healing, John Nichols for his knowledge and assistance with the texts of ancient Egypt, Gerry Kessler for his insights into early Christianity, and Vincent Bridges and Darlene for their astute work in the areas of the Egyptian mysteries and gnosticism. I also would like to express my immense gratitude to Darlene, sacred artist and priestess of Sekhmet, for the beautiful goddess illustrations and line drawings that adorn *The Path of the Priestess* and bring the sacred teachings to life. Thanks also to visionary artist Alex Grey for the use of his powerful images of the luminous energy body.

Throughout the writing process there were friends who nursed me through both the excitement and the frustration inherent in the creation of this work. I am grateful to Jill Bittinger, Dr. Kimerer La Mothe, Pedram Shojai, Annie Hickman, Lee Torchia, Simone Temkin, Laura Hungerford, Deborah Salt, Elena Johnston, Blanca Rose, Brian Beckenheimer, Cindy Hiller, Barbara Goldenberg, Shannon Dye, Amy Looker, Alex and Allyson Grey, John Major Jenkins, Jonathan Goldman, Laura Lea Cannon, David Tresemer, and Adelina Alva Padilla, for their support in this process.

For many years I have had great respect for the quality, focus, and artistic excellence of the books that Inner Traditions publishes. From the inception of *The Path of the Priestess* it was my wish to have it published by Inner Traditions. Needless to say I was delighted when my wish was fulfilled. I would like to thank those who I have had the privilege of working with during the birthing of this book: my project editor, Susan Davidson, for her questions and comments, which provoked deep contemplation in me; Jon Graham, for our fascinating conversations concerning the sacred mysteries; Jeanie Levitan, for overseeing all aspects of production; Robin Catalano, for her thorough copyediting; and publisher Ehud Sperling, who provided me with the forum to express myself through the medium of the written word.

Finally I would like to express my deepest gratitude to my teachers Sitara Devi, Chogyal Namkhai Norbu Rinpoche, and Dr. Robert Masters for their devotion to the preservation of the sacred knowledge of the ancestors. It is through their generosity and blessings that I, an American woman, have been able to enter into and drink from the fountain of their ancient lineages of transmission and directly experience the light, energy, and ecstatic bliss of the Divine Feminine.

I pay homage to the goddesses and dakinis who have filled my life with beauty and grace. May their selfless love, wisdom, and compassion continue to enlighten the hearts and minds of us all.

Preface

There is a sacred current of light that runs throughout time and space—the light of the Divine Feminine. It is a continuum. It arises at the birth of creation and forms a sacred path into the denseness of matter and back again. As we descend from the fullness of this light into the depths of the material world, this light is always present to nourish and sustain us. Flowing through all our lives and incarnations, it is the vital and transformative current of truth, virtue, and integrity, a shining stream of spiritual essence that leads us along the path of emanation to the path of return and reunion with the primordial source.

As women, as mothers, as teachers and guides, as emissaries of the Great Goddess, it is our sacred duty and privilege to hold this current of light in our hearts and carry it from generation to generation. This is our essential role as women: to hold this pure light of Divinity in our hearts, to keep the lamp of inner freedom burning in the darkness, to nurture and protect this light whatever the cost, and to transmit its radiance, its exquisite beauty, to our men and children.

Once upon a time, before the days of darkness and oppression of our sacred women's mysteries, we knew that we were living emanations of the Goddess, that as women, mothers, priestesses, and spiritual guides, our primary role was to be a conduit for her sacred current. Knowing that every thought, every action had a profound impact upon not only our own lives and those of our men and children, but on the very fabric of life itself, we created exercises and rituals to purify our bodies, minds, and hearts. In the midst of the forest, on the mountaintops, along the riverbanks and the shores of the sea, in the temples and monasteries, we would gather together to perform these sacred rites. We danced by the light of the moon, raised our voices in song and prayer, conversed with the myriad forms of divinity through our sacred gestures, and sat together in silent communion with them. Knowing the Great Goddess was our Primordial Mother and source of all life, we treated her with immense respect. As her priestesses, we offered our lives to her service. We gave her offerings. As her emissaries, we dressed in her image and emulated her extraordinary qualities.

With each heartbeat we attuned ourselves to her primal rhythms. With each inhalation and exhalation we opened ourselves to feel her divine radiance pouring through us, continuously cleansing and enlivening our bodies, minds, and luminous energy fields. Deeply in tune with her presence, we knew how to expand our senses and send out subtle waves of feeling-consciousness through the great matrix of interconnecting energetic paths that exist between her physical and numinous realms. With our feet firmly grounded upon the earth we would allow our awareness to extend through her vibratory dimensions as we monitored the ebb and flow of the visible and invisible landscapes.

Today, living in the midst of a society that has all but forgotten her, so few of us even know that the Goddess exists, let alone spend time conversing with her, feeling the power of her touch, reveling in the beauty of her myriad manifestations. For until we have a direct experience of her presence, how can we truly know her?

Like the vast majority of women growing up in America in the 1950s and 1960s, I grew up in a world dominated by patriarchal goals and values. As I moved toward adulthood I began to open my eyes to the multitude of problems that appeared to stem from the mental programming imposed upon us by this male-dominated, materialistic society. Inspired by the ideals of the feminist movement, my visionary capacity expanded through the use of psychedelics and my spirit enlivened by the teachings of the Eastern mystics, I began to wake up to the knowledge that I was living under the influence of a culturally-imposed trance that oriented me toward a way of life clearly opposed to my true spiritual nature. Confused by this dilemma I began to ask myself if this was the only path open to me. Or was there a deeper, more integrated path that I as woman could follow, one that was more conducive to my true feminine nature?

And so I embarked upon an amazing journey of discovery. At the heart of this journey lay a desire to discover and attune myself to the most sacred idealized vision of the feminine as it existed in cultures throughout the world.

This journey led me far from the shores of my birth, along strange pathways, deep into the heart of ancient civilizations. It led me to a time much different from our modern age, a time of grace, beauty, and sophistication, a time of harmony and balance. A time when sensuality was considered sacred and the female body the holy alchemical vessel of creation and transformation, when the sacred was expressed through dance, music, myth, geometry, art, and architecture. This was the age of the great civilizations of Egypt, Sumeria, India, Tibet, and Persia. What I have gleaned from this journey, this heartfelt quest for an understanding of the feminine in her human and divine manifestations, constitutes the essence of this book.

Part one, "Mystic Quest," describes my years of research and experience in these sacred mysteries. As I immersed myself in the teachings and practices of classical Indian dance, Tantra, Dzogchen, healing, alchemy, and gnosticism, I discovered that in ancient times there were sacred schools, societies, temples, and artistic traditions in which women, the Goddess, and the feminine principle were esteemed and venerated. As temple priestesses, yoginis, healers, prophetesses, and soror mysticas, women performed their essential and vital roles in society. Part one provides you with an intimate look at the living remnants of the sacred teachings and spiritual paths that support feminine values and provide time-honored techniques for self-awareness and spiritual illumination.

As a conclusion to part one, I offer you a very different view of history than the one taught in our schools and universities. This perspective concerns the cyclic flow of the four ages, or *yugas*, of humanity as revealed in tantric and alchemical texts. These teachings put forward an ancient yet powerful view of human history and the changing relationships between male and female, and between humanity and divinity. They also provide new insight into humanity's changing views toward nature and the feminine principle, the body and sexuality, and the fundamental and significant role of women in society.

From this introduction into the ancient mysteries, part two, "Awakening the Divine Feminine," begins with an analysis of the deep spiritual and cultural issues that face us as women of the twenty-first century. It is my belief that over the years our dreams for equality, respect, and acknowledgment of our essential feminine nature have been appropriated and distorted by the dominant forces of the modern world. Chapter 6 examines the issues and frustrations inherent in our current society's conditioning of and expectations for women, while contrasting them with the more spiritually attuned ways of the ancients. For many years now we have been living amidst a society that teaches us to constantly look outside of ourselves for answers to our problems, to numb our emotions through pharmaceuticals or forget our deep-seated concerns by losing ourselves in the superficial world presented to us by television and the media. But now, with all the horror and madness that surrounds us, many of us are beginning to realize that to find the solutions to the fears, uncertainties, and nightmares, like our ancestors before us we must look within. And when one looks deeply enough, she (or he) comes face to face with the Great Goddess. For without her divine animating presence, all life would cease to exist.

Therefore, in keeping with the teaching methods of traditional cultures, this book is designed to offer you not only an intellectual understanding of the role of woman and the Goddess but the means by which you can begin to look within and attune yourself to her powerful, integrative, and healing current. Beginning with stories and myths of the goddesses of strength and power, sensuality, and love and compassion, chapters 7, 8, and 9 are filled with meditations and visualizations designed to assist you in your own process of spiritual awakening. Each chapter focuses upon a particular aspect of female embodiment and includes sacred images and descriptions of the specific goddesses to be invoked and embodied; a visualization for perceiving and cleansing the luminous energy body that envelops and permeates the physical, freeing the mind of negative thoughts and feelings and filling you with renewed strength and vitality; and a comprehensive vocabulary of expressions and glances based upon the many moods, manifestations, and feelings of the enlightened goddesses.

If, like so many of us modern women, you have had little or no training in the ways of old, in the power of meditation, prayer, song, and dance, it does not mean that the doors to the sacred inner sanctum of the goddess are closed to you. You need only knock, and the Goddess will answer.

PART

1

Mystic Quest:
A Modern-day Odyssey
to Discover the Mysteries of
the Goddess and
Her Sacred Realms of Light

1

The Call of the Goddess

*Dancing is an ancient form of magic. The dancer
becomes amplified into a being endowed with supra-
normal powers. His/her personality is transformed.
Like yoga, the dance induces trance, ecstasy, the
experience of the divine; the realization of one's own
secret nature, and, finally, emergence into the divine
essence. . . . The dance is an act of creation. It
brings about a new situation and summons into the
dancer a new and higher personality. It has a
cosmogonic function, in that it arouses dormant
energies which then may shape the world.*

—HEINRICH ZIMMER, *MYTHS AND SYMBOLS IN INDIAN
ART AND CIVILIZATION*

ombay, 1983. As I stepped outside the crowded airport with
my three-year-old son, Ari, by my side, it was as if I had
entered a bizarre, almost nightmarish landscape. Twenty-
four hours ago we had left our home in Boston to travel
through New York and London, finally arriving at our destination. As I disembarked from the plane my nostrils were
assaulted by the smells of Indian life: the pungent odors of curry
and incense and, most of all, human sweat.

After making my way through the bureaucratic maze known as customs, where I
was asked a seemingly by never-ending series of questions concerning the nature of
my visit, I finally emerged onto the street. Taking Ari's small hand in mind, I looked
down to see his big blue eyes fill with wonder. It was still the early hours of the morn-

ing, before the dawn, yet the airport exit was filled with hundreds of people from all classes of society. Even though I had once lived amid the cultural diversity of New York, I had never experienced anything like this before. Wealthy women with golden bracelets adorning their wrists and colorful flowing saris draped around them ran up to greet their returning relatives. Men—some in Western-style business suits and others in more traditional dhotis and lunghis—hurried by me to greet their families, speaking words that were totally foreign to my ears.

All of a sudden I was surrounded by a large group of Indian men, all trying their best to address me in their broken English, wanting to be of some kind of assistance. Some tried to take hold of my luggage, others approached me crying out, "Taxi, Memsahib, taxi?" I was exhausted and overwhelmed, just trying to hold on to both Ari and my luggage. Out of the mass of humanity a thin twenty-year-old Indian man with a photo of me in his hand suddenly appeared, a welcoming smile on his face. "Sharron, are you Sharron?" he said. "I am Ravi, and I have been sent here by my aunt Sitara Devi to find you. Come, she is waiting to greet you." Ravi kneeled down to greet Ari face to face, saying "and you must be Ari. I'm going to call you Ari Krishna because you look so much like our lord Krishna when he was a little boy."

After Ravi deftly scooped up Ari with one hand and directed the baggage handlers to place our belongings on their motorized rickshaws, we stepped up onto the lead rickshaw. In a flash we were off into the Bombay night. As the colors, sounds, and smells of the strange city enveloped us I began to reflect on the remarkable circumstances that had led me to this strange place and time.

I was born in 1949 into a middle-class Jewish family in Baltimore, Maryland. As I was endowed with a sensitive and passionate nature, my mother, a highly educated woman who had received extensive artistic training, believed that the best way to harness the waves of deep emotion that flowed through me was through the performing arts. During this time most middle-class Jewish parents in America felt that a thorough education in the arts would enable their daughters to develop the sophistication and grace that would make them more attractive to their prospective husbands. But my mother sensed that like her, I had an innate gift for theatrical expression, and so she nourished my creative potential by enrolling me in singing, dancing, piano, and acting classes. Through this immersion in the exacting disciplines of classical ballet, opera, and theater I was not only given the tools with which to refine my physical body but a means by which I could pour out my feelings and insights.

By the time I reached college it was the late 1960s, when the winds of change were sweeping across the face of America. I had been born into a generation of

American women who rebelled against the seemingly subservient roles society offered them. In college and later in graduate school I became frustrated by the limited and one-dimensional theatrical roles written for women, and so I immersed myself in the literature of feminism—of women fighting for recognition in a world that was essentially designed to support male values, goals, and experiences. Fueled by this new expression of feminine power, I left behind my parents' dreams for marriage and family and came under the guidance of an extraordinary female dance teacher named Maida Withers. Later in Manhattan I studied under dance luminaries such as Twyla Tharp, Merce Cunningham, and Louis Falco, immersing myself in the intellectually stimulating world of American modern dance. This was a world in which I found great creative freedom, and a world in which I was encouraged to choreograph my own roles, work together with other artists and musicians, and create innovative dance-theater productions that spoke of the issues of our times.

In the mid-1970s I left the intensely competitive artistic atmosphere of New York City and made my way to Boston, where my training helped me find work as a teacher of modern dance, improvisation, and choreography. At this time I became inspired by the modern Western science of psychology, particularly the symbolic work of Carl Jung and the energetic body-oriented work of Wilhelm Reich and Alexander Lowen. I encountered this work after many years of training in theater, in which I had learned to read and interpret people's thoughts and feelings by observing their movements, facial expressions, and tone of voice. Not only had I learned to be aware of this aspect of people's energetic displays, but I also had become aware of the manner in which the expression of emotion by one person would trigger a wave of response in someone else. I had spent my life observing; I had just watched everybody. I had watched how people walked, how they used their bodies and their gestures, how they sent subtle messages through their eyes and hands. Through my studies of the work of Jung, Reich, and Lowen, I found confirmation of my insights into human nature and systems by which I could enhance my knowledge of the relationship between the mind and the body. Consequently I began to create fairly large-scale theatrical productions that often dealt with the profound relationship between the physical and psychological dimensions of life.

As the rickshaw abruptly jerked to the right I was jostled out of this wave of remembrance. The driver had made this sudden maneuver to avoid running into a cow that was silently making her way through the center of the street. What a strange and exotic place this is, I thought.

As we continued to speed through the outskirts of Bombay toward the heart of the city, my eyes took in a world and a way of life that was very different from any that I, as a sheltered American, had ever experienced. Huge concrete apartment buildings were surrounded by what appeared to be hundreds of dwellings made of tin or even cardboard boxes. People were everywhere. Some, like the street people of Manhattan, appeared to be sleeping in the entranceways of buildings. A number of women dressed in brightly colored saris stood outside before their cooking fires, making an early-morning meal for their families. Others walked through the streets carrying baskets of fruit on their heads. Men scurried about, some moving slowly, others rapidly making their way through the increasingly crowded byways. As I turned my head to view more of this wild atmosphere my weary eyes beheld the familiar sight of the sun rising in the hazy morning sky. I closed my eyes for a moment in an attempt to shut out all this stimulation, but my mind was suddenly filled with the memory of another remarkable experience, one that would dramatically change my life.

As a young woman of the psychedelic generation I was always seeking out new doorways to creative expression, and I had heard tales about the visionary power of psilocybin mushrooms. For years friends had encouraged me to experience the mysteries of the mushrooms. I had purchased a large bag of these purple fungi and boiled them into a cup of tea, which I quickly drank while seated on the edge of a rocky cliff overlooking the beach on Martha's Vineyard.

I suddenly fell into a swoon. As my senses expanded my body trembled uncontrollably, and my heart beat rapidly in my chest. Waves of energy washed through me, filling me with a sense of restlessness and fear. My neck and throat felt unbearably constricted, my mouth dry and pasty. I wondered, *Have I poisoned myself by taking too many of these?* My once firm grasp of reality was rapidly fading. Lost in the wild intensity of the experience, I felt as though I was dying. Everything around me was slowly dissolving into blackness, and the familiar being who called herself Sharron no longer existed. I was overwhelmed by the power and potency of the sacred plant, and I became consumed with the fear of death. I felt as if I was being flung headlong into a great empty void from which there could be no return.

In the midst of this terror a small voice within instructed me to close my eyes and focus on my breath—to concentrate on the simple process of breathing in and out. As I followed the instructions I began to relax and the knot of fear that gripped my solar plexus loosened. At the moment that I surrendered to the endless well of darkness, the scene changed and I found myself floating on a vast primordial ocean of light and energy. A great streaming current of light began to flow up my spine, rushing upward and pouring out from the top of my head like a fountain. Swirling vortices of light emerged and spread out around me, forming what appeared to be a radiant, multicolored cocoonlike web. Aroused by the subtle beauty of this astonishing play of light, the dancer in me awoke. I began to automatically move my hands and arms in intricate patterns that seemed natural to me, as if I had repeated them thousands of times. I opened my eyes to behold the image of a great luminous male deity seated in the sky before me, bearing witness to my dance. It seemed that I was performing this dance for him. The dance was incredibly intricate, its focus being the perfect harmony of gesture, posture, and expression. It felt as if each movement or expression was creating that moment of awareness. All I perceived, and the entire world around me, seemed born from this fluid, all-encompassing dance of life.

As the journey continued, what I later came to know as the sacred ritual dance of India flowed through and out of my being. Simply, naturally, as easily as breathing in and out, a wealth of subtle and sophisticated movements and expressions I had never seen or experienced came through me. As the profound joy of the experience pervaded my body, light emanated from me. Each inner feeling, each blink of the eye or movement of the hand, seemed to imbue the world around me with ripples of multicolored light and energy. I was transformed into a goddess, weaving this magical display and performing a dreamlike dance for the powerful deity seated before me. Every movement, every feeling, and every glance was done for both his delight and my own. Only later, when I began the work that would eventually lead me to this wild ride through the smoky streets of Bombay, did I understand the nature of what had occurred. In those moments, overtaken by the power of the magic mushroom, the veils between the worlds had parted and from the depths of my being—beyond the boundaries of time and space—a path much different from any that I had ever imagined opened for me.

In the course of a lifetime there are moments when magic happens, when outer circumstances and events seem to spontaneously arise like signposts that lead you into new levels of experience and awareness, beckoning you to a deeper realm of knowing. Like the odd pieces of a puzzle fitting together perfectly, these situations and experiences build on each other, mysteriously propelling you toward a new direction and destiny.

After this breakthrough experience my world suddenly shifted. I was amazed to discover that one of the instructors in the same school in which I taught modern dance was the former director of the National Dance Company of Pakistan. A generous warm-hearted teacher who had spent his life immersed in the classical dance forms of India, Dulal Talukdar introduced me to the technique and beginning repertory of the three main schools of Indian classical dance: Bharat Natyam, Manipuri, and Kathak.

I found all these styles fascinating, but I was especially drawn to Kathak. Dulal, a

Muslim of Bengali origin, focused on the secular technical aspects of the form, which was a unique part of the court entertainment of the Moghuls, whose invasion and rule of northern India had begun in the twelfth century. The Moghuls were from Persia, a land whose music, dance, poetry, and architecture retained influences from the ancient Zoroastrian and Egyptian cultures. Amid the elegant and sumptuous atmosphere of the Moghul courts, dances were created that celebrated individual expression and the technical virtuosity of the artist. Focus was placed on rhythm, line, form, and the expression of emotional states, particularly those of passion and seduction. Throughout my training Dulal always alluded to the fact that Kathak's deeper spiritual import sprang

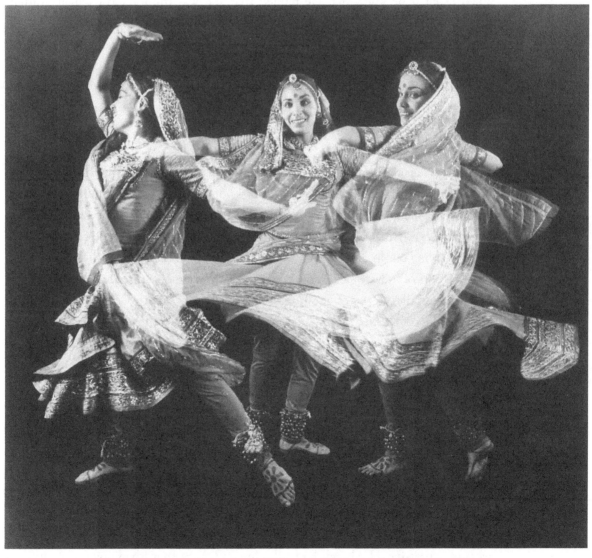

The author as a dancer in the Moghul court. Photograph by Christopher Harting.

from the ancient Vedic tradition of India.[1] As my lessons intensified, it became clear to me that in order to fully experience this ancient art form I must travel to the source, Mother India, and learn directly from a Hindu woman.

A rapid succession of events occurred to make my trip possible. I had told Dulal of my intention to apply for a fellowship to study in India, and that I needed to find a teacher. Since I was always searching for texts and other references to help me more clearly understand the nature of the Indian culture and its myths, legends, and art forms, Dulal loaned me a book titled *The Dance in India* by Enakshi Bhavani. When I took the book in my hands it fell open to reveal a series of photographs of a beautiful female Kathak dancer named Sitara Devi. I was captivated by these images, and asked Dulal if he knew her. He replied that she was the foremost female Kathak dancer in India and the only one with whom he would want me to study.[2]

Good fortune then caused me to meet one of India's most renowned musicians, Ustad Imrat Khan, who, after watching me dance, recommended me to both his longtime friend Sitara Devi and the American Institute for Indian Studies. I was on my way to meeting the amazing woman who was to become my guide, mentor, and guruji.

The streets became more and more crowded as we drove through Bombay. Every time we stopped at a traffic crossing we were surrounded by downtrodden and forlorn-looking men, women, and children—some missing an arm or a leg, some with bandaged leprosy-ridden hands, all bringing their hands to their mouths in the gesture of eating and crying out in desperation, "Bakshish, bakshish." Ravi, who was familiar with these beggars of India, quickly shooed them away. Then he continued to ask both Ari and me an endless series of questions about our life in America. Ravi entranced Ari with his tales of Krishna, whose picture was one of many that adorned the dashboard of the rickshaw.

After what seemed like an eternity we arrived at the apartment of Sitara Devi. As we approached Sitara's door I was extremely nervous; my hands were clammy and shaking and my whole body was covered with sweat. I had left behind my husband, who was continuing the blossoming law practice that made it inconceivable for him to accompany Ari and me on this journey. Looking down at Ari and thinking about my family's concern for his welfare I wondered if I had really made the right decision. But as soon as Sitara Devi opened the door and welcomed me into her life, I knew I had made the right decision.

What I remember most about our initial meeting were her hands and eyes; they were so expressive. Her hands had a fluidity and grace that I had never encountered before. When she spoke, every thought she conveyed was being transmitted to me through her words and through the exquisite language of gesture she called *mudra*. Her eyes were so alive and filled with fire, her every expression adding to the power and beauty of her story. As I watched her the magnetic power of her eyes seemed to reinforce the eloquence of her gestures, evoking deep inner feelings in me.

Sitara introduced me to the members of her family: her son, Ranjit, a handsome twenty-one-year-old jazz drummer who had grown up in both London and Bombay; her elder sister, Tara, who sat on the couch with an orange sari draped around her; and her sister-in-law, known as Mommy, who was Ravi's mother. Then she took me to the room that Ari and I would share. Finally she showed me her own room, which she shared with Ranjit when he was not away on tour. As I looked at the room I was instantly taken aback. Sitara quickly sat me down and asked me what was the matter. I looked into her eyes, took a deep breath, and considered what I was about to reveal.

I had always been quite a dreamer. Throughout my childhood and into my adult life I had experienced what I came to know as lucid dreams. I would fly through the air, meet with friends, or speak to a relative who had passed from this world. In my college days, inspired by the symbolic dream work of Carl Jung and the out-of-body experiences of Robert Monroe, I began to consciously work on my dreaming. I even gained the ability to occasionally leave my body and travel into other dimensions where I met odd beings with wings or glowing eyes, and sometimes a special silver-haired woman whose body was covered with breasts. As I related these experiences to Sitara she closed her eyes and smiled knowingly, as if to her they were a very natural part of life. I was filled with joy that I had found a woman who might be able to understand these abilities and even help me to enhance them. I began to tell her the unusual tale of how I had first met her in a dream.

As sometimes happens in my dream state, I found myself flying through the starry blackness of the night sky. Conscious that I had left my body sleeping in the bed below, I knew that I was free to journey beyond the usual boundaries of space and time and that I could choose my destination. I consciously focused my mind on my desire to meet Sitara. Immediately I became a tiny ball of light traveling with great velocity through a dark womblike tunnel. After a few moments my consciousness came to rest in Sitara's room. There she was, lying on the very same bed I now beheld in my waking life. Sitara quickly looked up, her eyes flashing. It was as if she instantly recognized that someone or something was there. Her expression was immensely powerful, unlike any I had ever seen from a woman before. I was so startled by its beauty and intensity that I instantly awoke.

I stopped speaking for a moment, overcome by the strange magic of this experience. I slowly surveyed the room, taking in every detail. Then I looked into Sitara's receptive eyes and in a voice filled with emotion said, "Now I see that I really did make my way here. I saw this whole room in my dream: the bed with its white sheets, the dressing table, and cupboard. Most important of all, I saw you. I really did find you in my dream. It must have been the power of your eyes that called me."

After listening intently to my tale Sitara looked at me with that same powerful expression I had seen in my dream. This was an expression that I soon discovered transmitted the rich fiery energy of the goddess Durga, the strong and powerful goddess whose energy so dominated Sitara's life. I later came to believe that Sitara was a living incarnation of Durga, whose myth is included in chapter 7.

"It is clear to me," Sitara said, "that the Goddess has brought us together. Take rest; you have had a long journey. You need your strength. We have much work to do."

As a young American woman, a scholar, and a dancer, I had arrived in India with a mind full of preconceived notions about what I would encounter. I had been imprinted with the American media's version of Eastern spirituality, and I imagined that my teacher would be an exceedingly peaceful, serene woman who when not dancing would sit for hours on her meditation cushion in a constant state of bliss. But all my preconceptions were turned upside down. Sitara was a wild and free-spirited woman. Through the first days and nights that we sat together and she told me the story of her life, I came to recognize that unlike most women of her time Sitara had pushed herself beyond every boundary that modern Indian society had built. Sitara had been recognized for her artistic abilities from early childhood, and by the age of sixteen she had been given the title "Queen of Kathak" by India's Nobel prize-winning poet laureate Rabindranath Tagore. Within the next few years Sitara had become a rising star in India's early film industry. But as with many modern women, her fame came with a price. The passionate Sitara married and divorced twice. Both husbands desired her for her fire, beauty, and artistry, but as soon as she married, each one tried to stop her from performing, wanting her to leave dance behind and become a dutiful servant and caretaker. Sitara tried, but her devotion to her calling was stronger than the restrictions that the society placed on her. Clearly this conflict caused her much pain. When I met Sitara she was sixty years old and totally fed up with the repressive nature of her society, and so she gave herself fully to her art and her goddess. As she sat on her sofa reminiscing about her life and her sacred tradition, with her two small fluffy white dogs by her side, she reminded me of a Hollywood movie star from the silent film era.

One evening as Ari and I sat together with Sitara in her living room, I looked up

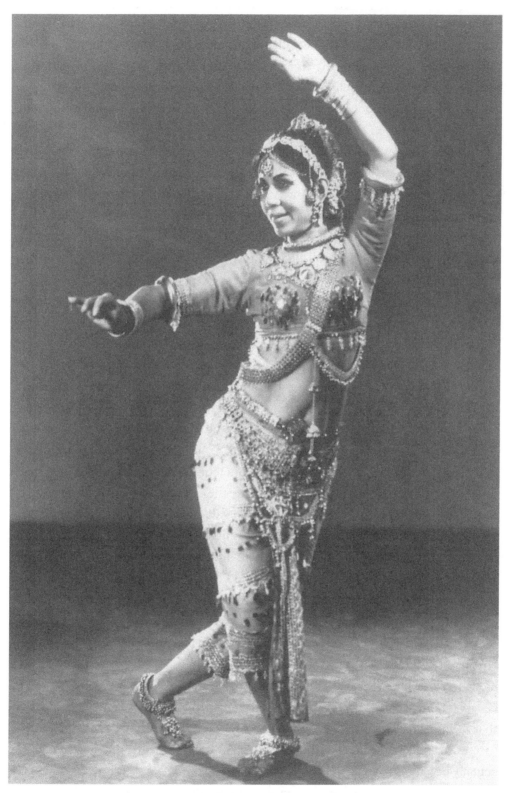

Sitara Devi, photograph courtesy of Sitara Devi.

to see a very prominent and powerful image of a beautiful goddess with many arms who was dressed in red and seated gallantly astride a lion. "Please, Guruji," I asked, "tell me about the Goddess. She seems to be so important in your life. In the Jewish tradition of my birth, as well as the Christian religion that dominates the West, we are told that there is only one God and he is definitely male. In our world, your Goddess does not even exist."

Sitara closed her eyes for a moment and quieted her breath as if going into a deep meditative state. The atmosphere of the whole room seemed to change. The power and energy that flowed through Sitara was so strong that chills ran up my spine. She began to speak, her voice filled with passion. "There is a sacred current of light that flows throughout all of creation," she explained. "It is the animating and nourishing force of life itself, the supreme all-illuminating power and energy in every thing and every being. We call this light and energy Shakti, or the Great Goddess. Once, at the beginning of time, before the world was created, Shakti was at one with her divine consort, Shiva, and they dwelled together in a state of constant bliss. But with the beginning of what we Hindus call the yugas, or cyclic ages of humanity, Shakti separated herself from her beloved to create the forms and forces of this world. As the creative power of Shiva, Shakti is the vital force in all beings; there is nothing in this world that is devoid of her presence. She fills all space with her brilliance, and whatever we perceive is only her manifestation. It is she who binds atom with atom, molecule with molecule. Comprising all knowledge, Shakti is the colors and shapes of the world in all of their shades and gradations. Inherent in gods, animate and inanimate beings, rivers and electricity, you and I, she is the self, the universe, all that exists. She is bliss itself and gives bliss to all. Shakti is life and gives life to all. She is the mother of the universe and the universe itself. Even though she is essentially one, in order for us to know her she manifests herself in many forms. She is the voice, light, and energy of what you in the West call the Godhead. Many of our ancient texts known as the Vedas, Upanishads, Puranas, and Tantras sing her praises. Watch carefully, and I will reveal her to you."

After Sitara spoke these words she went through an almost unbelievable series of physical transformations before my astonished eyes. As she named each goddess and brought her to life, it seemed as if she could magically alter the shape and size of her body. Not only could she shape-shift in this remarkable manner but also it appeared that she had the ability to transform her very flesh, so that with her depiction of each successive goddess the small wrinkles around her eyes magically disappeared and she actually became a younger version of herself.

First Sitara manifested as the fierce and powerful goddess Durga, whose image adorned the wall. Riding astride a lion Durga held in her many hands the weapons with which she destroyed the terrible demon Mahisha. The energy that exuded from Sitara was so compelling, her movements and gestures so powerful, that I could actually see these multiple hands as if they were real. In the blink of an eye Sitara then transformed herself into the warm sensuous Lakshmi, goddess of fertility and abundance. Light seemed to radiate outward from her body as her breasts appeared to swell and brim over with life-enhancing nectar. In one hand she held a lotus flower while sparkling gold coins poured out of the other hand. Sitara looked at me and laughed with delight as she became the youthful and serene Saraswati, goddess of music, singing softly to herself while playing her sacred instrument, the *vina*. Finally Sitara transformed into Kali Ma, the great wrathful goddess who with her shining sword destroys egotism and ignorance. The skin of Sitara's face tightened until her face began to resemble a skull. Her ancient all-knowing eyes were wild with fire, and her red tongue hung out of her mouth. A third eye suddenly appeared between her two eyes, as she looked at me with great ferocity. I gazed into its depths, and for a moment it was as if I was looking into the fiery core of creation itself. I was overcome with awe and amazement. This was a spectacle unlike anything that I had ever witnessed.

But this was only the beginning of Sitara's teaching, for she told me that in the ancient tradition of goddess worship, known as Tantra, every woman in the world is perceived as an incarnation of Shakti. "For so many centuries we have kept Shakti's teaching alive," Sitara said. "More centuries than you can imagine. According to our teachings the age in which we live is only one period of a much greater cycle of human experience known to us as the yugas. These yugas extend through vast passages of time, from the birth of creation to the very death of time itself. I know that you Westerners think that human beings evolved from apes and have only been civilized for five thousand years or so, but from our perspective this is not the case. Beginning with what we call the Satya Yuga, or Golden Age of truth and grace when we are totally at one with the light of Shakti and her shining realms of spirit, we travel through three other ages known as the Treta, Dvapara, and Kali Yugas, or the Silver, Bronze, and Iron Ages. During this journey we fall farther and farther away from the knowledge of Shakti's light, until we reach the time when most of humanity has not only forgotten her but has forgotten that it even has a connection with the spiritual world at all. This is the age in which we live—our modern age, the Kali Yuga, or Age of Iron, when the forces of darkness and repression have become so powerful that many people in this world can no longer see the Goddess or feel her divine presence." (See chapter 5 for a detailed explanation of this teaching.)

Sitara stopped speaking for a moment to pour herself a drink and let the import of her words sink into my consciousness. "Still," she continued, "there are some even in this dark age of human experience who have never strayed from Shakti's powerful path of love and light. We know that this is the final phase of her great cycle. Soon in the same way that the sun rises out of the darkness of the night sky, the goddess will return and a new Golden Age of spirit will be born."

Once again, before my eyes Sitara began to physically transform herself. But this time she molded herself into the radiant devotees of the Goddess. Sitara began as a village maiden dancing blissfully in the moonlight, and then transformed into a courtesan of the Moghul courts. In this role she performed exquisite mimetic gestures for her emperor while singing beautiful lines of love poetry. Next she became a wild yogini, or female yoga practitioner, her body adorned with ornaments of bone as she performed ritual practices amid the lush forest. From a graceful devotee of Krishna lost in the pleasure of her song, to a beautiful temple priestess preparing her ceremonial offerings for Shakti and Shiva, and a mother lost in the ecstasy of giving birth, Sitara embodied and transmitted to me a full range of feminine archetypes and spiritual role models.

Sitara's father, Acharya Sukhdev Maharaj, a great poet, composer, and Sanskrit scholar, had trained his daughter in this magical transformative art. He came from a lineage of artists who had lived for many generations in the holy city of Benares and had been instrumental in reviving what Sitara called Katha Nritya, an ancient form of Kathak dance. The name of the dance was derived from the Sanskrit *katha*, meaning "story" and *nritya* meaning "that form of dance-storytelling comprising movements of the body, hands, limbs, together with facial expressions and filled with emotion or sentiment."[3] Sitara's father had told her that the practices and teachings of Katha Nritya first took written form with the Vedas, or the sacred texts upon which all Hindu culture is based. But Katha Nritya existed as an oral tradition prior to that time; it appeared in northern India many centuries ago with the coming of the Aryan invaders from the West, and was instrumental in the transmission of the Vedic tradition to the indigenous people of India. Its proponents were known as Kathakas, and they traveled from village to village and temple to temple, transmitting the legends and epics of this ancient tradition that later came to be known as Hinduism. The Kathakas trained from childhood in the arts of physical and spiritual transformation. They worked with highly developed and exacting yogic techniques that had been handed down through the yugas that enabled them to embody the goddesses and gods, heroes and demons, of the Hindu pantheon. In this way they kept the sacred myths and memories of their tradition alive. The Kathakas played an essential role in the spiritual growth and sustenance of their ancient sacred society by enacting the great epics of the Vedic times, such as the *Ramayana* and *Mahabharata*, and transforming into the river goddess Saraswati, the great god Shiva, the ten-headed demon Ravana, and many more. Training in this sacred art of transformation became an integral part of the education of the priestesses and priests who directed and served in the holy temples.

I will never forget the day that I began my formal dance training. It was a Wednesday, the day of the great elephant-headed god Ganesh, the remover of obstacles. We had just completed the Sanskrit ceremony officiated by Sitara's priest, during which I became her disciple and was therefore initiated into her ancient artistic lineage. Even though Sitara and the priest spoke in a language that was foreign to me, there was something about the energetic frequencies of these sacred sounds that touched a place deep within my heart. It was as if some hidden memory from a distant age was being reawakened in my consciousness.

Respect and reverence for the ancestors, one's parents, and the deities themselves lie at the base of this sacred art form and of Hindu life, and so before I took my first

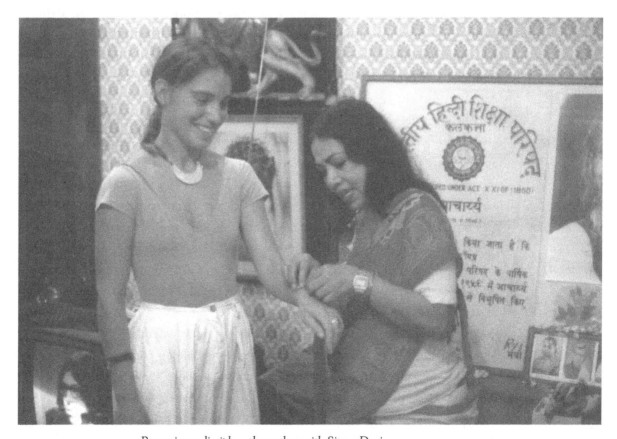

Becoming a disciple—the author with Sitara Devi.

step, before I placed the tinkling bells she called *gungaru* around my ankles, my guruji began her instruction. "Your bells are your sacred instrument," she said, "and the dance is the vehicle through which you can perceive and encounter the divine realms. Before you put on your bells you must focus your mind on me, your teacher, who has introduced you to this path. It is through my blessing that you have been able to become a disciple in such a powerful and ancient tradition. I am opening the doorway for you to a lineage that has remained alive for centuries. Therefore you must pay homage to the many gurus who have come before me, to the countless generations of ancestors, to all the magical dancer-storytellers, priestesses, and priests of this sacred art, who have devoted themselves to its preservation. You must consciously ask them to be present and assist you in your practice.

"You must then call upon the divine Shakti, the spiritual light and energy of all the deities who you will have the honor to embody. You must request that these deities, whose stories and energies will flow through you, be present and support you as you learn to embrace every aspect of their appearance, qualities, and teachings. You see, to really become a Kathaka, or one who walks the ancient path of the priestess, you must understand that when you are dancing Durga you are not just acting as if you are Durga; you *are* Durga. The stage around you becomes the fiery battleground on which you encounter and defeat the evil demon Mahisha. Since this is a solo dance form in which you will play all the roles, when you shift from Durga to Mahisha you then become the terrifying, shape-shifting buffalo demon who in his overwhelming desire for power has challenged and defeated many of the gods themselves." Sitara looked at me sternly and said, "This is not acting, this is not pretending; this is real. This is the mystical art of transformation. Open your body, mind, and spirit fully to allow the divine Shakti energy of these deities to enter you. Cast aside your own ego and merge completely with the radiant nature of these luminous beings. This is the essence of sacred dance; this is the timeless art of Katha Nritya."

Sitara continued, "If you are serious, from this day forward you must fully devote yourself to this art, attuning yourself to every nuance of *tala* (rhythm), *mudra* (hand gesture), *karana* (posture), and *bhava* (expression). For these are the sacred languages of these divine beings. This is not some fantasy; you must make a personal and intimate connection with them. A profound and delicate interplay will take place between you. Believe me, this is not an easy path. It is fraught with peril. It is purification and reweaving of your entire personality and way of perceiving reality. It takes lifetimes of commitment and sacrifice. But once you are on the path, there is no turning back.

"Before you begin, you must pay homage to your parents, for they are the beings that gave you birth, loved you, and gave of themselves to raise you. After this you may put on your bells. Then you must touch the floor and your heart to acknowledge and pay homage to the earth goddess herself, the Great Mother, who cares for and supports us all. And you must then pay homage in the same way to the musicians and their instruments, the tabla, harmonium, and sarangi that support you in your practice. Finally you must pay homage to your guru, who is your teacher. You must touch my feet and place your hands together at your heart in the sacred gesture of *namaste*, a gesture that means 'the divine Shakti in me greets the divine Shakti in you,' for it is through my love and devotion to the transmission of this sacred art that I have agreed to guide you on this path."

My dreams that night were filled with images of the Goddess. I saw myself walking through ancient temples, performing offerings before glittering golden statues, dancing and singing for audiences of copper-skinned, almond-eyed men, women, and children. In the next few days, whenever I was in my guruji's presence it was as if my own perception had expanded to new levels of awareness. In the time between our conversations and instruction, I read to Ari from the richly illustrated books of Hindu myths and stories that Sitara had given him. My son and I were both captivated by the vivid accounts of the magical feats of the gods and goddesses.

Only a few days after my initiation Sitara called me to the living room, where I received my dance instruction. Impatiently she motioned for me to take my usual place at her feet. As I looked up at her she seemed to grow in stature. In a somber tone she told me that since my arrival she had been watching me. She said that in my dress, mannerisms, expressions, and movements I appeared to be more masculine than feminine. She said that this was not my fault, but it was a problem stemming from the fact that I had grown up in a culture that had forgotten the Goddess. At that moment images flowed through my mind of how I had been raised to admire and emulate the ways of men. I remembered how in my youth I was considered a tomboy who loved to compete with boys in athletics or leap across the floor with them in dance classes. I also thought about how I generally preferred their company to that of females.

"For example, look at your clothes," Sitara noted, "They are not graceful and flowing like those of Indian women. Look at your body, so thin and muscular." She began to laugh. "If you didn't have breasts I might mistake you for a boy." I began to realize that she was right, and tears welled up in my eyes. Sitara's eyes filled with warmth and her voice became soft and soothing. She said, "I realize, Sharron, that you have sacrificed much to come here. I know the journey must have been difficult for you. But if you want to learn the ways of the Goddess all of this has to change." She informed me that I must give away my Western clothes and dress only in a sari.

How could I know what it felt like to be an Indian woman, let alone a goddess of the Hindu tradition, if I didn't even know how to dress like one? With great trepidation I surrendered to her the Danskin leotards and expensive Versace clothes that I had brought with me. Then she told me to grab my purse. We were going shopping.

Sitara led Ari and me out into the street and waved her hands to call a taxi. She ushered us into the backseat and jumped in alongside the driver. In a commanding tone she directed him to our destination. Soon after we arrived at the bazaar, where cows meandered along the sidewalks and teams of oxen slowly pulled wagons full of wares alongside honking automobiles and darting rickshaws. Sitara took control of the situation, and many saris were brought out for our inspection. Some were made of cotton, some of silk. Before long we had chosen several rich and colorful lengths of fabric, which would become my favorite mode of dress for many years. For from the moment when Sitara first wrapped the sari around my body I was moved by the beauty, simplicity, and elegance of this ancient style of feminine dress.

Now that I had the proper attire Sitara began my training in earnest. She encouraged me to read about the origins and significance of the sacred language of gesture. I discovered that in India, mudras play a primary role in the transmission of ancient sacred knowledge. According to the *Tantraraja Tantra* of the sixteenth century, the word *mudra* derives from the Sanskrit root *mud*, meaning "bliss," "rejoice," or "that which pleases the gods." In the ancient Vedic and later tantric rites, mudras were considered a magical code for communicating with the deities and forces of nature that sealed a ritual act of invocation or offering and endowed it with mystic power. With the creation of the *Natya Shastra*, an ancient text on the sacred science of drama and dance attributed to the Hindu sage Bharata, these symbolic gestures were used not only for ritual activity but also as a means of describing the qualities, moods, and actions of the deities.[4]

Sitara informed me that the gestures were only one vital aspect of this ritualistic training. She said that in the days of the temple, when the priestesses still performed their rites, training in all aspects of the sacred yogic science of theatrical expression was fundamental to their education. It developed awareness of the subtle powers of their bodies, minds, and emotions to such a high degree that they became perfect vessels for the clear untainted light of Shakti. As caretakers of the spiritual life of the people, these priestesses and temple dancers were responsible for the continued transmission of the sacred myths, legends, and stories of their heritage.

"Today, the temple priestess is but a fading memory," Sitara said wistfully. "Like a delicate shadow she dances across our vision. Many of us women faced with the difficulties of modern society long for the days when we could spend each waking moment in the service of the goddess as her emissaries on Earth." A trace of a smile swept across Sitara's beautiful face. "But all is not lost. As dancers we are fortunate to retain these precious remnants of her mysteries." She motioned for me to stand before her. "Come," she said. "Let us begin."

Because I had extensive training in ballet and modern dance Sitara began by teaching me a dance-story of the tantric god Shiva, whose powerful movements and strong expressions were closer to the athletic styles with which I was familiar. I began to learn what I later came to recognize as the "outer" or beginning stages of tantric practice: comprehension of the iconography of the deity, the many layers of meaning encoded in her or his form, what the dimension of the deity looks like, and the purification and offerings performed to invoke the deity. Sitara translated from the Sanskrit to introduce me to each karana and mudra of Shiva, the river goddess Gunga, and the other characters in the story. Sitara patiently demonstrated the movements and expressions for me, explaining the significance of each—how Shiva's four arms represent his multiple powers, how the drum he holds in one hand represents the beating of the rhythm, and how the primal power of sound itself, the first element, and the voice of Shakti vibrating through the ether in the first act of creation. In another hand, positioned in a half-moon shape, Shiva holds a flame, symbolizing the burning away of all evil. He dances upon the prostrate demon of ignorance with one hand directed to his upward-pointing foot, a symbol of release and salvation. Shiva's fourth hand is the hand of protection, offering his strength and guidance to those on the path. Surrounded by flames of energy and wisdom, he is the cosmic dancer, dancing the cyclic dance of creation, preservation, and destruction.

As in all the compositions of the ancient Katha Nritya repertoire, this dance was not only a dance of Shiva, but also an entire episode from the *Ramayana,* an epic said to have taken place in the beginning of the Golden Age, when goddesses and gods dwelled upon the earth. This episode described the manifestation of the holy Ganges River in our earthly realm as personified in the goddess Gunga, whose stainless waters purify the earth and the entire cosmos. I found it fascinating that my guruji chose to begin with this dance, as it depicts the influx of the holy river of feminine grace upon the earth from the celestial realms. According to the *Bhagavata Purana* this is a river of immense spiritual power. It is the luminous pathway over which the great sages travel from dimension to dimension.[5]

The flow of this river is so strong that if left unmitigated it would envelop the earth. In the tale, Shiva, lord of the yogis, sits in deep meditation on the summit of Mount Kailash. He agrees to receive the full force of the river's powerful flow into his matted locks. By doing so he becomes a transducer, reducing the current to the level

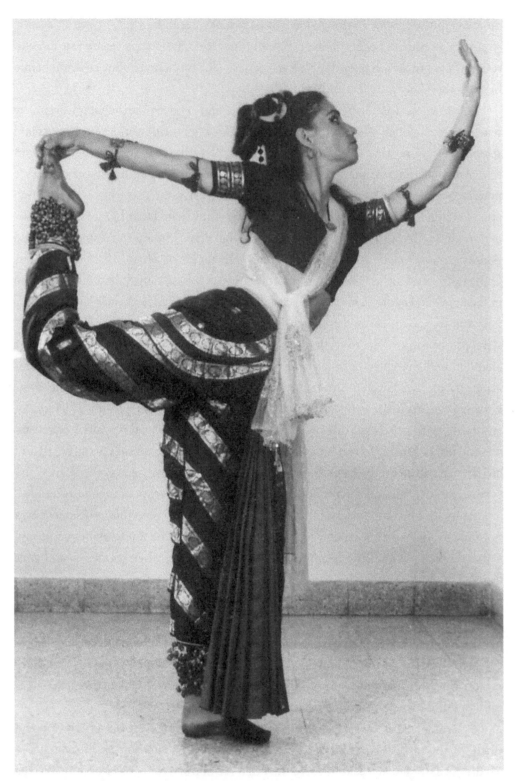

The author as the tantric god Shiva, photograph courtesy of Shantilal Somaiya.

at which it can be received and utilized by humanity. He does this so that every being can have the opportunity to bathe in Gunga's purifying waters and experience her revitalizing touch. As the consort of Shakti, Shiva is at one with this force. I wondered if by teaching me this dance first my guruji was attempting to shower me with the subtle energetic current of this goddess of purification. But this was not the only aspect of the dance that amazed me; as I began to study Shiva's image and allow his Shakti to flow through me, I realized that it was to this great tantric yogi that I had made my offering on that fateful mushroom-induced trip.

Clearly this training was worlds away from the outer technical display I had once regarded as dance. Here was a culture in which the art of dance was seen as emerging from the very act of creation itself. Rather than being merely a display of technical virtuosity, the movements of the Kathak dancer were a magical presentation of the many facets and forms of creation that contained the vital energy of the Goddess herself. I had been raised in a Western society that was imprinted with the Puritanical mind-set that the body, especially the woman's body, was inherently evil. After all, according to the Judeo-Christian tradition, it was Eve's sin—woman's desire for knowledge—that had led humanity out of paradise. To many Western people dance was some kind of lurid sexual display rather than a true art form; according to this view dance had no link to the transcendent realms of the spirit. Now I was being offered a completely different view. Here was a tradition in which the female body was seen as a sacred vessel, an expression of and receptacle for divine energy.

Sitara began to teach me the Saraswati Vandana, or dance of invocation and offering to Saraswati, the great goddess of learning, music, poetry, the arts, purification, and refinement. According to the *Saraswati Upanishad* this graceful goddess is "faith, the retentive power of the intellect incarnate. She has her home on the tip of the devotee's tongue. She is the river of nectar that removes the stress of worldly existence."[6]

Sitara taught me the Sanskrit prayer I would bring to life, translating each phrase and teaching me the corresponding postures, gestures, and expressions. Since I was now consciously working to relax and soften what Sitara referred to as my masculine style of movement, I was delighted to discover that when the sage Bharata encoded centuries of oral transmission into the text of his *Natya Shastra* he included teachings that were specifically designed for women. These teachings consisted of "gentle gesticulations and movements of the limbs, emotional sentiments, states, moods, and activities," and were characterized as "the charmingly graceful," with erotic sentiment at their base. Bharata states, "This style cannot be adequately portrayed by men. Excepting women, none can practice it."[7]

Through the study and practice of this dance something deep inside me began to relax. Perhaps it was the nature of the goddess herself mixing with my own being; perhaps it was the softness and grace with which my guruji transmitted the energetic current of this elegant goddess. It was a dance of purification, embodiment, and devotion, and I was taught the underlying significance of each movement. My hands weaved the atmosphere that surrounded me and my eyes transmitted the inner knowing of the goddess. The dance was a prayer, an invocation, and a realization all at once. The words of this dance-story were:

Oh, goddess Saraswati,
You who are born in the white lotus,
Pure white as the snow garlanding the mountains,
Whose face is as radiant as a hundred full autumn moons
Surrounded by thousands of shimmering stars.
Shining white is your raiment.

In your hand you hold the sacred vina
Upon which you play the celestial sounds of the universe.
As you sit ever peaceful upon the white lotus
Gentle waves of love and compassion pour forth from the
    depths of your heart.

Even Brahma the creator,
Vishnu the preserver,
Shiva the destroyer,
And all of the hosts of deities of the three worlds
Pay homage to you.

Oh, gracious goddess,
Shower me with your blessings.
Purify my soul.
Fill me with your divine nectar.
Let it flow down from the heavens, suffusing my body in an
    endless river of celestial grace.

Take my hand.
Lead me on the sacred path to enlightenment.
For the sake of all beings,
Open my heart.
Lift these veils of ignorance.
Wake me and the world from slumber.

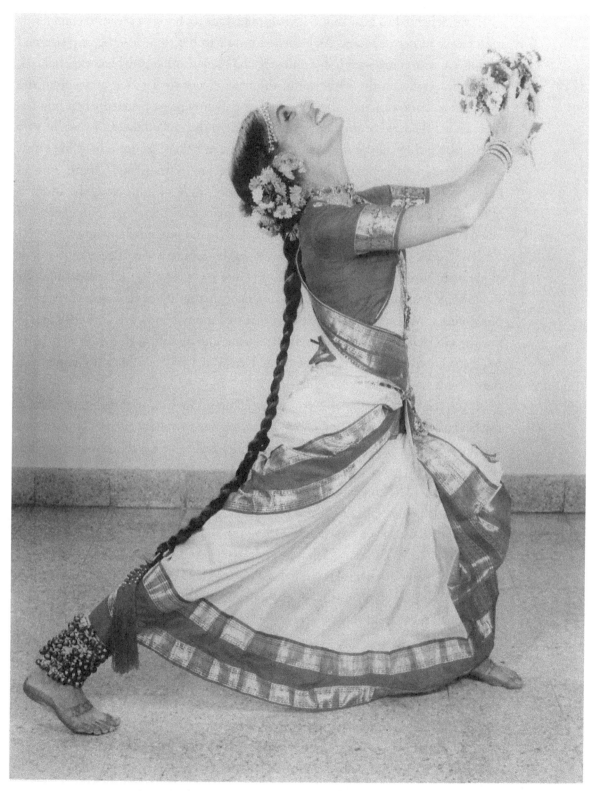

The author performing the Saraswati Vandana, photograph courtesy of Shantilal Somaiya.

I was delighted to hear that Saraswati, like Gunga, brings a cleansing and fertilizing power to her devotees. As I opened myself to her flow, a sense of peace and serenity came over me—a sense of quietude and silence unlike any I had experienced. Sitting peacefully on the white lotus, the magnificent flower that grows from the black muck, Saraswati embodies the state of enlightenment reached when one has transcended the hold of the dark passions.[8] She is the embodiment of wisdom who was worshipped by all the male gods and by human beings. In her role as the Great Mother, Saraswati exhibits many qualities, not just softness and serenity. In an instant she could transform into a great warrior of truth, clearing away the shadows of negative thoughts and provocations. It was incredible to me that in the course of one dance I could encounter and convey such rich and profound teachings.

The Goddess had entered my life. Every waking moment was filled with the study of her many aspects, and she now began to enter my dreams as well. Sometimes she would appear as my guruji, clarifying a mudra or rhythm that I had recently learned. Sometimes it was Saraswati herself who appeared in my mind's eye. At other times I saw the Goddess as a great river of light flowing into and through my body. When I told Sitara of these experiences, she treated them in a very nonchalant manner, as if they were a very natural part of life.

"You see," Sitara said, "this power to call upon the hidden dimensions, such as the land of dreams, visions, or feelings, lies at the heart of all sacred art. Through this training you begin to have access to the subtler realms of existence. Connected to these realms, the great priestesses, priests, and dancers of old were what you might call magicians. They had a vital awakened sensitivity to the energetic and symbolic character of these realms. With this profound knowledge of the elements, of nature, of the subtle language of vibration, they had the ability to communicate in ways that seem miraculous to us today. Each tala, each *raga* (melodic framework that gives birth to musical composition), each mudra and karana, held a specific energy, feeling, or vibration that had the power to shape both the invisible and visible realms. These women and men could sing or play or dance to bring the rain, call the animals, or help the plants grow. Through the vehicles of their ritual performances they could elicit the deepest of feelings in their audiences, and move them to the lowest of depths or the highest of heights by transmitting divine energy with such clarity that the people in attendance were transported beyond the limitations of their ordinary reality into the shining dimensions of the gods."

Sitara continued, "Your essential role as a dancer is to depict the play of light and energy that is the creative power of the Goddess. This role has many, many levels. In order to be able to depict the play of her energies and forces, you must be willing to travel very deep within your own psyche and ride on the waves of energy that some-times threaten to overtake you. Observe yourself first in all of your experiences; do not run from them but feel them. Become aware of how they rise and manifest. If you cry notice how you are holding your body as the pain overwhelms you; when you laugh be aware of how that emotion moves you.

"Remember every experience and weave it into your personal book of knowledge. Keep your eyes constantly open to the movements, gestures, and expressions of those around you. They are the foundation of your craft. Just as the mudras, karanas, and bhavas I teach you are sacred symbols designed to strike a responsive chord in the heart of your audience, so is every action that is taking place within the human being. Learn to read, understand, and focus the energy of these signs and symbols that are poured out from the inner depths of every one of us in every moment of our lives. Be aware. Work with this constant flow of information. Become a living vessel for the sacred art of the Goddess."

To implant these teachings more deeply in my psyche, to transform me into a more refined and receptive vessel, Sitara took me to temples, introduced me to the symbology and ritual of *pujas*, or religious rites, and showed me how intimately these sacred activities were embedded in the dance. She fully opened herself and her life to me, constantly instructing me not only in the art of dance but also in the art of being a woman.

In addition to my training in Katha Nritya, Sitara continued my instruction in the later Kathak dance style of the Moghul emperors. One afternoon as we sat together in her living room drinking some delicious spiced tea known as chai and munching on samosas, which looked and tasted like spicy fried dumplings, Sitara told me that over the centuries the Moghuls were profoundly influenced by two great spir-itual movements: Islamic Sufism and Hindu bhaktism. Both of these traditions broke away from the constraints of their societies and priesthoods. Islamic Sufism and Hindu bhaktism highlighted the universality of human experience and taught that the light of the divine was immediately accessible to all, regardless of caste or culture. For practitioners of these traditions, love, and devotion were the fundamental means through which one could achieve spiritual awakening. Exquisite poetry, songs, and dances were created to transmit these teachings. While the writings of Sufi poets such as Rumi, Attar, and Hafiz metaphorically depicted humanity's relationship with the Divine as the lover and his beloved, bhakti poets such as Mirabai, Kabir, and Surdas wrote tales of the milkmaid Radha and her beloved lord Krishna. Rich with sexual innuendo and filled with passion, these poetic tales became a major part of the Moghul Kathak repertoire.

Later that day when Sitara began to teach me the playful seductive expressions, mudras, and movements unique to this realm of sensuality, I felt like she was opening Pandora's box. She was asking me to reach inside and bring up my personal experience of sensuous pleasure, which was both exciting and terrifying for me. Sitara saw this inner conflict begin to arise within me, and she asked me to speak to her about these feelings.

"Guruji," I said shyly, "my sexual experiences have always seemed to create utter confusion in me. On one hand, I feel that as human beings we were born to experience pleasure, and at times I have experienced states of incredible bliss. I believe that somehow, somewhere deep within me, I innately understand the immense potential for power, beauty, and empathy that exists within the intimacy of lovemaking. But at the same time this experience of bliss is constantly undermined. It is as though at the moment that I feel the highest bliss I am filled with memories of my Western suburban upbringing, in which I was told that only 'bad girls' let themselves fully indulge in pleasure. Since my first sexual experience a part of me has always felt guilty and ashamed that I allowed myself to let go to that extent. I remember only too well the turmoil that arose within me during my teenage years when I would get lost in the pleasure of the sex play we referred to as 'making out,' only to suddenly realize that I had allowed my boyfriend to touch me in places I had been told that I shouldn't. Feelings of fear would overwhelm me, and I would begin to cry uncontrollably. I am married now and past this point, but still these feelings and memories haunt me."

Sitara looked at me, her eyes filled with compassion. She told me, "This is a problem that stems from the repression of the Goddess in your society and in mine. It is a problem endemic to this dark Age of Iron, when men who have forgotten the Goddess's beauty rule the earth. In ancient times every woman was seen as an aspect of the Mother and was worshipped as such. Sex was considered a sacred act whose mysteries were held and transmitted by women. Instead of sex being looked upon as merely a means of procreation, the physical union of woman and man was seen as a powerful means by which one could feel the presence of the Divine within oneself. In the more recent era of the great temples the priestesses, known as *devadasis*, retained and transmitted these mysteries. They learned to control and regulate their sexual energy. This knowledge was crucial to their significant and divine role as initiators, for it was their appointed responsibility to ignite and channel the spiritual fire, or Shakti, of the male and teach him how to transform this physical desire into spiritual bliss."

Sitara paused and closed her eyes for a moment, as her sister Tara entered the room and circled around us chanting prayers, a tray of incense in her hands. Then Sitara continued, "In our tantric tradition this spiritual fire is known as the Kundalini

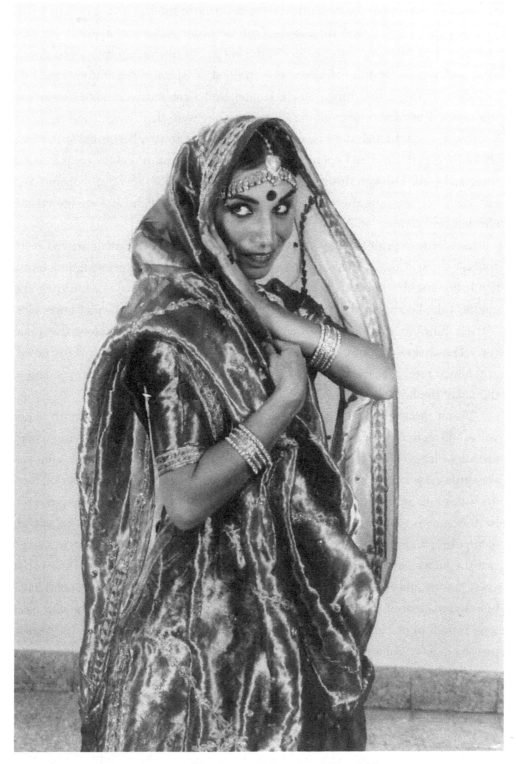

The author as Radha, photograph courtesy of Shantilal Somaiya.

Shakti, and it is symbolized by a coiled serpent sitting at the base of the human spine. This serpent sleeps coiled three-and-a-half times around what we call the base chakra, or the visionary energy center at the bottom of the human spine. The priestesses and yoginis of this tradition were trained in specific meditative practices, including rhythmic breathing, mudra, karana, and visualization designed to arouse this mystic Kundalini energy of the Goddess. They were then taught how to direct her flow upward through their bodies, for as she begins to rise, beginning at the base chakra, she permeates and opens the seven subtle chakras, or energy centers along the spinal cord. Through this powerful process the mystic or inner eye is opened and one begins to see how the Goddess's flowing currents of light and energy create, envelop, and connect all living things."

In order to imprint this teaching in my mind more clearly, Sitara illustrated every concept through the ancient symbolic language of gesture. Her graceful undulating hands became the serpent on its path upward through the chakras. Utilizing the mudra of the budding and growing lotus flower, Sitara gave me a distinct impression of these spinning, whirlpool-like energy centers and their placement along the spinal cord. The chakras are located at the base of the spine, four fingers below the navel, at the solar plexus, at the heart, at the throat, in the space between the eyes, and at the top of the head.

"As my disciple you are on a new path now," Sitara said with great warmth in her voice, "the path of the priestess, the path of the Goddess. I know that it must be hard for you to let go of all those beliefs that you were raised with, beliefs that give you very little knowledge of your true power as a woman. Having lost their mysteries, having little or no awareness of these subtle energetic teachings, so many modern women have begun to use the power of their sexual energy merely as a means to attract, manipulate, and control men. I have seen so many foreigners looking at our sacred text the *Kama Sutra* as some kind of pornographic material. Little do they know that every posture and embrace performed by the priestess and her consort was considered holy and was carried out in conjunction with a specific configuration of the stars after long periods of preparation on both internal and external levels. Today the average person longs for amusement, diversion, and entertainment more than true knowledge or spiritual sustenance. To so many, lovemaking has become devoid of love, devoid of spirit, and is merely an expression of animal lust." Sitara stopped for a moment, closing her eyes contemplatively.

"Still, today you are here," she said with great feeling, "leaving the comforts and lifestyle of your world behind to learn from me the ways of the ancients. Come now, let us continue your training. As you learn to embody Radha and Mirabai and feel the sensuous dance of the Goddess within you, you will gain a clearer understanding of the true nature of these teachings."

Over the next months I discovered that Sitara and her elder sister, Tara, were masters of the realm of female sensuality. Physically transforming before my eyes from shy young virgins to women longing for union with their beloved and women sated by the divine nectar of union, the sisters demonstrated glances and gestures that were incredibly rich, filled with nuance and innuendo. Even though Sitara was my acknowledged guruji, Tara sensed my hunger for knowledge of their art and also shared her unique gifts with me. Tara would sit on the floor playing her harmonium, and in a deep and evocative voice she would sing to me the songs of the milkmaid Radha. Tara sang of Radha's longing for her divine lover Krishna, and the immense joy she felt at their moment of union. As Tara sang she demonstrated sensuous glances—a rich display of erotic energy from a woman in her seventies!

I tried my best to copy Sitara and Tara's expressions and gestures, but in the beginning, as soon as the true feeling would rise to the surface I would start to giggle with embarrassment. Since this experience of shyness appears in the course of love play, Sitara taught me how to use it in portraying Radha, who upon beholding her lover, Krishna, is so overwhelmed with desire for union that at the sight of him she becomes exceedingly shy. After glancing in his direction with a heart full of joy, Radha slowly lowers her head and eyes and smiles demurely.

This was but one of a wealth of expressions designed to exhibit what I came to understand as the natural feelings of receptivity, bliss, passion, and mystery that Sitara said should be an integral part of every woman's vocabulary. This was not just a dance of worldly seduction and manipulation; it was a dance in which the sexual and spiritual aspects of life were completely interwoven. It was a dance of union and separation, of lover and beloved, of the divine love play between goddess and god. Encoded in these dances and their mudras, karanas, and bhavas was the key to understanding and experiencing every subtle gradation of love and longing, from wonder and delight to deep sadness and frustration, from the pain of loss to the joy of reunion.

As the days passed I went deeper into the energies of female sensuality. Part of me was elated but another part was terrified. Learning to feel and express these energies gave me a new sense of feminine power and magnetism, yet I had not gained the maturity to transmit the energies with discernment. As I learned to awaken, control, and direct these sensuous energies men were attracted to me more than ever before. I found that by working with this aspect of the Shakti energy I could affect men's moods and emotions to a great extent. I soon began to realize that I had been handed the emotional equivalent of a stick of dynamite. These were the very expressions, gestures, and movements that had played a major part in the symbolic teachings of the temple priest-esses as they performed their roles as initiators into the sacred mysteries of sexuality. To them lovemaking was a holy act that mirrored the divine union of Shakti and Shiva. The priestesses had been trained since childhood to understand the nature of these energies and use them with wisdom and intelligence. But I was an American woman of the twentieth century who had years of false imprints about her body and sexuality to break through. When I spoke to Sitara about these problems she merely told me to have patience, a quality that she felt was very lacking in Western women. To her, Western women appeared to have completely lost their feminine qualities and were turning into men in women's bodies. This was because modern women had forgotten the Goddess and her teachings for so long that they now had no proper role models.

In order to clarify what she meant Sitara taught me the dance of Mirabai, the great visionary poet and saint of India who was a role model to all female seekers on the path of spirit. Mirabai was a sixteenth-century princess of Rajasthan who was so in love with her divine lord Krishna that she begged her father-in-law, the king, to allow her to leave the palace and become a *saddhu*, or wandering holy woman.[9] Heeding the internal call of the Divine, Mirabai cast aside all the limitations placed on her as a royal princess. She left behind the sumptuous life of the palace and became a disciple of the great bhakti yogis and later a renowned poet and teacher of both women and men.

Mirabai lived a life filled with love and grace. She constantly experienced the living presence of Krishna within her.[10] In order to adequately portray her I had to open my own heart to the path of bhakti, the path of devotion and surrender to the immense power of the divine Shakti that flows from the heart of God. In Mirabai's own words:

> From my body, I will make an instrument to sing your praises. I drink the nectar
> of your name. In every moment, with every action, I will worship you. My beloved
> Krishna, I lay my heart at your lotus feet.

I would sit, close my eyes, and meditate on the words, opening myself like Mirabai to the pure untainted light of divinity. As I felt this light pour into and per-meate my being, a sense of deep relaxation would come over me. It was as if every cell of my body was drinking in this delicious and radiant nectar of Krishna. I longed to fully relinquish all my fear and all my earthly pain and confusion and bask in the warmth of his divine embrace. The overwhelming desire for love, the longing for union, and the need for release that I carried all my life flowed outward from my heart into the movements of the dance. Sitara perceived the deep connection between Ari

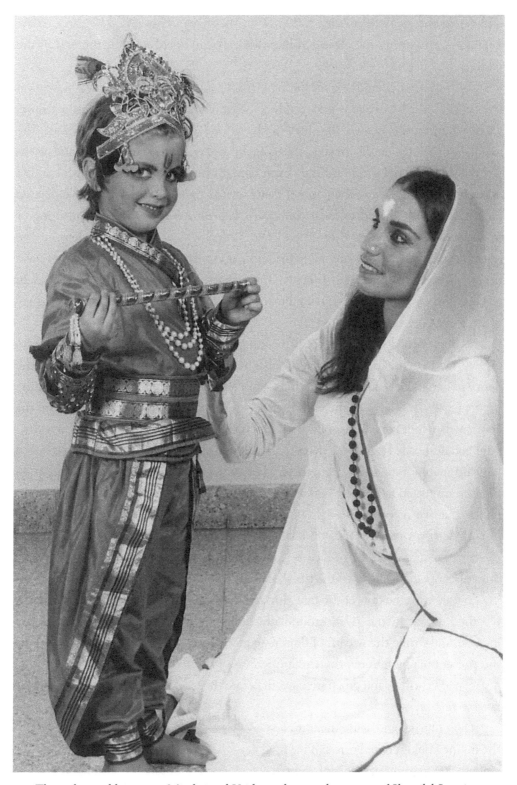

The author and her son as Mirabai and Krishna, photograph courtesy of Shantilal Somaiya.

and me, as well as Ari's growing fondness for the playful Hindu god Krishna, so she taught Ari to portray the child Krishna, who appears to Mirabai at the end of the dance.

Contrary to my family's expectations, Ari loved India. To him it was a magical wonderland filled with gods and goddesses, demons and kings. Living in a culture where children are treated like little gods, he was given constant attention. The members of Sitara's family loved to dress him up and enact the great stories and myths with him. When Ari was four Sitara even brought him up on the stage with her and asked him to demonstrate the poses of many mythic figures. Living amid an extended family that still adhered to their traditional values, Ari never lacked nurturing or attention. When he cried there was always someone to care for him, when he was hungry there was always someone to feed him, and when he wanted to play there was always someone to play with him. At the same time he was given the lessons in respect, appropriate social behavior, creativity, and compassion that are increasingly rare for most American children.

Having opened me to the sensitive aspects of myself, Sitara felt it was time to present me with a dance that would utilize all I had learned from her. This was the dance of her goddess, Durga, the quintessential tantric goddess who embodied all the mystic power, or Shakti, of the gods themselves. In her myth Durga emerges from the combined energies of all the gods to rescue them from the near domination of a powerful buffalo-headed *asura*, the demon named Mahisha. Moving from inner states and outward manifestations of strength and power to sensuality, love, and compassion, Sitara transmitted her knowledge and experience of the radiant Durga. The Sanskrit phrase that we repeated throughout the dance as a refrain was *Jai, Jai Juga Jnanani Devi* ("Victory, victory to the goddess of wisdom, mother of the world").

Sitara taught me a dance that began as an invocation to Durga. Like the temple priestesses of old, I performed the ritual activities of purification, invocation, and offering. In time with the flow of the tala, through the graceful actions of mudra and mime, I bathed myself in the river, ground the sandalwood paste, lit the oil lamps and incense, and strung the wreath of flowers to place on the statue of Durga. I performed the rite of puja by miming the ritual offerings of the five senses (sight, smell, taste, touch, and hearing), and prostrated myself before the Goddess and asked her to bestow her blessing on me.

Then I arose, and as the nectar of the divine Shakti poured through me I entered her pure dimension of light.

The author as Durga.
Photograph by Christopher Harting.

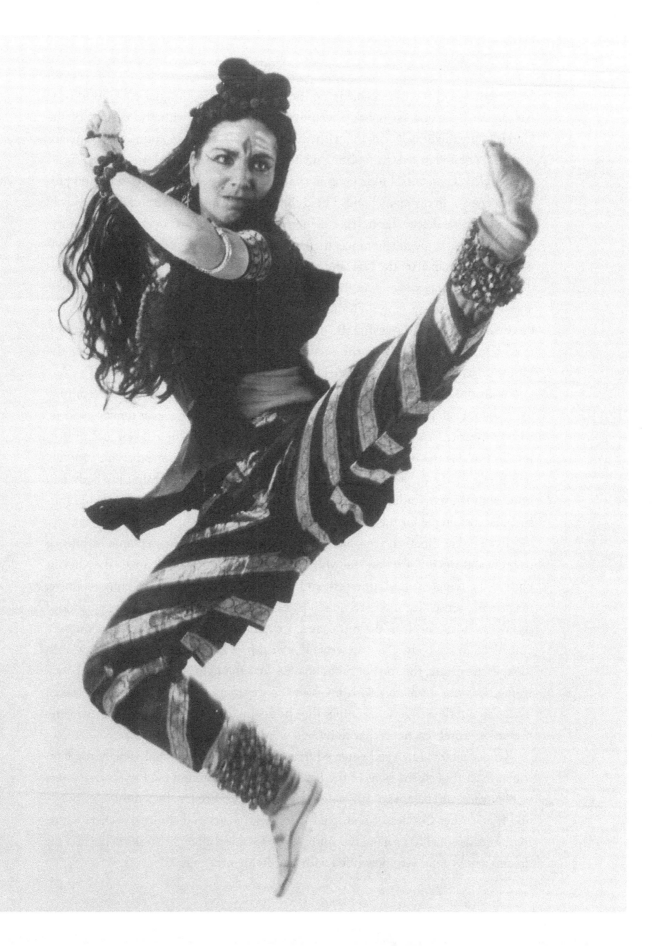

Instantaneously I was transformed into the resplendent Goddess herself, transmitting her divine light and energy to the universe. I was filled with the ecstasy of the Goddess, my ankle bells ringing with the beauty and sophistication of the ancient rhythms. Dressed in red, symbolizing my feminine essence, and adorned with flowers and jeweled ornaments, I rode upon my valiant lion, the symbol of my wild and protective energy. In my many hands I held the sacred weapons given to me by my male counterparts to defeat the horrific demon who threatened to overcome them: the sword that cuts through ignorance; the lasso or noose, symbols of the supreme knowledge of impermanence; the bow and arrow, symbols of the power of the will; the trident, symbol of my power over the three worlds; the discus, symbol of God's highest authority; and many more. Through the course of the dance I merged with the Goddess, feeling and displaying the distinct energies of her countless manifestations, from the fierce protector to the sensuous consort and the loving Mother of the Universe, as she enters the battlefield to vanquish the demonic Mahisha.

With this dance I was trained to embody and transmit the fullness of feminine expression. Each phrase brought forth yet another aspect of the great tantric goddess, who was created and worshipped by the gods themselves as their savior and protector. To this day the performance of the dance is a deeply moving experience for me. It was one of the most profound gifts my guruji gave me, imprinting my body and mind with the extraordinary power and energy of her goddess, a gift that would nurture and sustain me for the rest of my days.

Even today, nineteen years after I first met her, the seeds Sitara planted continue to grow and ripen, for it was she who opened my eyes and my heart to the ancient path of the temple dancer, priestess, and wise woman. Her lessons in grace, courage, magnetism, sensuality, modesty, quietude, kindness, and compassion were embedded in my psyche as deeply as the intricacies of rhythm, movement, and expression were embedded in my body. Over the years the wealth of knowledge transmitted by each look, each gesture, the tone of Sitara's voice, and the light in her eyes has deepened in me, merging intimately with my own life experience as a woman and a seeker. These are subtle energetic teachings that lie at the heart of Sitara's ancient women's mysteries, secret teachings that transcend words and the written language.

Under Sitara's tutelage I emerged from my Western patriarchal view of the feminine. Even though the signs of the Kali Yuga were all around me I knew that there were women and men who still had respect and reverence for the feminine principle and the Mother Goddess. I had lived with great artists and spiritual seekers whose lives were devoted to keeping the spirit of the Goddess alive. My waking life and my dreams and visions were now filled with her divine presence.

As I left my new family to return to my husband and former life in America, I was filled with trepidation. My eyes had been opened to a different way of life, a more graceful way of being. Would my husband, now caught up in the fast-paced superficial world of his successful music-business clients have any understanding of what I had experienced? Would my friends or family? Would there be anyone with whom I could share these extraordinary teachings and insights? As I said my goodbyes, I bent down to touch the feet of my guruji in reverence and gratitude for all she had given me. In her usual manner Sitara placed her hands gently on my head to offer her blessing. But this time she lifted me up, took me in her arms, and gently whispered, "Do not be afraid, Sharron. Remember, the Goddess is with you in every moment. If you feel fear or anxiety, if you become troubled by the fact that your old life appears to be in conflict with your new one, just stop for a moment, turn your mind inward, and sense her presence within you. Take a deep breath and feel the powerful rhythmic beat of your heart. This is the sound of the Goddess's voice resonating through you. Do not hesitate to ask the Goddess for her guidance and assistance. Then, as you quiet your thoughts and open your eyes once again to the outer world, never forget that no matter how much we as human beings who live amid the darkness of the Kali Yuga are taught to deny the Goddess, it is her light and energy that sustains us all. Cast aside the veils that your culture has placed over your vision and seek out her spirit in all things. Have faith. She has led you to me. I have opened the door for you to her ancient mysteries. Now she will lead you onward."

2

The Dance of the Dakini

Our body is from the very beginning a mandala.
Our state of consciousness is from the beginning
divinity. When one has perfectly entered into this
knowledge of that which one is, then one is what one
is, and that is what we call true initiation.
—ARAGA, TIBETAN KAGYDPA MASTER

eturning home was more difficult than I had ever imagined. Yes, it was pleasant to once again experience the material comforts of American life and to be back in a country where the vast majority of people spoke my native language. Part of me was elated to be away from the staring eyes of the Indian men that had seemed to constantly follow me through the streets of Bombay. In Boston I no longer had to make my way through swarms of people or had beggars run up to me crying out for alms. But at the same time, back in this culture of my birth I felt like a complete stranger. It seemed that there were very few people in my life who really wanted to hear about the depth of what I had experienced. My husband, who was immersed in the material seductions, time constraints, and social expectations of his burgeoning law practice had little time or energy to give much attention to Ari and me. He was beginning to make serious money now. Even though he had encouraged me to go to India and had even visited Ari and me there during the five years we spent traveling between India and the United States, once my grants were completed it was as if he expected me to forget everything I had learned and become the stereotypical outwardly attractive yet inwardly superficial music-business wife, who would adorn his arm at important social events. I was deeply saddened by this turn of events. When we first met, he had told me exciting tales of how in his hippie days he had spent a year traveling through India. He had even given me books to read about the Hindu and Sufi traditions. We had even dreamed of living in India and exploring her wonders together. Now caught up in a whirlwind of activity, he never even asked to see me dance and took little interest in what I had learned or experienced. Like the husbands of my guruji, Sitara, this beloved father of my child who had originally been attracted to me because of my artistic capabilities and spiritual leanings suddenly seemed obsessed with the need for constant demonstrations of my skills as a housekeeper, caretaker, and socialite.

My friends were not much better. So many of them seemed to be caught up in the need to live up to parental expectations or the desire for professional advancement, with its corresponding financial rewards. They seemed to believe that if one had enough money every problem could be solved. They thought I had gone a bit daft, as I walked around in my saris with a diamond adorning my left nostril, singing devotional songs and dancing with Ari, and constantly trying to speak to them about the Goddess, her priestesses, and devotees. To many of them India had turned me into one of those bizarre Hare Krishna types who assaulted them at airports, telling them that their lives would be better if they purchased and read the teachings of their lord Krishna.

I was alienated from the secular materialistic orientation that appeared to me to be the signature of Western culture, and I felt so lost. I watched as the people around me became trapped by their consumer lifestyles. I noticed how the women and young girls at music-business events worked extremely hard to live up to the media's expectations of how they should act and appear. Dressed in skin-tight black attire that exposed their muscle-bound legs and phony implanted breasts, and clinging onto the arms of rich executives three times their age, these women clearly thought sex was a way to advance their positions. All around me I saw women doing their best to mold themselves into what I now considered to be a completely distorted image of feminine expression that was imposed upon them by popular magazines, television, and, of course, the dream weavers of Hollywood.

I was deeply saddened as I also began to realize that my former sisters in the feminist movement had increasingly begun to take on what I now considered to be masculine modes of dress and action. Nowhere did I see the kind of grace, serenity, courage, or sense of mystery that I had seen in the Indian women I had known. Having been opened to the ways of the Goddess and schooled in her mysteries, I was disturbed by this clear distortion of feminine expression. I did my best to follow the advice of my guruji—to look for the Goddess in all beings—but that only seemed to intensify my suffering. Yes, I knew that her divine spark was in each and every person, but it seemed to me that no one else could see it or even knew that it existed.

Then one night, in the midst of what was becoming a deep depression, I had an unusual dream. I was in a dark forest surrounded by snow-covered mountains, seated among a circle of women. We were all dressed in red saris. Necklaces and earrings of turquoise, silver, and carnelian adorned our bodies. Our hair fell in thick braids down our backs. We were singing together while performing beautiful mudras. Our eyes were closed but our facial expressions bespoke delight and rapture. I woke up feeling blessed by the presence of the Goddess.

Not long after this dream a friend I had met in India visited me. Jean Finney was an American poet, performance artist, and wild woman who had spent many years living in India seeking out the ways of the Goddess. She saw how difficult it was for me to reintegrate myself within the American culture, so she asked me to accompany her to a retreat organized by the Tibetan tantric master Namkhai Norbu Rinpoche. Jean said I would find a place of refuge there and would meet others who would understand and appreciate my training in the sacred teachings of the East. When I asked if Ari could accompany me to this retreat, she smiled and said, "Of course. Tibetans love children as much as the Indians. Lots of Norbu Rinpoche's students bring their children to his teachings. Usually there are teenagers who hang out and play with the younger ones. They can even come and participate in the rituals. Ari will have a wonderful time."

On the two-hour drive from Boston to the retreat center in the Berkshire Mountains of western Massachusetts, Jean told me of the intimate relationship between the spiritual teachings of India and Tibet. "Tibetan Tantric Buddhism developed late in the eighth century," she said. "With the teachings of the Indian sage Gautama Buddha as its base, Tibetan Tantric Buddhism's development was also greatly influenced by the indigenous Bon Shamanic tradition of Tibet, the tantric teachings of India, and Cha'an from China. However, at the heart of Tibetan Tantric Buddhism are the teachings of a great spiritual adept named Padmasambhava, also known as the Lotus-Born Guru. The legends say that this great magician was born spontaneously on the earth out of the heart of a lotus flower. Even as a small child he was filled with a knowledge, wisdom, and the capacity to interact with the visionary dimensions and manifest miracles that transcended those of the most powerful adepts and magicians of his time. He was born in India, but he felt that his mission was to bring the great teachings of the ancient masters to the people of Tibet."

Jean handed me a snack of a rice cracker covered with peanut butter and continued, "Secluded by the highest mountains in the world and isolated from the materialistic focus of the West, throughout the ensuing centuries Padmasambhava's followers have continued to study, compare, and preserve these sacred teachings. At the same time they looked inward, seeking answers to the fundamental questions of existence. While we in the West strove to conquer the outer realms of nature and journey to the stars, these Tibetans—like the priestesses, priests, yoginis, and yogis of India—traveled the inner realms seeking the subtle pathways and landscapes of spirit. For them the shining lights of the energetic dimensions have not faded."

Upon hearing about this intimate connection to Hindu Tantra, I was very excited. Was it possible that I could continue my tantric training right here in America? It was almost too good to be true. As Jean and I continued to speak, she told me that the tantric transformational practices transmitted by Norbu Rinpoche would expand on the teachings I received from Sitara. Jean said that these teachings had not only given her tools for understanding and depicting the outer iconography and manifestation of the deities, like the ones I had found in the temple dance tradition. But in addition, the Tibetan tantric practices transmitted by Norbu Rinpoche would help me enter into, more deeply experience, and therefore express the inner visionary dimensions of the deities themselves.

"You have told me about your experiences with Sitara and your longing for greater understanding of the path of the Divine Feminine," Jean said as we turned off the highway onto the beautiful countryside that led to the retreat center. "I'm sure Norbu Rinpoche's teachings will give you further insight into and experience of the yogic practices that were so essential to the training of the temple dancers and priestesses."

From the first moment I entered the tent created to house the teachings of Chögyal Namkhai Norbu Rinpoche, I knew I had entered a magical realm. About a hundred Buddhist practitioners, mostly of American and European origin, were seated with Norbu Rinpoche, performing an ancient tantric ritual of offering, transformation, and protection. The power and energy that pervaded the place was palpable. Norbu Rinpoche, an intriguing man in his late forties, sat on a dais in front of the assembly, the extraordinary power of his presence radiating through the room. Behind him were exquisite paintings of what looked like Hindu goddesses and gods. Some, like Shiva and Kali, had flames of fire exuding from their dancing figures; others, like Lakshmi and Saraswati, were seated or standing on a lotus flower and adorned with exquisite jewels and flowers. Some of the figures that looked to me like yoginis dressed in ornaments of bone were pictured in the flexible yogic postures that I knew as karanas and yogic asanas. One image even showed a female and male deity seated together in sexual union. Streams of rainbow light surrounded this blissful couple.

The whole scene was astonishing to me. The actions of Norbu Rinpoche and his students so clearly reflected the movements I had performed in my dream of the circle of women in the snow-covered mountains. I wondered, *Has the Goddess answered my prayer and led me to others like myself, whose lives are devoted to walking her shining path of spirit?* Tears of gratitude welled in my eyes. I closed them for a moment and in my mind's eye I saw my guruji, Sitara, in the form of the Great Goddess bestowing her blessing on me. Her eyes were filled with love and radiance. *Yes, the Goddess has brought me here*, I thought.

As I watched the group of practitioners chanting, performing mudras, and playing ritual drums and bells, it became clear to me that this community of women and men was focused on an ancient means of communication and interaction with the invisible realms of light and energy that were the domain of the Goddess. The primal beauty of the sound, the grace and fluidity of the gestures, and the passion and focus with which they performed the rite fascinated and attracted me. From my previous training with Sitara, I knew that this was no ordinary display but a living spiritual expression that had been handed down through generations.

The members of the *sangha*, or community, welcomed me with open arms. I discovered that Norbu Rinpoche had attracted a fairly eclectic and international group of students. There were many artists, scholars, psychologists, teachers, and others like me who had been raised in the Judeo-Christian tradition. Many of them had spent time in India, and so they had firsthand knowledge of the difficulties I was experiencing. Having lived among the spiritual teachers of India, a culture that still retained vital links to the teachings and values of their ancestors, these people had also experienced culture shock upon their return to the West. They felt that my training with Sitara would be of immense benefit to me, providing me with a base from which I could appreciate the value of Norbu Rinpoche's powerful teachings. In fact, they told me that his teachings had helped them to more thoroughly comprehend what they had learned from their Indian gurus.

Norbu Rinpoche, they said, like many of his fellow countrymen, had fled to India to seek refuge from the political turmoil that had erupted with the invasion of Tibet by the Chinese. In 1960 at the age of twenty-two, Norbu Rinpoche was invited by Guiseppe Tucci, the great scholar of Oriental studies, to collaborate with him in his research. A few years later Norbu Rinpoche became a professor of Oriental languages at the University of Naples. Here he began extensive research into the origins of the Tibetan culture and the streams of influence that had joined to form the foundation of the spiritual teachings he had received throughout his life. Not long after he began to receive requests to give teachings throughout Europe and America. Having now lived for half his life in the West, Norbu Rinpoche had developed great insight into both the advantages and disadvantages people faced when they left their native culture and then tried to reassimilate.[1]

My curiosity was aroused, and I continued to question the group members, who called themselves the Dzogchen community, about the Tibetan lineage of spiritual transmission and Norbu Rinpoche's connection to it. They told me that the Tibetan lineage, like that of the Hindus, is one in which great caretakers of the spiritual transmission reincarnate throughout the yugas in order to assist human beings in their realization and liberation from the pain and suffering of the material, or *samsaric*, world. Norbu Rinpoche, they said, was one of these spiritual masters.

From a talented and verbose tabla drummer named Paul Leake, who had spent many years in India and Nepal studying this classical Indian instrument and the teachings of the Tibetan masters, I learned that in Tibet when a great master left his

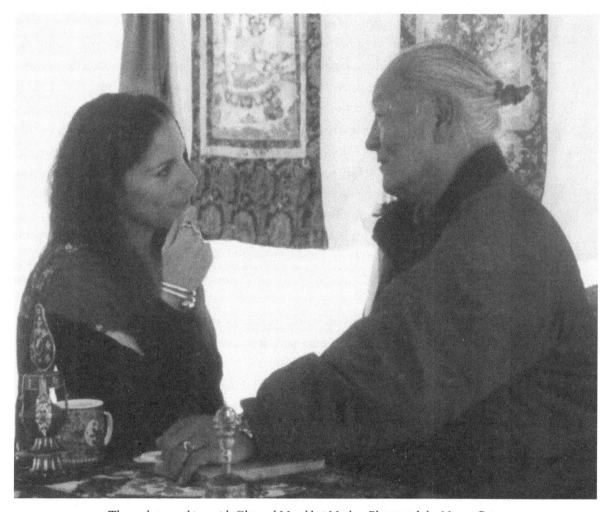

The author speaking with Chögyal Namkhai Norbu. Photograph by Naomi Zeitz.

or her body at death, students and other great masters waited for signs and portents of his or her return or new incarnation. These signs often appeared in dreams and the natural world. In many cases the master had even left prophecies of this future appearance. Through the masters' and students' ability to understand the significance of these prophecies and signs, the reincarnated teacher would be discovered. The practitioners would then travel to the home of the newly incarnated master to test whether the signs were authentic and this actually was a genuine *tulku*, or reincarnation. Often the followers brought the personal items of the former master, particularly implements connected with ritual practices. These items would be placed before the small child along with similar items of other teachers and practitioners. In many cases the child would immediately pick up the implements that had been familiar in his or her former life and even recognize his or her former students. These actions were considered authentication of the master, and he or she would be given the honorific title *Rinpoche*, meaning "precious jewel."

Paul, who later became my primary accompanist and creative partner in the world of classical Indian dance, told me that at the age of two, Namkhai Norbu Rinpoche was recognized as the reincarnation of Adzom Drugpa, one of the great masters of the ancient Tibetan lineage known as Dzogchen. At the age of eight Norbu Rinpoche was also recognized as the mind incarnation of the historical founder of the state of Bhutan. From childhood Norbu Rinpoche was trained to enhance his natural perception of and ability to interact with the supersensory realms. He sat at the feet of many great masters and received numerous initiations. In this way both male and female teachers transmitted to him their own direct perception and experience of the luminous realms and assisted him in the realization of his own innate capacities. Through this age-old process of learning, Norbu Rinpoche not only received initiations into the transformative deity practices of Tibetan Tantra, but also into Dzogchen.

To clarify my questions about the nature of this transmission, one of the senior students, a warm empathic woman with intelligent blue eyes, offered this metaphor: "Imagine, Sharron, that we are seeds emerging from the formless heart of emptiness, or the void, the very core of creation itself. Each of these seeds contains the potential for its own spiritual growth and enlightenment. When the time is right, perhaps after lifetimes of lessons, one meets a teacher who introduces her to the true nature of the mind and the luminous nature of reality itself. Through this direct mind-to-mind transmission of knowledge she is given a genuine experience of what we followers of Tibetan Buddhism call the original or primordial state of awareness. This is the essential awakened and unified state of consciousness that transcends time and the conditioning of the mind. It is what those of us raised in the West would call our divine spiritual essence.

"The teachings tell us," she continued, "that through actions taken in the course of the endless cycles of birth and rebirth, we have accumulated negative karma, which blinds us to the pure untainted radiance of this primordial state of being that we all once knew. This primordial state of awareness is like a pure stream flowing outward from our hearts, the spiritual core of our beings. Through the results of negative actions taken over these lifetimes, the stream becomes so muddied and thick with painful thoughts and emotions that we lose all knowledge of its essential clarity."

Jean, Ari, our new friend, and I walked together toward the small lake where Norbu Rinpoche and the students were swimming. As we watched them playfully splashing each other, the woman continued her explanation of the concepts that are so essential to the Tibetan spiritual teachings. "When you receive this introduction to the primordial or unified state of being," she said, "it is as though in that moment you have awoken from a dream. In that pristine instant of awareness you can see the illusions of the world with great clarity. The lamp of your own spiritual awakening has been lit in the darkness. From that moment on, through the implementation of specific practices given by the master, the essential seed is nourished. The radiant light of one's original primordial state, or spiritual essence, which is symbolized by a luminous ball of light we visualize in our hearts, now becomes a beacon. One then begins to tread the pristine path of spirit that leads out of the suffering of samsara, or this world of pain and suffering. This is the path of Tibetan Tantra and Dzogchen, of which our teacher Norbu Rinpoche is a living master."

On that day as I sat at the feet of Norbu Rinpoche, whose presence and teachings I found so compelling that I hung on his every word, I was directly introduced to the remarkable path of integration and enlightenment that I would follow for the rest of my life. It was a path that would lead me to deeper understanding of the inner yogic training and visionary world of the temple dancers and priestesses.

That evening I continued to question the gracious members of the sangha. From a tall American man named John, who was dressed in Indian attire with a turban wrapped around his head and who was a scholar of Tibetan culture and language, I learned that when the great sage Padmasambhava came to Tibet from India, he brought with him knowledge of the ancient yogic path of spiritual liberation. Padmasambhava claimed that he had come to Tibet to tame the hearts and minds of the Tibetan people and lead them onto the valiant path of *dharma*, or righteousness. The great Tibetan king Trisong Datsen came to value Padmasambhava's teachings so highly that he made them the basis of the spiritual life of his people and even entered his own wife, Yeshe Tsogyel, in instruction and initiation. Yeshe Tsogyel became the consort and primary student of Padmasambhava, and together they practiced the path of Tantra, communed with the larger dimensions, and developed a body of teachings and practices that came to be known as Tibetan Buddhism. These teachings and practices gave students the means by which they could attune themselves to the path of spirit, purify their negative thoughts and actions, and live lives filled with generosity, love, and compassion. The teachings and practices also assisted the students in understanding the true nature of their minds, the power of their emotions, and the luminous nature of reality itself.

From my previous training with Sitara, I understood that this luminosity was a visible expression of the Goddess energy, or Shakti, flowing out from the heart of creation. It was the voice of the Divine expressing itself as the multitude of forms and forces of this world. From the ancient Tibetan perspective, these forms pour out from the original void or primordial source of creation in ever-densifying waves of frequency. From sound they merge into light, then become rays of light, and finally become the forms that make up our physical reality.

After my failed attempts to convince my friends and family of the existence of the realms, I was thrilled to discover that for Norbu Rinpoche and the Tibetan masters these normally unseen dimensions of the Goddess were as real as the physical world is to most of us. Unlike those of us schooled in the modern scientific method of inquiry, which only takes into account what we can discover with our physical senses, Tibetan masters teach that every human being has the innate ability to perceive and interact with these nontangible luminous dimensions. After all, every being in this world is fundamentally composed of light. The Tibetan masters believe that infinite manifestations of enlightened beings, or beings who have realized their luminous nature, exist in the universe in all dimensions, beyond time and space as we usually experience it.[2]

As the group sat together around the dinner table with Norbu Rinpoche drinking Italian wine and singing songs, the master told us that fully awakened beings were once ordinary beings like us who have used their own rituals and practices to attain the state of enlightenment. Known as *dakinis* (female) and *dakas* (male), these luminous beings, or deities, appear in the form of a human or animal—or a combination of the two—so that we in our concrete human dimension can recognize them. "These beings," Norbu Rinpoche said, "are our spiritual ancestors and our inspirational role models. They are beings who out of their great compassion have remained active in the subtle realms of our energetic landscape to inspire us in our practice and assist us as seekers on the path."

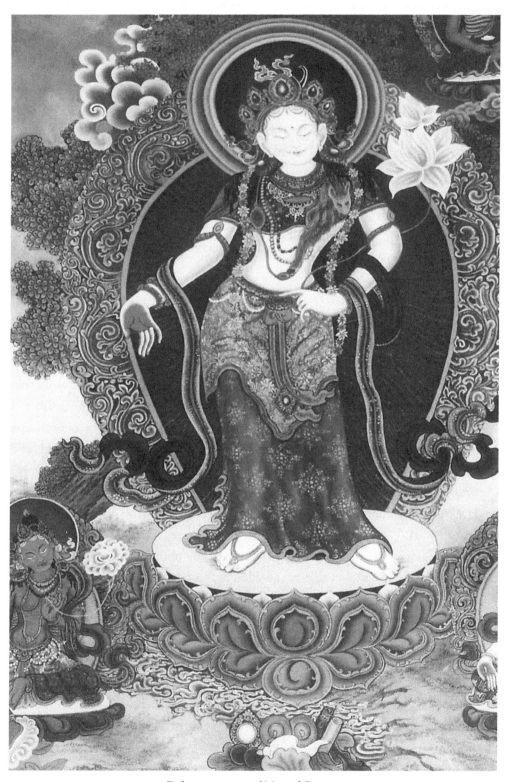

Dakini, courtesy of Nomad Design.

In keeping with this teaching, the next day Norbu Rinpoche spoke to us about the fundamental goals of the higher tantric practices and Dzogchen. "Essentially the goal of both these methods of Tibetan spiritual teaching is to realize your rainbow body, or immortal body of light. If you are diligent and committed to your practice, by the end of your life it is possible for you to exhaust your karma and develop the capacity to enter into the essence of the five elements, which is light, and transform your physical body into pure radiant energy and vanish like a rainbow in the sky. On a physical level, when the person who has accomplished this transformation passes from this material world his or her material body dissolves into this light of the elements, and all that is left of it is hair and fingernails, which we consider impurities. Once this transformation is effected the cycle of reincarnation is complete and one can choose to reappear in a luminous rainbow body whenever one chooses in order to help and teach sentient beings."

Norbu Rinpoche then told us tales of how his ancestors—the yoginis, yogis, and spiritual adepts who have followed this path—were able to accomplish the ultimate level of their practice: transmuting the dense material of the physical body back into its true nature of light. "Once we achieve this fully unified state," he explained, "we no longer see the world and all of its components from a subject-object, I and other dichotomy, but in its true original radiance." He informed us that throughout Tibetan lore we can find evidence of the manifestation of the rainbow body by masters and highly developed practitioners. (The "Legend of Mandarava" presented in chapter 8 offers the story of a princess of India who realized this level of illumination.) According to Norbu Rinpoche, his own uncle, a devoted Dzogchen practitioner, realized this fully illuminated state that exists beyond time and the dualistic nature of our everyday reality.[3]

After receiving this teaching I was stunned. The ability to manifest a rainbow body seemed almost unbelievable to me. Here was a teaching that could help me to purify my body, mind, and spirit to such an extent that I could realize the very essence of Shakti herself. As I continued to reflect upon this teaching, I remembered the story of Christ's resurrection that I had been told by a Catholic friend. My friend had said that three days after his death on the cross, Christ had appeared to Mary Magdalene in a shining "body of glory." I wondered, *Was the magical transmutation that Christians referred to as Christ's transfiguration akin to this Tibetan manifestation of the rainbow body?* If the Eastern teachings were right and we are all made of light, why couldn't we have the innate ability to return to light? Perhaps Christ, like these Eastern adepts, had come to this earth as a divine role model to demonstrate to us that through love, devotion, and right action this magical transmutation was indeed possible. Perhaps

Christ's mission, like those of the Eastern adepts, was to help us purify and reattune ourselves to these more subtle dimensions so that we could enter the mystical path of the light.

In the days that followed I learned about the processes by which I could further refine my awareness of what I knew as Shakti's subtle realms of light and energy. Through the application of specific tantric practices transmitted by Norbu Rinpoche, I was taught how to transform into these luminous dakinis and dakas. During the first retreat with Norbu Rinpoche, I discovered that in a similar manner to the goddesses of the Hindu tantric tradition, the dakinis, or feminine personifications of enlightened energy, were generally placed into three categories. Some, such as the lion-headed Simhamukha, were fierce and wrathful like Kali and Durga. Some, such as the blissful Mandarava, were fertile and sensuous like Lakshmi, while some, such as the graceful Tara, were loving and compassionate like Saraswati. However, just like the Hindu goddesses, each one essentially contained all aspects of Divine Feminine expression.[4]

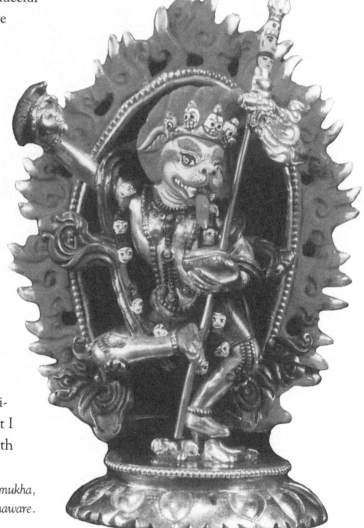

To most of us Westerners, whose perception has been conditioned by the prison of materialism, the tantric deity practices seem wild and phantasmagoric. But for centuries, if not aeons, spiritual masters, priestesses, yoginis, shamans, and healers have utilized methods such as these to balance and harmonize what I call the psychic-energetic-emotional landscape of our reality. This is the fundamental realm of divine energy, or Shakti, and her radiant sisters the dakinis. It is a realm that I discovered is intimately connected with

Dakini Simhamukha,
courtesy of Dharmaware.

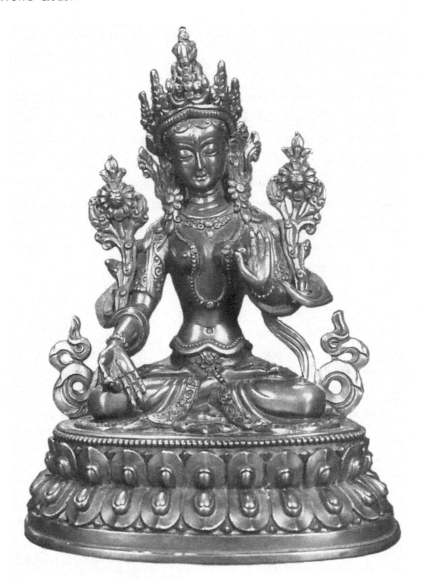

Statue of Tara, courtesy of Dharmaware.

the feminine experience—a realm dominated by feeling, intuition, creativity, imagination, dreams, visions, magic, and miracles.

Because I had learned to embody the goddesses of the Hindu pantheon the dakini practices came easily to me. Visualizing myself as a blissful or wrathful dakini dancing in a realm of light was a powerful and ecstatic experience for me. Having seen me perform the dance of Durga for the community one evening, Norbu Rinpoche even told the members of the sangha that I was a very talented artist who had the capacity to bring these wild, sensuous, and loving dakinis to life. He spoke about how the

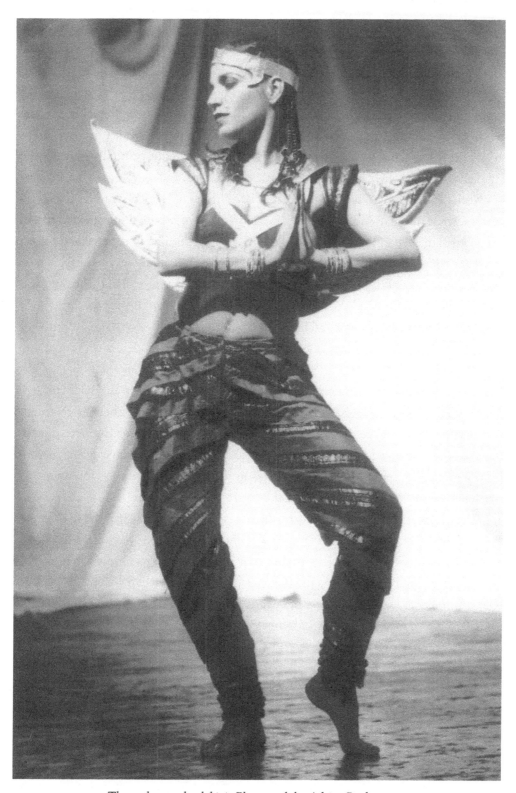

The author as the dakini. Photograph by Adrien Buckmaster.

temple dancers' great discipline, sensitivity to the flow of breath and subtle energy through the body, and extensive training in the art of transformation gave them the ability to accomplish profound levels of yogic practice. "In fact," he said, as he smiled encouragingly at me, "many great Tibetan masters sent their male students to live with and learn from these temple dancers of India." What a powerful acknowledgement of the training my guruji, Sitara, had given me, and the work I had done! For this praise came from a tantric master who was in intimate communion with the divine dakinis and their luminous energetic dimensions.

Norbu Rinpoche is what is called a *terton*, or finder of hidden treasures known as *termas*. These hidden treasures come in the form of teachings transmitted by an enlightened master and then concealed in order for them to be discovered and taught at a later time, when the conditions are ripe for their rediscovery on earth. These teachings were generally written in the language of the dakinis called the *twilight language*. Most of the principle termas discovered in our time are linked with the great Tibetan sage Padmasambhava and his consort, Yeshe Tsogyel. Prior to her attainment of the luminous rainbow body, Yeshe Tsogyel is said to have hidden these termas and entrusted them to the care of the dakinis. Legend even states that the finders of the hidden treasures are the reincarnated disciples of Padmasambhava himself. Through their visionary clarity they have the capacity to discover and decipher the treasures, whether the termas were concealed in the earth, the elements, or the pure dimensions of light.[5] I was told that Norbu Rinpoche had received and revealed to his students a number of termas. Most often it was in the realm of dreams and visions, in a clear state of awakened presence, that they were revealed to him.

What a joy it was for me, a woman who was actively searching for the living remnants of the path of the Divine Feminine, to encounter Norbu Rinpoche's teachings on the dakinis. For in the ancient tradition of Dzogchen the teachings are transmitted, protected, and preserved by the dakinis. The next day when I went to speak to Norbu Rinpoche, I told him that whenever I visualized the dakinis in my mind's eye they started to dance. He stared with great intensity into my eyes, as if he could see into the depths of my soul itself. Then he smiled and said, "That its very good. You are understanding their fundamental energetic nature.

"As symbolic beings the dakinis can be perceived on many levels," he continued, as other students gathered around to listen. "In addition to their role as an expression of enlightened energy in feminine form, dakinis are seen by us as personifications of wisdom and the subtle flow of psychic energy that we practitioners of Tantra and Dzogchen work with to become enlightened. The Sanskrit word *dakini* is translated into English as 'sky-dancer' or 'she who dances in the sky.'

"You see," Norbu Rinpoche added, as he motioned for one of the female students to massage his feet, "in the Tibetan teachings energy is generally thought of as feminine and matter or substance is considered masculine. Therefore, as beings in feminine form, dakinis are linked with the manifestation of energy. This is why they are most often shown in dancing postures." Norbu Rinpoche stopped speaking and turned his gaze toward the patch of clear blue sky that lay beyond the confines of the tent. It seemed to me that he was looking beyond the material realm directly into the subtle realms of the divine dakinis. After a few minutes he continued, "Emanating like beams of sunlight from the primordial source of creation, from the Dzogchen perspective these enlightened beings are a symbolic representation of the fundamentally lucid nature of our minds, free from emotional and mental conditioning."

To give us a clearer picture of this teaching, Norbu Rinpoche used a beautiful metaphor. "The nature of our minds," he said in his heavily accented English, "is like the sun that continuously shines with great clarity and luminosity. But the clouds of our negative karma, dark passions, and grasping ego-centered personalities have obscured this original clarity. With our eyes we can perceive that even though clouds cover its face the sun still shines underneath. In the same manner so too does our essential light constantly shine forth. To remove these dark clouds we must remove these obscurations and illuminate our inner sun—lift the veils of confusion and discover the luminous beings we really are."

During the entire time Norbu Rinpoche was speaking, it was as if I had entered a more lucid state of reality. Everything around me, including Norbu Rinpoche himself, appeared to be glowing. As I gazed into the sky, images of sensuous, peaceful, and wrathful dakinis danced through my consciousness with greater clarity than ever before. It felt as if Norbu Rinpoche was magically transferring his understanding of their divine nature directly to me. At the end of this amazing manifestation, the illuminated images appeared to coalesce into one glowing ball of rainbow light, which then dissolved directly into my heart. The experience was so strong that afterward, even though it was the middle of the day, I was so exhausted that I had to lie down and take a nap.

In the tantric practices transmitted to me by Norbu Rinpoche, I was taught how to directly enter the vibratory dimension of the dakinis and dakas. I also learned how to use mudras, visualizations, and mantras (sacred sounds) to mix my own energy with the deities' more subtle energies.[6] During the next day's teaching, as Norbu Rinpoche sat on the dais dressed in his typical American-style T-shirt and sweat pants, he told us that in the tantric practices the mantra is the key that opens the door to the experience of the essential qualities of the dakini or daka. "There is a plethora of mantras," he said, "each relating to the specific energies and manifesta-tions of a deity. They are akin to a frequency signature that attunes the student to the frequency of the deity's pure dimension known as a *mandala*. Mantras contain a spir-itual power that is transmitted directly from the master to student. Based on what are called seed syllables, the sacred roots of all language, these mantras are said to have originated from the original, primordial source of all becoming."

According to Norbu Rinpoche, when we sound the seed syllable of the deity, in a flash of luminosity the visual form of the syllable arises in our minds. Instantly we feel ourselves transform into the deity, manifesting in its mandala. Everything we see, hear, smell, touch, and taste becomes a part of this luminous dimension.

As I began to chant the sacred mantras I felt as if every tree, every animal, and all the manifest world around me was glowing, nurtured by the power of the sound and the energy of the manifestation. From Sitara I had received an understanding of how to allow the Shakti energy to flow through me and outwardly manifest as a god-dess or god. Now I was learning how to work with mudra, visualization, and mantra in tandem to enhance this transformative training.

Since this first retreat, as I traveled the ancient path of the yogini, I have become intimate with a body of sacred ritual practices that were linked to a primordial tradi-tion that had been nurtured and handed down throughout the ages. These practices helped me to work with and refine the powerful energy of emotion, attune myself more fully to the dimension of dreams, and develop qualities in myself that at one time were not only intrinsic to the character of the temple priestess and yogini but to all women. These are qualities such as fearlessness, commitment, right use of power, generosity, humility, patience, serenity, empathy, and compassion.

Over the years the dakini, like the Goddess herself, has filled my life with her divine energy. Free and fearless, the dakini flies through the empty sky of my aware-ness, her magical luminous body shining brightly with the colors of the rainbow. Dancing playfully through the invisible landscapes of my world, the dakini transmits her divine wisdom to me not through the coldness of intellect but through the warmth of emotions, sensations, visions, and dreams. In this way the dakini embod-ies the essence of the Divine Feminine. As she manifests in her wrathful, blissful, and peaceful forms, she is my fierce protector, joyful and sensuous teacher, and loving mother. As she appears in dreams to instruct me, rescue me from fear, or help me through difficulties, she is my constant attendant. The dakini is receptive, alert, and compassionate and filled with a magical spiritual force that is present and palpable. She is my inspiration, my deepest insight, and my divine teacher. Whenever I begin to feel the shadowy tendrils of negative emotions take hold of me, I sound the dakini's seed syllable, recite her mantra, and visualize myself as the enlightened dakini seeing through to the energetic essence of the negative provocations, until they loosen their hold on me. As my divine role model, the dakini, like her beautiful goddess sisters from cultures around the world, has helped me to grow into a more conscious and caring woman.

As I attuned myself to the more subtle frequencies of enlightened energy and as the wisdom of these illuminated beings began to delicately mix with my own day-to-day experience, I began to perceive the distinction between actions that resulted from these pristine moments of clarity and actions that resulted from the neurotic, compulsive, ego-centered motivations of my deeply imprinted personality. Too often, as challenging situations presented themselves I would not react with subtlety and restraint but rather I would automatically react with anger or frustration. From my studies in psychology I knew that these reactions were often carried over from painful experiences in childhood. Because of the power of these early experiences, I would feel and react to the "residue" of the early imprints. In most cases I was unconsciously responding to unresolved conflicts with parents, teachers, friends, or relatives. I also discovered that my actions frequently stemmed from the powerful mental programming I had received as a child growing up in America's modern consumer culture—programming designed to motivate me toward materialistic self-centered goals and actions.

I have often equated my work in this energetic-emotional aspect of the teachings with what I call the dark night of the soul. Through my research into the tantric practices I discovered that these transformative techniques have always come with a warning: DANGER AHEAD. In the literature the tantric path itself is equated with walking the razor's edge or playing with fire. Why? Because it leads you beyond your imprinted dreams and fantasies of spirituality to discover your true nature. It takes you into a process of mental and emotional purification in which you learn to acknowledge and free yourself from those irrational, savage, grasping, narcissistic impulses—those judgmental thoughts and subtle urges that support the survival of your precious ego at all costs.

When I first began to encounter these issues face to face, they were overwhelming. I wanted to think of myself as a pure angelic being of light, beauty, and endless serenity. I wanted to fly into the mystic realms, transcend the harsh and painful aspects of human experience, conquer all of my dark self-centered impulses, and learn how to repress those impulses. But what I discovered was that I was nothing more than a mortal and vulnerable human being, in denial of my true self. The techniques I learned under the tutelage of Norbu Rinpoche forced me to observe myself, to uncover all my cleverly concealed ego-driven problems and bring them to light. I had to fully embrace these problems and then release them. These are the techniques through which I not only learned to understand the energetic play of my passions but also to experience their power and intensity.

During this self-discovery we were taught that rather than renouncing or suppressing a feeling we should recognize it for what it is: merely the dance and play of energy itself. Norbu Rinpoche gave us numerous practices for seeking, experiencing, and mastering the mental distortions of what he called the five elemental passions: anger, ignorance, lust, jealousy, and pride. Through the application of these practices I began to work with my emotions, using them as implements for spiritual growth. As a person who has always been so overcome by the power and energy of emotions, I often felt that I was drowning in them, so the fact that I found these teachings was a great blessing. Since I had been brought up in a culture that believed that because of their highly emotional nature women were somehow inferior to men, I was amazed to hear Norbu Rinpoche reveal that an important root text of Dzogchen known as *Beyond the Limits of Sound* states that twice as many women as men will be realized through the ancient practice of Dzogchen. Over the years I have come to believe that this is in part due to women's innate receptivity, their ability to keep a commitment once they have made it, and their innate familiarity with the psychic-energetic-emotional landscape.

Dzogchen, also known as the Great Perfection or the Vehicle of Ultimate Union, is considered the highest and the most ancient and revered of the Tibetan teachings. Tsultrim Allione, a vital member of our sangha who has devoted her life to the preservation of these teachings, offers an excellent description of the essence of this path in her book *Women of Wisdom*:

> Dzogchen teaching is based on the idea that we are fundamentally already enlightened. Through transmission from an empowered teacher, and by working together with our energy, luminosity and vision are reawakened and the primordial state of illumination shines through.[7]

Introduction to this primordial state is transmitted from the mind of the master to the mind of the student. In the Dzogchen teachings a master such as Norbu Rinpoche enters into the original primordial state of pure lucid awareness known as *rigpa*, or contemplation. He then directly transmits his realization of this clear, limitless, natural state of mind to the student. The transmission is a telepathic and energetic awakening. During the initiation the student opens herself to receive the energetic vibrations of the teacher, and through the transmission she enters into knowledge or a directly felt perception of the fully awakened state that is beyond karma, conditioning, or the ravages of time itself.[8]

Transmission of the teachings is also accomplished through oral and symbolic means. Oral transmission exists on an intellectual level. To me oral transmission is like preparing the ground for planting a seed. For example, during the many retreats I attended through the years Norbu Rinpoche would clearly explain the methods of practice through which we could attain awakening. Using metaphors, readings, and explanations of the meaning of the texts, he would prepare us to receive his more subtle energetic transmissions.

Symbolic transmission works on a deeper level, as the teachings transcend the spoken word. In the symbolic transmission the master uses ritual objects such as a crystal, mirror, peacock feather, or mudra to convey the inner workings of the universe and the essential nature of the mind. For instance, one sunlit morning during a retreat, Norbu Rinpoche held up a mirror to transmit a simple yet profound teaching concerning the nature of the mind. "The mirror," he said, "demonstrates the pure luminous quality of the mind. It possesses an innate capacity to reflect any object that is placed in front of it. But the mirror itself is never affected by these reflections; it always maintains its pure essence." Then he asked rhetorically, "From this perspective, what is the symbolic purpose of a mirror?"

He answered, "The mirror is both a tool for perceiving the nature of mind and a symbol for the act of self-observation. It is not just an accessory to utilize in order to notice whether your image and attire are in accord with some conditioned societal program. Rather the mirror can be used to introduce you to some of the fundamental aspects of your own being. Its nature, which represents the nature of mind itself, is crystal clear, impartial to any object that it may reflect. Its reflections, which can be seen to represent all of our conceptual thoughts, all of our mental dogma, our convictions, assumptions, and judgments, are just those: reflections.

"But although a mirror has the capacity to reflect, it does not become conditioned by its reflections. It does not display emotion, and it does not judge; it just reflects. And it reflects all with the same degree of clarity; it has no partiality toward one object or another. For the mirror everything that it reflects is the same. And it's the same for the mirror if it doesn't reflect anything. The mirror reflects simply because it possesses the capacity to reflect.

"Our imprinted way of gazing into the mirror," he continued, "is by looking from the subject toward the object. We, the subject, focus our eyes upon the object: our own reflection. In that instant of objectification our minds, conditioned by the overwhelming influence of cultural values, parental persuasion, media inducements, and sociopolitical policies, begin to make judgments. But when traveling the path of liberation judging ourselves in this manner has no real merit. Rather than use the mirror to judge ourselves we should use the mirror to observe ourselves, to understand the inner workings of our own minds.

"When you look around you," he went on, "all that you perceive, whether beautiful or ugly, good or bad, happy or sad, can be likened to the reflections in a mirror. If an individual is found in the state of the clarity and purity of the mirror, in that moment all that one is reflecting—beautiful or ugly, whatever it may be—manifests as one's own nature and qualities. For the true practitioner these reflections—beautiful or ugly, pleasant or unpleasant—don't condition, don't disturb, or cause confusion. One simply remains in that awakened state of clear and instant presence that is the fundamental nature of the mind itself. But instead most of us are found in the condition of the reflections, and without knowing what the reflections really are, become a slave of the reflections. If one can remain in the clear, lucid state of the mirror," Norbu Rinpoche noted, "she or he has realized the essence of the practice."

From my perspective as his student, Rinpoche has fully actualized this profound teaching. Whenever I have had the opportunity to sit at his feet or speak to him about my life and practice, it feels as though all my passions and all my thoughts, both positive and negative, are being reflected back to me so that I can clearly experience their gentle or tumultuous nature.

As I continued on my path I found myself living what I called a dual life. Half of my life was spent as a sacred dancer, Buddhist practitioner, and mother. The other half was spent as the wife of a successful music-business attorney. I was happy that my husband's financial success gave him a measure of respect and acknowledgment in his field. I was also pleased that it gave me the freedom to nurture and care for Ari, as well as to continue my training and studies. But at the same time the disparity between these two worlds was almost unbearable; it was as if they were polar opposites. The world of contemporary pop music appeared to be vain, ostentatious, contrived, and filled with the most up-to-date technological wonders. The other world of sacred dance, Tantra, and Dzogchen was ancient, beautiful, and timeless, filled with teachings that were laden with mystic power. One world was dominated by teenage pop-music idols and their hysterical screaming fans; the other was ruled by spiritual masters, great artists, and their students. One used the term *artist* to describe the members of performing groups manufactured by cunning executives and producers. In many cases these performers, who were chosen merely for their outward appearance, didn't even know how to play their own instruments or even carry a tune. In the sacred world an artist was someone who had spent his or her life devoted to the preservation of the ancient and sophisticated languages of the spirit.

Even though we tried to find ways to keep our marriage together, the conflicting values and goals of our individual pursuits were inexorably pulling my husband and me apart. At times I felt that he was actually jealous of my relationships with Sitara and Norbu Rinpoche. I suppose this was because he saw me devoting more and more of my time to the study of their teachings and because he felt that these teachings would inevitably lead me away from the materially-dominated lifestyle he was trying so hard to maintain for us.

I eventually became very sensitive to the motivating factors that lay at the root of both my own actions and those of others. At this time I became even more deeply aware of the media's intrusion in my family life. Attending social events like the Grammys and MTV award shows which once would have thrilled me, now became a living nightmare. I did my best to maintain the clear mirror that Norbu Rinpoche spoke of, but all I could see and feel around me was a haze of emotional insecurity and mental confusion. People seemed to be fashioning themselves after some media-contrived version of how they should dress and behave, their eyes always darting about to see if there was anyone more important than I that they could speak to. They desperately tried to advance their careers or hold on to their moment in the limelight, making it seem like these people were merely programmed automatons trying to live up to someone else's expectations of them. I did my best to listen to and sympathize with their incessant tales of how they were being taken advantage of by record companies, producers, and the media, or how excited they were about their new Mercedes, expensive condos, or new sex partners. It was as if they were caught up in an endless whirlwind of activity designed to keep them in a perpetual state of craving and anxiety. As I listened to their stories I would remember Norbu Rinpoche's beautiful teachings about the nature of mind and wished that I could share them with these needy restless souls. But I knew from past experience that it is better to share these precious teachings with those who ask; otherwise people think you are either a bit mad, proselytizing, or both.

Fortunately, by this time I had students, friends, and fellow Indian-music aficionados with whom I was able to share the teachings I had received from Norbu Rinpoche. Some of them were also students of the same master. Others were so inspired by the teachings that they even joined me on retreats. One hot and sticky afternoon as a group of us sat together in the incense-filled tent that sheltered us from a powerful thunderstorm, Norbu Rinpoche began to instruct us in the art of self-observation. He gave us this instruction so that we could individually gain a clearer understanding of the difference between the conditioned mind and the nature of the mind. He asked us to observe how and from where our thoughts arose and disappeared, and how these thoughts were linked with emotions. He asked us to become cognizant of the cycles and patterns of their flow and how they obscure the clarity of our minds. Then he sent us off to follow his instructions and report back to him.

As I sat in the shade of a tall tree with the smell of the rain-washed earth wafting through my nostrils, I began to apply this powerful method for perceiving the true nature of mind and emotions. Over the next few days I continued this practice. I discovered that when a wave of emotion arose, rather than perceive it as energy to be acknowledged, employed, or released I often allowed it to take hold of me. That spark of emotional energy ignited a process in which my thoughts appeared to build upon each other. I found myself constructing scenarios based on memories of the past or visions of the future. I could easily see how my mind became trapped in repetitious thought patterns that obscured my clarity and even affected my health and well-being.

I continued to reflect on the energy of these thought processes, and I realized that for most of us the patterns seem to alternate from one extreme to the other. In one moment it seems that the world is full of beauty and radiance, but in the next the world is full of horror and confusion. We hope, we dream, we long for success, for love, for security, for power, or for freedom. We fear sickness and death, loss, pain, chastisement, and brutality. Depending on what manifests as the outer circumstances of our lives, our moods swing back and forth—one minute joyous and filled with enthusiasm, and the next depressed and devoid of energy and inspiration. We vacillate between hope and fear, attachment and aversion, exertion and exhaustion.

One afternoon I walked into the tent that housed the sacred teachings and discovered Norbu Rinpoche sitting on the dais braiding bits of multicolored string to make protection cords for some of the students. I knew that these were given as a kind of blessing from the master, and many people felt that they contained a magical power that would protect them from harm. I thought it would be good for me to have one also, and so I went up to Norbu Rinpoche and requested that he make one for me. With that direct, incisive glance of his he said, "What do you need this material object for? You know that the best protection, the only true protection, is to be fully present in the primordial state of lucid awareness itself."

It is one thing to know this concept on an intellectual level, but it is another to actualize it. I continued to observe myself, and I could feel the restlessness of my mind, how my thoughts constantly fluttered about. It also seemed that the more anxious I became, the more problems I created in my life. Like many of the singers and musicians who populated the music business, I too had grown up with a deep insecurity complex. Desire for acknowledgment, love, intimacy, celebrity, material security, and power seemed to lie at the heart of this restlessness. Like these sensitive and impressionable performers, I was too often looking to the outer world to find some sort of personal validation. Because Norbu Rinpoche understood these tendencies, one afternoon I asked him which practices would be best for working with these issues. He recommended that I focus on the *chod*, a powerful practice for overcoming attachment and the self-clinging machinations of ego.

When Norbu Rinpoche was fourteen years old he was instructed to seek instruction from an accomplished yogini named Ayu Kandro, who, through her devotion to her practice, had realized a high level of inner luminosity and visionary clarity. She lived and practiced in a simple, tiny windowless stone hut under a cliff in the region near Norbu Rinpoche's family's home. Ayu Kandro was 113 years old at that time, although she looked much younger. Perhaps this was because of the power of her practice and the fact that she had lived in this hut in almost total darkness for more than fifty years.[9] During the time Norbu Rinpoche spent with her, she transmitted the chod practice to him, as well as one of the most important and secret Dzogchen teachings: the practice of the dark, or dark retreat.[10]

Chod is a practice that works with images and appearances that arise in both the physical and psychic-energetic-emotional landscapes. By recognizing the original purity and luminosity of the primordial state of awareness beyond the limitations of the ego, the student of chod can cut through the dominion of the ego, attachment, and desire and free herself from the prison of the samsaric, or material, world of illusion. This is a practice that had been realized and brought forth by a great Tibetan yogini named Machig Lapdron, who lived around A.D. 1000. An inspiration to all women on the spiritual path, Machig Lapdron lived a full life as a practitioner, teacher, wife, and mother. In fact, she had many children, as well as numerous disciples who became great chod practitioners. Chod, culled from her personal integration of the wealth of teachings and transmissions from masters of Hindu Tantra, Tibetan Tantra, and Dzogchen, became one of the most widespread teachings in both India and Tibet.

Machig Lapdron understood that at the root of our suffering was the grasping self-centered ego and its material manifestation, the physical body. She recognized that in our three-dimensional reality, dominated by a dualistic mode of perception, we are separated by I and other, subject and object, and blinded from our innate knowledge of the primordial state of union. Therefore we attach supreme importance to our own sense of self and its visible symbol, the body. As Lapdron went deeper into her practice and as her experience of the world grew, she realized that we humans are obsessed with our bodies. She also realized that the passions or emotions that arise from our attachment to these bodies—coupled with the ego's desire for dominion—are at the root of our problems. So she developed a practice designed to assist her students in recognizing this attachment and working with the manifestations of their minds, in order to cut off problems at their source. She felt that by abandoning our attachment to the body and perceiving reality as merely the external display of the mind, we could conquer the demons of the ego, whether they arise as mental obscurations or external energies.

During my graduate studies I had worked with the teachings of Carl Jung and other psychologists who used the symbols and impressions of dreams, visions, and the daily circumstances of one's life in the process of making their clients conscious of the causes and conditions that had formed their irrational fears and neurotic tendencies. The chod gave me an even greater understanding of these issues, helping me to become aware not only of my own fears but also of the powerful energetic nature of fear itself.

Chod is a practice that works with the psychic-energetic-emotional landscape. It is an active dynamic practice that combines singing, playing instruments, visualization, and contemplation. In this practice both female and male practitioners begin by visualizing themselves in the wild and fearful domain of the cremation ground. The cremation ground is a place of great power. It is a place where human beings are forced to confront their deepest fear: death. Metaphorically the cremation ground represents a place of supreme sacrifice where the ego and its self-seeking tendencies is offered up to be purified and transformed. Through this process the veils of illusion are lifted. One is then able to more clearly distinguish between compulsive, habituated patterns of behavior and those arising out of true awareness and integrity.

Chod is a highly symbolic rite. The practitioner uses a bell, which symbolizes the dimension of sound and vibration, and a two-sided drum whose beads simultaneously strike its two faces, which symbolizes the ultimate union of subject and object. After performing the preliminary invocations, she transforms into wrathful dakini. In this illuminated form she visualizes herself dancing with wild abandon before the false masks of her own ego, which she visualizes as demons, deities, animals, and humans. Imagining that the physical body that once housed her consciousness is now transformed into life-enhancing nectar, she offers this luminous elixir to the enlightened beings, guardians, and demons, as well as to the human beings to whom she owes karmic debts. Once this offering is made the chod practitioner reintegrates into the clear, fully conscious primordial state of awareness and dedicates the fruit of her practice and the precious teachings themselves to the benefit and spiritual liberation of all beings.[11]

Chod is a powerful method for working with the mind and emotions. In Tibet these teachings were offered at what we might call chod "colleges," where both women and men spent seven years dedicating themselves to the clear understanding and realization of the chod teachings. After that these nomadic practitioners, or spiritual adepts, traveled alone or in groups throughout the countryside with only the instruments needed for their practice. In remote and forbidding places such as cremation grounds, cemeteries, dark forests, caves, and mountain peaks the adepts practiced the chod. The powerful energies of these places served to intensify the visions and sensations they evoked. Working directly with the psychic-energetic landscape, the practitioners used chod to call up, deal with, and overcome their fears. As a result of their commitment and high level of integration they were able to transcend their attachment to body and ego. Evidence of this level of spiritual realization can be found in the fact that whenever an infectious disease, epidemic, or plague arose in an area, the adepts would come to assist, nursing the sick, burying the dead, and so forth. Norbu Rinpoche told us that chod practitioners were even capable of stopping infection, whether it was carried and manifested among humans or among animals.

As modern-day practitioners living amid the hustle and bustle of Western culture with its increasing demands on our time and energy, we are fortunate that we can even find time to devote ourselves to the realization of such a practice. Because we are caught in the Kali Yuga and imprisoned in the cage of materialism, one of the most difficult issues we are dealing with is the immensity and subtlety of our own egos. Our culture glorifies the outer achievements of the concretized self, and so we have been imprinted to actually reinforce the machinations of ego. As you will see in chapter 6, I have discovered that for us Westerners this is one of the most difficult lessons on the path.

Since dreams were such an important part of my life, I was pleased to discover that in addition to the tantric transformational practices Norbu Rinpoche also focused on what is known as *dream yoga*.[12] This is a potent practice that is connected to both the ancient Tibetan death rites and the practice of dark retreat that Norbu Rinpoche had been given by his female master, Ayu Kandro. In Tibet, as in India, physical existence is considered part of a great cycle of experience that includes birth, life, death, and rebirth. Our innate consciousness is believed not to disappear at death but to travel through a great cycle of incarnations. As we journey through this cycle our actions cause us to create negative karma. This karma obscures our vision so that we cannot see the fundamentally clear luminous nature of reality.[13]

I knew from my training with Sitara that throughout the unfolding of the yugas, direct knowledge of the supreme all-illuminating power and energy of the universe—

Shakti—becomes covered by these karmic veils. Having been bound by the chains of our karma and caught in the visceral thrills, mental cravings, desires, and attachments of material reality, we lose sight of the fact that we have the innate potential to awaken from this karmic dream and see the world with total clarity. The Dzogchen teachings and practices that were transmitted to me by Norbu Rinpoche were designed to assist me in the process of purification and liberation from this distorted karmic vision.

I had often heard Norbu Rinpoche say that life itself is like a dream. "One day you are alive," he would tell us. "You see the world around you as the manifestation of your karma. The next day you could pass away. When this happens your consciousness leaves its physical shell and enters into what we Tibetans refer to as the *bardo*, or intermediate state between death and rebirth where you exist in merely a mental body [similar to the Judeo-Christian soul], without a physical frame of reference. This mental body, like our physical bodies, is fundamentally composed of light. But until the moment of total illumination and reintegration with the primordial state the light of this mental body is like a polluted stream that has been contaminated by our karma."

Norbu Rinpoche informed us that in Tibet, as in other shamanic cultures throughout the world, community members are trained not only to purify this stream but also to maintain conscious awareness during the transitional period between death and rebirth. In this way they have a modicum of control over the bardo experience and the circumstances of their next incarnation. This training even offers practitioners the possibility of attaining the fully awakened state of enlightenment and the immortal rainbow body at the moment of death, or even during their journey through the bardo itself.[14]

Since the cycle of wakefulness, sleep, dream, and wakefulness so resembles the experience of the bardo (life, death, intermediate state, rebirth), it is used as a training tool for maintaining the much sought after continuity of consciousness. During one retreat Norbu Rinpoche transmitted teachings and practices to assist us in maintaining conscious awareness in dreams. He told us that the dream practices not only help prepare us for death but also help us perceive the seeds of our karma and the illusory nature of reality. "By recognizing dreams as dreams while we are yet asleep," he explained, "we become aware of the illusory nature of the dream state, and during the waking state we become more conscious of the illusory nature of everything in daily life."

As I listened to him speak I remembered how I had heard him say that as one performs the dream yoga practices he or she learns to become fully aware in the dream state. In the same way that a playwright scripts the situations surrounding and actions of his characters, the yoga practitioner develops the capacity to consciously script and direct his or her dreams. It follows, then, that by learning to develop and maintain clarity in the dream state one can understand how to maintain this clarity during the waking state as well. Daily life and dreaming life begin to intermingle. Like a sparkling stream snaking its way above and below the ground, the innate light of one's conscious awareness maintains its continuity no matter whether one is awake or asleep, embodied or intangible.

Having developed competence in the art of dreaming, I asked Norbu Rinpoche if there was a practice I could use to further develop this capacity. He questioned me intently about the nature of my dreams. After hearing what I had to say he recommended that I go into dark retreat. In this practice one spends time in total darkness, performing specific techniques and visualizations linked with the transmission. "In the dark," Norbu Rinpoche related, "separated from the distractions of the world, whatever appears in the form of visions is clearly perceived as your inner nature manifesting externally. Not only will you find this to be a remarkable practice to enhance your capacity for dream yoga, but for purifying your impure karmic vision. When this happens you will continue to ascertain the differences between your conditioned mind and the essentially free and luminous nature of mind itself."

I must say that I was a bit nervous when I entered into a ten-day period of total darkness. I had been going through difficult times with my husband. It was as if my entire thought process was a storm of disappointment, discontent, and frustration. The swells of anger, self-doubt, and depression were so intense that I felt as if I had lost all sense of clarity. But I had made the commitment to do this practice. Perhaps the barrage of emotions had been designed to cover the fear I felt in having to face myself without any of my usual day-to-day distractions.

I performed the dark retreat at a simple cabin in the woods that had been specially constructed for this purpose. It contained a number of rooms whose doors opened out to a common hallway, which led to an area containing a sink and a toilet. The handrail that ran through the building made it easy for me to find my way in the darkness. Twice a day, Kathy, a warm and loving student of Norbu Rinpoche's, came by and left food outside the door of my room. The ingenious design of the cabin let in not even the faintest glimmer of Kathy's flashlight when she came to the door.

For the first few days I mostly slept. I did get up occasionally to make my way to the bathroom or eat some food, but it was amazing how exhausted I really was. Living a typical modern existence filled with constant stimulation, expectations, and distractions made my whole system need rest. During this time I began to have many dreams in which I seemed to be trying to work out the problems I was encountering with my husband. Every now and then I would have one of those dreams where I was flying, speaking with Norbu Rinpoche about some part of my practice, dancing with Sitara, or being rescued by a dakini. I even had a repetitive dream in which I was leaving the retreat by swimming in a river that flowed through a dark underground cavern. Throughout this voyage I felt the presence of some shadowy reptilian creatures swimming around and alongside me, but somehow I was not concerned. I seemed to know that if I paid them no mind they would not bother me. In the dream when finally I emerged from the cavern into the light of day I said to myself, "What am I doing here? I'm supposed to be in the dark retreat." As soon as this flash of awareness crossed my mind, I woke up into total darkness. It was an odd experience, as though day and night had been reversed. My dreams were filled with nonstop action and color; my waking life with darkness and silence. It felt as though I had returned to the womb.

The next few days were increasingly difficult. The memory of every negative experience I had over the years with my husband seemed to be replayed over and over in my mind. I could also feel the energy of every argument, every moment of anger or confusion, taking hold of my body. From my early days I had a very emotional nature. Even in my daily life I was very sensitive and overly dramatic. I seemed to be able to feel everyone else's emotions, and somehow I would feel personally responsible for any sadness or pain experienced by the people around me. It was as though I had no boundaries, no protection, and therefore could tap into the ocean of feeling that constantly surrounds and pervades us. My dance training combined with my emotional sensitivity helped me develop a refined kinesthetic sense. Too often in my interactions with others I could not only feel the energy of my own emotions but the energies of others' emotions as well, and they overran my nervous system, creating knots of pain and fear in my stomach or moving me to break down in tears. Alone in the dark, it was as if every one of these incidents was reccurring.

As personal dramas continued to play themselves out, I struggled to remember Norbu Rinpoche's instructions and let my mind relax into its natural spaciousness. I tried my best to harness my concentration and visualize the luminous ball of light in my heart, which symbolized my essential or divine being, free and pure from the beginning of creation. As this radiant symbol of my own enlightened state arose within me I began to relax. Then I remembered Sitara's instruction that in moments of extreme anxiety, I should focus on my breath and ask the Goddess for assistance. Quickly, I called upon Tara, the loving and compassionate dakini and divine protector of Tibet. (The story of Tara, along with exercises to attune oneself to her graceful energetic current, can be found in chapter 9.) As I recited her sacred mantra, *Om Tare Tutare Ture Svaha*, to myself and visualized her in my mind's eye, the speed of the mental images that had plagued me began to slow down. (This powerful mantra of Tibet's divine protector can be translated as "I pay homage [Om] to Tara [Tare], the swift and courageous liberator [Tutare] who removes all fear [Ture] and bestows good fortune. I bow at your lotus feet and experience unity with your divine nature [Svaha].") As I relaxed even further it felt as if Tara, in the form of the Great Mother herself, was weaving a glittering web of light around and through me. I magically began to see the very threads that wove the fabric of my nervous system. Along my spinal cord appeared three subtle channels of light: one that ran parallel to my spinal cord, which I knew from my yogic practices was called the *uma, Shushumna,* or central channel; one to the right of the spine called the *Ida,* or solar channel; and one to the left called the *Pingala,* or lunar channel. Along the central channel whirling radiant funnels of light—my chakras—emerged. Like the spokes of a wheel, out of the chakras glittering lines or threads of light began to spread and interconnect through my body in a pattern similar to the branching of a tree, creating a glowing egg-shaped nebula around me. As the dramas continued to play themselves out, now in a kind of slow motion, in my mind's eye I could see this web of light around my husband's image. I also began to see that as we argued swirls of dark energy emerged from one of us and attached themselves to this luminous energy body of the other. When this happened the area where these dark patches of energy had attached themselves became dimmer, as if suddenly drained of light. As I looked closer at the structure of my own luminous body I noticed that there were even darker spots in my chakras that appeared like deep wounds. When I focused my attention on them new scenes began to flash across my inner vision—scenes from my childhood, scenes in which I had been ignored or emotionally wounded by a parent or friend. These scenes started to mix with those of my more recent dramas with my husband. I slowly began to realize how intimately connected these childhood and adult dramas were, and how in many cases I had been responding not to the incident that I was experiencing with my husband but to unresolved issues in my past. During this whole experience I could simultaneously sense the presence of Tara and the luminous ball of light in my heart, which was a constant source of comfort and refuge for me. Finally I became exhausted, and as I began to drift off to sleep it seemed as if the thoughts, images, and the web of light slowly dissolved into the core of the glowing ball of light in my heart. With the clear essential light of my own radiant spirit still shining within me, I fell asleep.[15]

As the days of the dark retreat continued, I became more and more relaxed. In fact, my mind had a new sense of clarity; my body had a new sense of vitality. On the evening of the tenth day, I emerged from the darkness to discover that even though it was night the world around me was shimmering with light. As I looked at Kathy, who had guided me out from the retreat into this glittering luminescent world; it was as if I could see the light of her subtle energy body forming a kind of cocoon around her.[16] Everything around me was glowing with radiance, and I could see the subtle currents of light that penetrate and interconnect us all. I now understood that the physical form was merely the concretized or material version of this sacred current of light, or Shakti. It was a moment of great realization for me, one that would have profound implications for the rest of my life.

I returned home with new insight into the nature of the problems that existed in my life. I did not know whether I could resuscitate my failing relationship, but I knew that I had been given another key to unlock the secret doors of the sacred temple of light where the dakini danced and the divine Shakti wove her brilliant tapestry of life. How was I to know that the next step on my mystic quest would lead me toward the West to discover that our ancient ancestors in Egypt also possessed information concerning the immortal body of light? And this information would further authenticate the precious teachings I had received from Norbu Rinpoche.

3

Opening the Mystic Eye

*The Temple (for the Egyptians) was a center of the
learning and dissemination of a psycho-physical and
spiritual science whose purpose was to reveal and
develop symbolic, intellectual and physical techniques
which might effect perceptual, behavioral and
physiological changes in the human organism—a
science having the purpose of gradually leading
towards humanity's highest conceivable evolutionary
potential, towards the appearance, that is, of a
Divine or Supra-Human, an organismic being who
had mastered the contingencies and dualities of
mortal existence.*

—ROBERT LAWLOR, SACRED SCIENCE

What was it that led me to the next phase of
my journey—karma, outward circumstances conforming to inner desires, destiny,
or the great healing power of the Goddess herself? Why did it seem that as I opened each new door
into another culture and I began to learn its sacred rituals and practices, they felt so familiar to me? What was it
within these ancient teachings that resonated so deep within my being?

In the healing practices of many traditional cultures there is a powerful technique
known as soul retrieval, a practice in which the healer travels into the visionary landscape to retrieve energetic aspects of the patient that have been lost or stolen or that
have dissipated in this and past lives. As I traveled through life and immersed myself

in the sacred practices and teachings of ages past, I have often felt that I was constantly performing this process of soul retrieval, working to rediscover and reintegrate the knowledge and experience gained in former lifetimes. Through this process, I have been able to develop greater insight into the nature of mind, material reality, and the glittering dance and play of the divine Shakti herself.

What actually triggered my search into the sacred mysteries of the West and the traditional feminine domain of healing? My body.

I had returned home from the dark retreat filled with renewed hope for my marriage. But I quickly came to realize that the new insights I had received into the energetic nature of my relationship with my husband had come too late. My husband was totally entrenched in the day-to-day dramas of his clients, as he had become attorney for the producer and manager of the now world-famous teen pop group the New Kids on the Block. He was spending most of his time either on the telephone negotiating million-dollar contracts or traveling to high-level meetings in Los Angeles and New York. There was little time to attend to our relationship. For a while I moved into a separate room in our huge loft, but finally Ari and I moved into a separate house. Once we were there the strain of the separation began to take hold of me. My body, which had functioned so effortlessly for so long, began to speak to me in ways that I could not ignore. It began to ache all the time as a result of the distress I felt over the failure of my marriage, as well as the fact that I had been dancing since the age of three. Living the life of a dancer, training and pushing myself continuously day after day, year after year, to lift my leg that much higher and to open my hips that much farther while pounding my feet into concrete floors and trying to make my footwork and turns that much faster—often without adequate time for warm-up—it was obvious that sooner or later my body would rebel. Like most dancers and athletes, throughout my life I had minor injuries from which I easily recovered, but now there were constant twinges, aches, and irritations that were crying out for attention. In searching for physical release from the nagging pain I began my exploration of the powerful world of what is referred to in our contemporary jargon as alternative healing.

From my training in the sacred arts of India and Tibet I knew that the physical body is but an external manifestation of more subtle internal, psychic, and metaphysical forces. Therefore I was aware that much of the pain and irritation I was experiencing in my muscles, tissues, and nerves was caused by not just physical injury, such as a fall or car accident, but also a multitude of intangible factors, including karmic traces, genetic propensities, and societal conditioning.

The practices of Tantra and Dzogchen had provided insight into the inner workings of the mind, the subtle landscape or etheric channels and chakras of the luminous body, and the power of the emotions. My visionary experience in dark retreat had indelibly imprinted itself upon my consciousness, affecting both my dreaming and waking life. In this new stage of my journey I wanted to find a healing technique through which I could free myself from pain and more deeply understand the relationship between the anatomy and physiology of the body and these energetic-emotional realms.

I sought out the therapeutic benefits of healing modalities such as massage, rolfing, and acupuncture. Each of these techniques gave me some relief and insight into the relationship of the body and the mind. However, there was one modality, craniosacral therapy, that had a powerful effect on me. Once a week I would travel through the madness of Manhattan traffic for treatment from a highly trained and gifted healer named Margaret Ann Markert.

With every craniosacral session waves of deep emotional memories rose out of the tissue of my body and into my consciousness. I began to perceive where and how these deep-seated emotional patterns, which had been maintained since childhood, had been indelibly imprinted into my body. Yes, there was wear and tear from the years of physical strain, but this attrition was exacerbated by habitual ways of holding and moving my body that had been created in response to painful life experiences. Through the sessions with Margaret Ann I began to discover that in order to energetically protect myself I had locked my body into repetitive patterns of behavior that were often fear based. Now these patterns had locked me into the energetic equivalent of a suit of armor from which my spirit was crying out for release.

One evening after a session, as we sat together in the small garden Margaret Ann had created behind her apartment on Manhattan's Upper West Side, I asked her to speak to me about the history and theories behind this subtle and powerful mode of hands-on healing. She poured us each a cup of chamomile tea and began, "Craniosacral therapy is a diagnostic and healing technique practiced in modern times by cranial osteopaths such as A. J. Still, William Sutherland, and my teacher Dr. John Upledger. This therapy combines concrete knowledge of anatomy and physiology with the development of a sense of intuitive knowing in the practitioner. Like master artists, we craniosacral therapists are trained to directly perceive the subtle rhythms and movements of the craniosacral system, the network of membranes that surround and support the brain and spinal cord and that reach from the cranial bones to the sacrum, forming the outer covering of the coccyx at the base of the spine. These membranes house cerebrospinal fluid, the fluid that protects and nourishes the nervous system.[1]

"Since I know from our work together that you are sensitive to the subtle energetic aspects of this work," Margaret Ann continued, "you will be interested to know that the cerebrospinal fluid is made up of biomineral substances that conduct electromagnetic energy in and around the body. In fact, Hippocrates, the ancient Greek physician, claimed that cerebrospinal fluid carried and transmitted what he referred to as the 'spark of life.'"

These words were like music to my ears. "No wonder I have responded so well to these treatments," I said excitedly. "It seems to me that there must be an intimate connection between the tangible flow of energy in the craniosacral system and the more subtle luminous flow of the Kundalini Shakti, or vital spiritual fire and energy of the Goddess."

Margaret Ann was clearly intrigued and asked me to explain what I meant. Over the course of the evening, as we sipped our tea and watched the boatlike sliver of the crescent moon rise above our heads, I told her tales of my training in the sacred arts of the priestess, temple dancer, and yogini. Then, in the same manner that Sitara had transmitted her knowledge of the Kundalini Shakti, or serpent power, to me, I used the ancient art of mudra to transmit my own experience of the luminous energy body to Margaret Ann. "This is incredible," she said, her eyes glowing with enthusiasm. "Through your symbolic mode of expression you are showing me the very waves, flows, and lines of energy that I have learned to see through my own years of training in the healing arts." She quickly grabbed my hand and led me into her candlelit treatment room. There, under the loving gaze of the image of Tara that hung over the massage table, she taught me how to feel the gentle wavelike pulse of the cerebrospinal fluid that is the essential diagnostic tool of the craniosacral therapist.

She placed her hands together in a mudra that resembled a gesture I had often seen in statues and paintings of the Buddha. This mudra symbolized the Buddha's empty meditative state of mind, in which he was free from the disturbances of thought. Margaret Ann lay down on the table and explained, "Keeping your hands in this configuration, place them under the base of my skull. Then close your eyes and open your awareness. See if you can sense my cranial rhythm." I placed my hands under her head, closed my eyes, and began to tune in to her energy field. In a matter of seconds I could sense a throbbing current that seemed to flow through her body like waves in the sea. As I described these images and sensations to her she said, "It's just as I thought, Sharron; you know how to listen. *Listening* is the term we use for feeling and monitoring the craniosacral system." As I continued to tune into the subtle rocking motion of this current, it dawned on me that what I was listening to was the beautiful voice of the Goddess herself singing through the energetic landscape of

Margaret Ann's nervous system. In that instant, I realized that the Goddess had once again guided me to find yet another key to her mysteries: the key to her ancient art of healing. Once again my divine teacher was leading me on a journey beyond the limits of the rational mind and into the feminine domain of energy, emotion, and intuition. I shared my realization with Margaret Ann. She hugged me and said, "Sharron, I know that you have the ability to become an excellent healer. There are few who can tune in to the cranial rhythm so fast. I wholeheartedly encourage you to take some classes in craniosacral therapy."

Entering this world of healing was exciting but at the same time a bit daunting. Here I was, a dancer training alongside physical therapists, massage therapists, chiropractors, dentists, and physicians. At first I was intimidated by the wealth of their knowledge and experience. I spent night after night poring over books, working to memorize the names and locations of bones, muscles, organs, and systems. Yet it seemed that I had certain skills that would serve me well in this domain. My practice as a dancer had helped me develop strong kinesthetic and tactile senses, which gave me the ability to easily feel the subtle pulsations and rhythms of the craniosacral system and the organs themselves. In addition, my tantric training in the visionary realms of the psychic landscape gave me a base from which I could perceive energetic blockages and distortions in the body. As I gained a measure of confidence in my intuitive abilities, I became more adept in reading the signals of both the physical body and its luminous energy field. In this way I was able to obtain a glimpse of the factors and forces that had come together to create an energy blockage.

My teachers were excellent at helping me to refine the techniques upon which this healing modality was based, but they generally shied away from my pointed questions about the luminous body. "Don't get lost in visual phenomenon," they would say. "Keep your mind on the tissues; the tissues never lie. Develop a solid grounding in technique, and then you will have a base from which you can further develop your intuitive and visionary abilities."

A year and a half into my craniosacral therapy training, circumstances led me to a man who would not only help me to integrate these techniques with my intuitive faculties but who would also become my next teacher in the sacred mysteries of the Goddess. Dr. Robert E. Lee Masters was born into a Baptist family in the heartland of America and was named after the well-respected leader of the Confederate Army during the American Civil War. Like his namesake Dr. Masters was also a rebel. Over the years of my mystic quest I had heard many colorful stories about Dr. Masters's wild adventures in the realms of healing, psychedelics, and the occult mysteries. He, together with his wife, Dr. Jean Houston, had written the books *Mind Games* and *The*

Varieties of Psychedelic Experience. These two books had greatly interested me in my graduate-school days. I had also heard that Dr. Masters was a magician and a hypnotist who had great healing powers, which he attributed to his relationship with Sekhmet, the powerful lion-headed goddess of ancient Egypt. I was intrigued, and when—by karma, coincidence, or the hand of the Goddess herself—I happened to meet Dr. Masters's secretary, I asked her to introduce me to him.

On the day that I first stepped across the threshold to meet Dr. Masters and Dr. Houston, I knew that I had entered a world of myth and mystery. Every nook and cranny of their spacious home was filled with extraordinary statues and artwork of ages past. Gods and goddesses from India, Greece, Tibet, and Egypt sat side by side, creating what felt like an incredible energetic field. Each statue seemed to resonate with an inner life. As I listened to Dr. Masters speak about his healing work and his extraordinary relationship with the ancient Egyptian goddess Sekhmet, to whom he was ardently devoted, I felt as if I was in the presence of an ancient Egyptian priest or a wizard straight out of Tolkien's *Lord of the Rings* series.

After listening with great interest to the history of my metaphysical training with Sitara and Norbu Rinpoche and my more recent studies in craniosacral therapy, Dr. Masters suggested that we work together. He felt that my dance experience and my extensive training in the sacred arts and yogic disciplines of the East would make me an excellent assistant. I was captivated by the mystical atmosphere of his home and his strong presence, and I realized that this was an incredible opportunity for me to learn from a great healer and devotee of the Goddess, so I quickly agreed. As I closed my eyes for a moment to reflect on this decision, an image of my guruji, Sitara, rose before me. She had a beatific smile on her face, as if she was pleased with my new adventure. After all, Dr. Masters had spent the last hour questioning me in detail about the techniques and practices I had learned from her. I had even danced a little for him and his wife, Jean, after they had asked me to demonstrate my knowledge of the ancient tantric art of Katha Nritya. They were so pleased with my embodiment of the Hindu and Tibetan goddesses that they requested I once again manifest for them as Kali, Tara, Lakshmi, or the fierce lion-headed Simhamukha. After watching me dance Dr. Masters sat back in his chair and continued with his questions. He seemed particularly interested in my knowledge of Shakti, the dakini Simhamukha, the luminous body, and the serpent power, or kundalini energy.

After I had sufficiently answered his questions, Dr. Masters asked me if I would like to travel with him into the inner landscape of vision to ancient Egypt and meet the goddess Sekhmet. I eagerly consented. He told me that since this was the first time we would work together he would use a hypnotic induction method, but he suspected that soon we would have no need for this technique for entering into what he called a mutual trance state.

Before we began our journey Dr. Masters told me about the goddess Sekhmet. He said that there was an intimate connection between Sekhmet and Shakti. "Both the Sanskrit root for the word *Shakti* and the Egyptian root for the word *Sekhmet* are translated as 'power,'" he reported. "In fact, I believe that the Sanskrit word *Shakti* was originally derived from the name *Sekhmet*." He raised his eyes toward the huge wooden statue of the Sekhmet that stood next to him. "Look at the hooded serpent that sits atop her head. Sekhmet, like Shakti, is a kundalini goddess who awakens and transmits the serpent fire. In this form she is known as the great awakener. Sekhmet, like the goddesses and dakinis of India and Tibet, has a sacred mantra that attunes her devotees with her powerful energy." In his strong and sonorous voice he said, "Repeat after me: *Sa Sekham Sâhu, Sa Sekham Sâhu, Sa Sekham Sâhu.*" As I repeated the mantra with Dr. Masters I could feel the atmosphere of the room shift. It seemed that all the statues around us began to vibrate with energy. "We can translate this

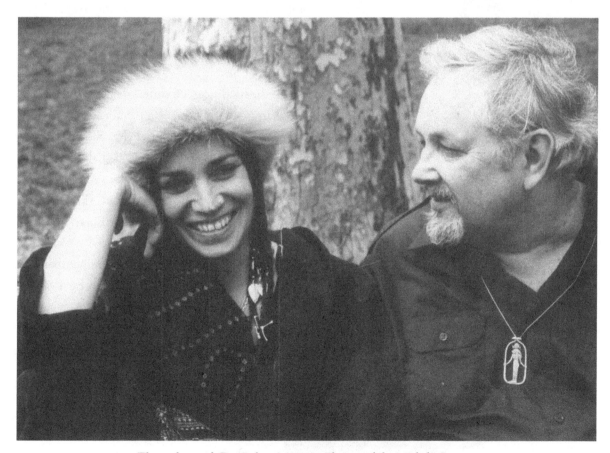

The author with Dr. Robert Masters. Photograph by Michele Carrier.

mantra from the ancient Egyptian," he added. "*Sa* means 'the breath of life,' *Sekhem* means 'the sacred power,' *Sâhu* means 'the realized human.' It is the first mantra to be practiced by all the initiates on Sekhmet's sacred path." With a gleam in his eye Dr. Masters said, "Come, let us journey to her sacred temple. I'm certain that she will have some surprises waiting in store for you."

Dr. Masters sat across the room in his oversized chair, peered at me with his dark mesmerizing eyes, and spoke in a slow hypnotic tone. I felt like I was being introduced to the teaching methods and ritual practices used in the mystery schools of ancient Egypt.

"Five . . . breathing slowly and deeply." My eyelids began to droop as my chin floated slowly downward toward my chest. "Four . . . sinking into a state of deep relaxation, every breath taking you deeper and deeper." The tips of my toes and fingers began to tingle with energy. "Three . . . with every passing moment going deeper and deeper." I felt my eyelids flutter as warm soothing energy radiated through me, seeping into my bones. "Two . . . falling deeper." My whole body was slowly immersed in a soft delicate sense of pleasure. "One . . . traveling effortlessly together across time and space . . ."

Out of the darkness of inner space a blue lotus flower rose from the depths of a primordial ocean, its delicate petals shimmering with light. Slowly, effortlessly, the petals spun open to reveal a shining solar disk that climbed into the dark sky, glowing with energy and power, illuminating the world. As this vision unfolded, I heard Dr. Masters whisper, "Witness the birth of the sun, Ra's emblem in the sky, source of life and light. Awaken, Shaha-Ra, and remember."

I opened my eyes and felt the radiant heat of the sun on my face as the sensuous touch of a gentle breeze wafted across my body. I was a tall, long-legged female of approximately sixteen years, dressed in a simple tunic of pure white linen. My long black hair flowed in waves down my back; my

Dr. Masters' ancient statue of Sekhmet.

almond-shaped blue eyes were ringed with kohl, powdered lapis, and malachite. My teacher and guide, Dr. Masters, whose name in this ancient setting was Nefer, stood beside me. He was a tall, regal, and powerfully built man with the wise and compassionate eyes of a healer. Dressed in priestly attire and with hooked staff in hand, he knew me well, and called me by the name Shaha-Ra. Perhaps it was the lost remnants of our vital energy that had drawn us back to this ancient time and place, or perhaps it was the longing that we both felt to walk the ancient path of the mysteries once again, but there we were on the fertile banks of the Nile River, basking in the warmth and energy of Ra, the sun.

As we walked through the tall reeds that grew in the rich black earth along the bank of the river, Nefer stopped for a moment. Reaching down through the high grass he deftly picked up a multicolored serpent and offered her to me. As she slowly wrapped herself around my olive-skinned arm, I felt the texture of her skin, her coolness, the fluid, supple, undulating nature of her motion. I held her up and looked deeply into her hooded face. I noticed the keen alertness of her fiery golden eyes and watched her long forked tongue as it flickered in and out of her mouth. Placing the snake next to my ear I heard her whisper the word *sekhem* to me in her soft hissing language. She spoke of the power of *sekhem,* the inexhaustible power and potency that gives birth to life; the overwhelming living presence that ceaselessly arises and overflows, spilling forth into the world in uninterrupted streams of energy.

I thanked the serpent for her teaching and released her onto the riverbank, where I continued to watch the rippling patterns of her movement. "Open your eyes to the wonders of the manifest world, Shaha-Ra," my perceptive guide instructed me. "Notice how closely the patterns of the serpent resemble the flowing patterns of nature, the undulating quality of the land, the flowing waters of the river." As Nefer spoke, the serpent made her way into the grass, coiling her body into a spiral configuration in the shade of a tall palm.

Watching her display, Nefer laughed and continued, "I see that she is offering you a great and auspicious teaching today, Shaha-Ra, providing you with an opportunity to see into the energetic forms and elemental forces of the Great Goddess herself. Here the serpent lies coiled about herself, demonstrating the geometric configuration of the potential, seed, or essence of life waiting to unfold. As you will soon discover, this circular pattern lies at the heart of manifestation and is the essential shape of the feminine force that nourishes and vivifies us all."

We walked along in silence for a while, lost in contemplation about the energetic qualities and geometric configurations revealed to us by the magical serpent. Soon we reached the outer enclosure of the great Temple of the Goddess. The walls of this magnificent structure appeared to be alive and glowing, a rich flowing tapestry of color and form. As we came closer I noticed that the walls were covered with images and glyphs painted in the bright, multicolored hues of the rainbow.

My wise companion turned and looked deeply into my eyes. I felt as if he was peering into my soul, questioning whether I was prepared to receive the next level of the teaching. Then he took my hand and placed it on the glyph of the serpent carved on this luminous yet solid wall. As my hand traced the outline of the glyph, I heard the sound *iaret*. Once again I saw the living form of the sleeping serpent coiled at the base of the tree. She slowly uncoiled herself and rose straight up before me, her sup-

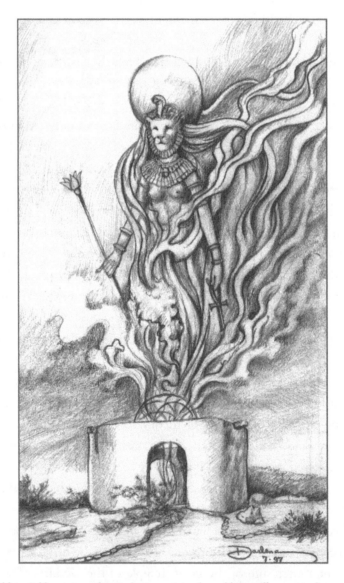

The goddess Sekhmet providing a doorway into the sublime. Illustration by DARLENE.

ple body moving in rhythmic, undulating, figure-eight patterns. When she had fully uncoiled herself she resembled a tall pillar or column of luminosity, and she once again lifted her glittering hood and spoke to me in the subtle vibratory tones of her hiss. "*Sa Sekhem Sâhu,*" she whispered. "*Sa Sekhem Sâhu.*"

Waves of energy began to course through me as the gates of my perception suddenly burst open. Images juxtaposed themselves upon my consciousness; sea shells, snails, pinecones, tree growth patterns, rose petal formations, hurricanes, and the heart of the galaxy itself appeared before my eyes in a vibrant exhibition of the circular, spiraling pattern of universal manifestation. From this central core of the galaxy scintillating waves of liquid light emanated in all directions, forming a vast pulsating network of luminosity. I saw the earth as a reflection of this same primal weblike pattern. Rivers and streams snaked through its dense body, weaving serpentine pathways that traversed both the inner and outer dimensions of the planet. I noticed that these fluid glistening streams of light were pulsating in synchronicity with the heart of the galaxy itself, as if they were in direct communion.

My kind mentor reached down and softly placed his hand on my heart. I felt my heart begin to beat at the same frequency as his. "Shaha-Ra," Nefer said in his deep and soothing voice, "feel the primal pulse of the Goddess—the source of all becoming, the lady of the place of the beginning of time—beating deep within you. Harmonize your heart with hers, with the center of the universe itself. Rest free and easy in the warmth of her boundless love."

We bowed together in homage to the Great Goddess of the universe and made our offerings as we entered the immense portal of the temple. Great stone statues lined the hall. They seemed to be silently inspecting us with their ancient ever-watchful eyes. Soon we entered the central chamber. Slowly and with great reverence we walked forward until we were standing before the immense living statue of the goddess Sekhmet. The whole room was alive with a powerful energetic presence. Sekhmet's lion-headed body glowed with an inner light. Aware of our presence, she lifted her head and roared with power and energy. Then she looked directly at us with the kind and generous eyes of the mother who nurtures and protects all.

As high priest of the goddess Sekhmet, Nefer made a series of ritual gestures and spoke the sacred incantation:

> *Sa Sekham Sâhu.* Oh, flaming one, goddess of fire, lady of the lamp, remover of shadows, opener of ways, lift the veil of darkness that surrounds your priestess Shaha-Ra. Illuminate her inner fire, awaken her heart, open her mystic eye, so that she may perceive the true nature of your shining kingdom.
>
> Beloved Sekhmet, gentle mother, powerful of heart who protects and heals all,

grant Shaha-Ra your treasured gift of inner sight. Allow her to enter and take her place among the priestesses who perform their life-enhancing craft amid the walls of your ancient temple of healing.

While holding the golden *ankh*, a symbol of life, in her hand, the great lion-headed goddess moved toward me. The serpent that sat upon her head reared up, its eyes alive, its darting tongue sending out multicolored flames of energy. As I bowed down before the goddess she lifted my head and placed her thumb between my eyebrows. In a blazing flash of light I once again saw the luminous sleeping serpent, but now she was coiled around the base of my spine. A searing sensation like liquid fire traversed my spine. Something quickened inside my body. The serpent awoke and began to make her way up my spine, moving, dancing, undulating upward to my navel, solar plexus, heart, throat, and the center of my head. Millions of glittering particles of light burst forth, merging into multicolored streams of luminosity. Wave after wave of energy radiated through me like flickering tongues of fire. I was filled with Sekhmet's fiery energy, and I awakened to a new level of light and life.

As I continued to stand before the primordial goddess, the one who was before the gods were, Sekhmet's whole body began to glow with an immense brilliance. Flames darted from her mane. The entire room throbbed with the electricity generated from her hands. Her eyes shone with power. She reached forward, ankh in hand. Pointing it toward my heart and turning it like a great key, she made the sacred gesture of opening. A vertical shaft of light immediately emerged from the center of my heart to link the earth and sky, followed by a horizontal line that intersected and crossed the first, reaching outward toward the horizon. Then, just as quickly, another line of light emerged traveling front to back. Upon this three-dimensional structure, a net of intersecting lines of light gradually materialized. A tiny vortex shone at each intersection, the brightest of them manifesting along my spinal column. The light danced and played and wove its way through the matrix that now surrounded me in what resembled a great oval-shaped ball of light. I immediately understood that this was the same pattern of energy that had appeared in my vision as the rivers, streams, and oceans of the planet—that this same luminous "cocoon" that now enveloped my body also surrounded the earth, the stars, and the universe itself.

Nefer spoke to me, the rich, deep tones of his voice resonating with warmth and wisdom. "The universe of your body, my child, is but a mirror or microcosm of the vast macrocosmic universe that encompasses us all. The great kundalini goddess Sekhmet has opened a doorway for you to a new plane of existence and awareness. You have seen the spiritual fire that assimilates the darkness and turns it into light, how spirit infuses and illuminates the flesh. This is a gift for you, my child, a gift of perception, insight, and healing. Do not use it in vain. Study well; conscientiously apply yourself until you know how to integrate and refine its magical force. Then you will live a life of service, using your craft not for selfish gains but for the benefit of all beings that walk upon this sacred land. Soon we will awaken and remember all that has happened here. It will be indelibly imprinted into our psychophysical bodies. We will remember this time and place so that we can return and receive further teachings from the great awakener."

Sa Sekhem Sâhu.

Over the months that followed Dr. Masters and I traveled together through the visionary landscape created by the interweaving of our experiences in the mythic and symbolic realms. We journeyed back in time to the ancient temples and domains of the Goddess to take teachings. From Egypt to India, Tibet, and Hawaii we flew on sparkling beams of light. Sometimes through light-filled tunnels, sometimes in luminous balls of light, we traveled together along the mystic currents of her divine light and energy. After some time Dr. Masters and I developed the capacity to link our energy and enter the psychic-energetic landscape together just by looking at each other.

Both Dr. Masters and I felt that it was the great lion-headed goddess herself who had brought us together. For years, transforming myself into Simhamukha, the Tibetan lion-headed dakini, had been a major part of my tantric practice. I felt that some portion of her powerful, fearless, and protective energy had been encoded in my cells. Dr. Masters, on the other hand, described himself as a priest of Sekhmet, who was "born out of" her and had been chosen by her for a special purpose.[2]

One afternoon in the early days of our work together, he brought me into his private study, which was filled with statues of goddesses, wizards, dragons, crystal balls, ceremonial daggers, books, manuscripts, and other mystical items from around the world. He showed me an ancient bronze statue of Sekhmet that he said served as a focal point for his healing and visionary work. While gazing at this statue I asked Dr. Masters to tell me about how he came to be a priest of Sekhmet.

"From early childhood," he said, "I was fascinated by all things Egyptian, especially statues and mummies. The huge statue of Ramses II familiar to many from frequently reproduced photographs resembled me very closely when I was in my late teens and twenties, and I felt a great affinity with and attraction toward Ramses II. The pharaoh, I would later learn, claimed Sekhmet as his actual mother.

"I was finally claimed by Sekhmet when I stood before a large granite statue of her in New York's Metropolitan Museum of Art. It was as if my soul rose within me

to proclaim its love for and dedication to Sekhmet. Soon, under unusual circumstances, there came into my possession this ancient bronze statue of her, which made
unnecessary the daily trips to the Metropolitan Museum and the monumental statue
of the goddess. I then embarked on a program of regular meditation that yielded an
unending flow of information that was important to me."

As he spoke, we continued to gaze at the statue, which he said was three thousand years old and was rumored to have been owned by Ramses II. This statue seemed
to possess a powerful energetic frequency. Having been enlivened by our attention,
subtle currents of light appeared to radiate outward from the statue toward us. "In the
temples of ancient Egypt," Dr. Masters related, "small statues such as this one were
kept in the most sacred chambers of the temple. Great care was taken in their construction, for they were said to house the living presence of the *neter*."

For the ancient Egyptians the realms of nature, the human body, and the cosmos
were completely intertwined. According to Dr. Masters the ancient Egyptians did not
yet experience the concretized ego-personality that we moderns do, but a vast interweaving of divine energetic forces that pervaded and enveloped them. To the ancient
Egyptians these divine all-pervasive forces were known as *neters*, or living deities.

At this point Dr. Houston came into the room to invite us to join her for lunch.
Overhearing the topic of our discussion, she eagerly read to us from the pages of the
manuscript of her forthcoming book on the teachings of ancient Egypt titled *The
Passion of Isis and Osiris*. "Of the forces contributing to the intense and complex
growth of ancient Egyptian civilization," Dr. Houston read in her rich and powerful
voice, which reminded me of an Irish bard or poet, "one of the most vital was the
notion of the livings gods, or the concept of *neters*. Egyptian gods and goddesses are
the divine impulses that reveal themselves in the natural world and in the body. The
neters of Egypt are the rock bed of our first spiritual longing."

What an amazing couple, I thought as I listened to the beauty of Dr. Houston's
words. How fortunate I am that the Goddess brought me here to learn from them. "If
we trace the Egyptian word *neter* through the Coptic and Greek, we arrive at the root
form of our word *nature*," Dr. Houston continued. "Male or female, the neters
revealed their divinity through nature, and the divine nature was present in all
things—animals, plants, moving water, the heavens, the earth."

Over a delicious lunch that Dr. Houston had prepared, she and Dr. Masters told
me about the worldview of the ancient Egyptians. First she directed me to the work
of the great scholars R. A. and Ischa Schwaller de Lubicz, a pair of Western
Egyptologists who had spent many years living in Egypt, decoding the symbolic
teachings of the architecture of the ancient Temple of Luxor. Dr. Houston then

informed me that these teachings, as well as those she had received from Dr. Masters, revealed that the laws, processes, structures, and systems of the human being were a fractal reflection of both nature and the larger surrounding universe. "In other words," she said, "what manifests in our outer world manifests also within the earth itself and on the inner realms within our own bodies. In the expansive worldview of the ancient Egyptians there was no distinct differentiation between inner and outer realities, but there was a constant energetic interconnection and communication between spirit and matter. Theirs was a world rich with symbol and metaphor, a world in which every organ and system, every feature and factor of the body, was seen to be a result of the divine forces, or neters, entering into and pervading the world of form."

I exclaimed, "This was the teaching I received in my initial journey with Dr. Masters, when the goddess Sekhmet introduced me to a new level of what I had previously known as the luminous world of Shakti! From what you are saying, the worldview of the Egyptians appears to be very similar to that of the Indians and Tibetans. From this perspective the neters, or divine energetic forces, can be seen as a manifestation of Shakti like the dakinis and dakas of Tibet."

Dr. Masters added, "There is one source, one light, from which all of these great teachings arose. That is why we find such similarities in the teachings." His dark eyes glowed with an inner light. In that instant he appeared to resemble a fire-breathing dragon from some medieval legend. Calling me by the name Shaha-Ra, which Dr. Masters said was a powerful name energetically linked with both Shakti and Sekhmet, he said in a commanding tone, "Let us continue our work."

We walked back into his private office and took our usual place before the magical statue of the goddess Sekhmet. " I have seen that through the ancient art of temple dance Sitara Devi has taught you one of the essential tasks of the priestesses and priests in the temples: attending to and caring for the statues themselves. Throughout the ancient world these devotees of the Goddess cared for statues such as these and communed with the divine forces that resided within them on a daily basis. They knew that these statues had the capacity to heal, to overcome enemies, to perform a great many other magical and miraculous feats, but most important of all, to teach."

Dr. Masters then described how during his years of meditation on and communion with Sekhmet, he was led through elaborate exercises and practices that taught mindfulness and ways to differentiate, experience, and make use of our subtle energy bodies for psychospiritual work and exploration. He related how over the course of several decades he had trained priestesses in this work, which he called the Way of the Five Bodies of Sekhmet. These teachings included ways of creating new neural pathways in the physical body so that the powerful energies made available would not be harmful, as, for example, kundalini is harmful when experienced by those not prepared for it.

"According to the ancient Egyptians," Dr. Masters told me as we sat before the powerful statue of Sekhmet, who seemed to be watching over us like a mother lioness, "the human being is composed of five bodies. Each of these bodies has a dimension in which it resides and functions. Beginning with the physical or material body, or *Aufu*, these five bodies and their dimensions become increasingly subtle. As the initiate becomes sensitive to these five bodies and their dimensions, she or he begins to make contact with increasingly subtle levels of awareness. The second body is called the *Ka*. Known as the double or body of experience, the Ka is what mystics generally refer to as the astral or etheric body. It is intimately connected to the physical body, and it is the energetic body that our minds perceive as our body image. The next body is called the *Haidit*, or shadow. This more subtle body is in contact with the reality generally experienced by us as mental and mostly unconscious. We work with this body during dreams, visions, trances, or drug-induced states.

"Contact with the next two extremely subtle bodies are only rarely consciously experienced by most individuals these days. These are the *Khu*, or magical body, which is used by highly trained priests, priestesses, yogis, and shamans, and the *Sâhu*, or spiritual body." He stopped speaking for a moment to commune with the goddess Sekhmet, whose presence filled the magical statue. I felt as if I was once again in the ancient temple of Sekhmet, receiving teachings from the high priest Nefer.

"It was these bodies, Shaha-Ra," Dr. Masters continued, "that the initiates of the ancient temples and mystery schools were trained to experience and work with. Knowledge of these bodies and the realms they come into contact with ultimately led these initiates to a direct experience of the realm of total or cosmic consciousness— what your Tibetan master Norbu Rinpoche would call the fully awakened state of enlightenment. The *Sâhu* itself corresponds to what you know as the luminous rainbow body: It is the totally clear and pure body of light that returns to the primordial or supreme source. Once you have reached this level you have gained the knowledge of how to fully integrate and interact with all five of your bodies." I discovered that Dr. Masters had integrated his knowledge of the Way of the Five Bodies into a system of healing he called the Psychophysical Method of Neurosensory Reeducation.

During the time we spent together Dr. Masters and I had often traded healing sessions. He was very pleased with my training in craniosacral therapy and felt that his psychophysical work would help me to develop an even greater capacity as a healer. He even said that he had found a connection between the craniosacral work I had been trained in and the work of the priests and priestesses of Sekhmet's ancient temple of healing. Dr. Masters explained, "There are many ancient Egyptian texts known as papyri that deal with the healing arts. The *Edwin Smith Surgical Papyrus* even mentions the healing work of a priest of Sekhmet. This papyrus was copied down by an Egyptian scribe in 1700 B.C.E., but it is considered part of an ancient scientific tradition that traces its roots back to the great sage and physician Imhotep, who lived around 3500 B.C.E. The text demonstrates that the Egyptians had intimate knowledge of the brain, spinal cord, organs, and systems of the body. The *Edwin Smith Surgical Papyrus* even describes the throbbing, pulsing current of the membranes that comprise your craniosacral system." This new revelation thrilled me, as I realized that in my search for a modern-day healing technique I had magically been led to one that appeared to be connected to the teachings and practices of the priestesses and priests of the temples of ancient Egypt.[3]

Dr. Masters and I spent a great deal of time working together in his treatment room, a large chamber lined from floor to ceiling with books. In the center of this room was a massage table that was watched over by an ancient bust of Athena, the powerful Greek goddess who was so special to Dr. Houston, and two huge colorful Balinese statues of wild and mythic creatures. I had been telling Dr. Masters about a problem I was having in my healing practice. "More often than not," I began, "when I finish my sessions with those who ask me to work with them, they feel refreshed and invigorated. They often remark how much clearer their minds are after the session, how it is like a weight has been lifted off them and they have received new insight into the issues they are facing. I, of course, am happy to hear that my work has been of benefit to them. But as soon as they leave my body begins to go cold all over and even to tremble. Usually I have to wrap myself in a blanket until I warm up again. It is as if I have been depleted of energy. Can you explain why this is happening and what I can do about it?"

Dr. Masters replied, "I have noticed this phenomenon in you, Shaha-Ra. It is due to the fact that when you work you are both not protecting your own luminous energy field and also giving away your vital energy to others. In fact, your empathic ability is so strong that you are actually, at times, energetically taking on their pain. This is a situation that happens to many beginning healers, and it is a situation that can easily be remedied.

"By now you must know that the Shakti energy is readily available to us all; we just have to avail ourselves of it." Dr. Masters looked at me sharply. "You must learn how to protect yourself." I told him about Norbu Rinpoche's instruction that the best protection was to be fully present in the primordial state, and how I found it difficult to maintain this awareness. Dr. Masters said that there were other techniques I could use for protection—in fact, these techniques had been given to me by my former teachers, but I hadn't realized that I could use them in this situation. "Come, I'll show you what I mean," he said with a big smile. "Let us begin by going to the Temple of Sekhmet to replenish our vital energy."

By this point in my training Dr. Masters and I were so energetically attuned to each other that within seconds our world had shifted and we were together once again in the Temple of Sekhmet. As we entered her sacred domain there was a greater feeling of power than on any past occasion. The very air around us seemed to crackle with electricity. The statue of the great lion-headed goddess was enormous, filled with a strength and magnificence that was almost overpowering. In rapid succession we became luminous energy bodies, then bodies of fire, then one body of fire—a cool but very powerful flame that seemed to purify and empower. This flame was inside a vast plane of energies that first opened horizontally and then vertically, expanding upward and downward simultaneously as a great spiral of energies, which became the enormous coiled serpent that we knew as the Kundalini Shakti herself.

From the top of this energetic vortex the eye of Sekhmet looked down. The mouth of the vortex kept expanding until it was of cosmic dimensions. It was moving, opening, expanding, until it seemed that the ultimate experience of the cosmos or divinity was there waiting to reveal itself to us—and all under the direction of the goddess Sekhmet. During this movement there were many rapturous feelings experienced by this one body of flame, including intense feelings of being linked with a primordial energy, of being fed, of drinking light, and of becoming intoxicated, as each cell was flooded with this vital fire of the Goddess.

As we continued the journey it seemed that both our voices spoke from within the one being. There was a sense of many beings present—figures from various religions of the world—with eyes looking in and eyes looking out, and *tigles*, or luminous balls of light, with buddhas, dakinis, and other figures inside. The experience assumed awe-inspiring proportions, with an overwhelming sense of sacredness, wonder, reverence, and the strong feeling that we had crossed over the boundaries of anything that could be called a strictly human experience.

I soon discovered that this powerful influx of energies was merely preparing us for the next session. Dr. Masters had told me that one way in which I could protect myself and not lose my vital energy was to transform myself into a goddess or dakini in the tantric way I had been taught by Sitara Devi and Norbu Rinpoche. He said that this would give me energy and insight into the nature of the luminous body as well as protection from taking on other people's negativity.

As I placed my hands under Dr. Masters's head to monitor his cranial rhythm, I relaxed and opened my proprioceptive faculties, feeling the subtle flow of his cranial rhythm and taking note of the rate and fullness of its expansion and contraction, as well as the imbalances that existed on the two sides of his body. Gently I brought both of us into the heart of stillness, felt his pulse relax, and sensed his whole nervous system begin to release. Tuning in deeper, I projected my kinesthetic awareness and feeling capacities down into his body. He had recently taught me to "see" more clearly into the luminous energetic landscape of the body, observing misalignments, imbalances, energy blockages, and restrictions.

Following his instructions I repeated the goddess Sekhmet's mantra, *Sa Sekhem Sâhu,* over and over in my mind. Soon I was filled with Sekhmet's powerful energy. I could feel her golden mane surrounding my head like a glowing corona. Transformed into the lion-headed goddess, I felt the sensation of my third eye opening and a large beam of golden light pouring forth, illuminating and expanding my inner sight. I was able to see Dr. Masters's skeleton and ligaments as if I had X-ray vision. The goddess showed me the places that needed attention and nurturing, such as Dr. Masters's right ankle, and instructed me to send light into them. She also showed me the dark patches of energy that appeared to envelop certain areas. Sekhmet, I discovered, particularly likes to work with these energetic disturbances at a core level. I began to see myself as Sekhmet either licking or chewing on Dr. Masters's bones, ligaments, connective tissues, and organs in order to cleanse them, removing toxins, tensions, and distortions. Or I mended these parts by directing at them beams of laserlike light. I later discovered that this work is different from the work of other healing deities, such as Tara, Kuan Yin, and the Blessed Virgin Mary, who work very gently to soothe inflammation, childhood emotional trauma, broken hearts, loneliness, and so forth. Both Dr. Masters and I believe that the goddess Sekhmet, like the divine Shakti, assists one in total transformation at the level of essence.

As the session continued, I, as the goddess Sekhmet, poured golden healing light into Dr. Masters. I felt that she loved him dearly and wanted him to be clear and healthy to serve her, and she wanted me to assist her in this process.

Finally, Dr. Masters and I alternately sent streams of luminous revitalizing energy into the subtle network of threadlike filaments that enveloped us. Waves of healing light poured forth as we wove a glistening cocoon of light and energy around ourselves. We emerged from this experience of the powerful healing abilities of the Goddess renewed and refreshed. I continued to integrate these transformative tantric practices into our sessions. This tantric method of protection, as well as the visualization I call "The Energy Field of the Strong and Fiery Goddess," which can be found in chapter 7, have been of great assistance to me not only in my healing work but also in my day-to-day life.

As I began my technical training in the psychophysical method, Dr. Masters and I continued to be guided and assisted by the goddess Sekhmet. All of Dr. Masters's work has at its base his deep love for humanity and the heartfelt desire to assist patients in releasing the psychological chains that bind them. In the same manner that a good detective searches for clues to solve a mystery, Dr. Masters had the capacity to piece together evidence from his observations and interactions with the individual. Like the priests and priestesses of ancient Egypt he perceived each and every human as an intriguing constellation of emotional, energetic, physical, and spiritual expressions woven together to create a unique tapestry.

As we sat together in his garden one late afternoon, taking in the warm rays of the sun, Dr. Masters explained, "The psychophysical work is first of all directed toward making changes in the brain—rearranging brain cells especially—and in the physical body. Musculoskeletal, sensory, and other changes follow the changes in the brain. It is thus not 'bodywork' as usually conceptualized and practiced. As you have seen, Shaha-Ra, this work can be greatly enhanced when done in the context of profoundly altered states of consciousness. When the healer is aware at subtle energetic levels, especially in altered states, she or he can then gain access to at least some subtle body levels of the person being worked on. In doing so changes can be made, for example, to occur in the unconscious with respect even to the potency of symbols and the effects of symbol systems and memories on the conscious mind of the person—and, by that means, on the physical body also."

From his many years of research into psychedelics, psychology, yoga, and the nature of mind itself, Dr. Masters believed that in an altered state of consciousness, free from the limitations of our ordinary waking realty, one could produce any kind of bodily experience, including healing, intensification of pleasure, and reduction of pain. As we continued to travel the visionary dimensions we were fascinated by the fact that we had the capacity to naturally experience altered states of consciousness that were indistinguishable from chemically-induced ones. It appeared that through the medium of this work we were able to tap into and reproduce any manifestation of energy, any experience or sensation that had been lived and therefore encoded in our individual mindstreams, which we could then make accessible to each other. Through the power of this work we were able to create a deep telepathic and empathic connection, mutually experiencing states of tranquillity and serenity, as well as powerful sensations of bliss and rapture.

Throughout the years of my mystic quest I discovered that much of the tension and pain we experience in life is a result of the distorted values, ideas, and expectations imprinted on us during childhood. Even though I had years of training in the sacred arts and craniosacral therapy, I had come to Dr. Masters's door still holding on to many layers of negative conditioning, particularly in my interactions with men. As the work we did together brought us to even deeper levels of awareness and communion, I discovered that I still possessed many contradictory and unresolved feelings toward men, including the desire to please men coupled with a fear of rejection; the longing for true spiritual connection with a man, which was shadowed by concern for being taken advantage of; the need to be acknowledged by them, and the anger and frustration when my insights and opinions were ignored.

Under the guidance of Dr. Masters I became keenly aware of the depth of my internal body-mind split. I came to realize that during the ecstasy of dance and performance, in my work as a teacher, in meditative states, and during healing sessions with my clients, I felt totally connected to my body and the present moment. In these shining crystalline moments, I would automatically enter a more vivid state of clarity and allow the pure light of the divine Shakti to flow through me. This type of experience had been essential to my training. However, in the midst of the tension and pressures of daily life I too often found that rather than stay in my body and work with my feelings I would often swallow my emotions and "fly off" to the visionary realms I loved so much. Desiring what I thought was love and afraid of the magnitude of my own feminine power, rather than face the lesson of the situation I would run away from any type of confrontation, particularly with those of the opposite sex. Now it was time for this negative pattern to be liberated.

Because of his extensive research and experience in the healing arts, Dr. Masters was always cognizant of the profound impact of parental and societal conditioning, as well as the power of the emotions to shape the physical body. From the book *Listening to the Body*, which Dr. Masters had written with Dr. Houston, he read, "Much that happens in the body is clearly a product of emotions, which are more or less unconscious and which are themselves conditioned by attitudes which may be unconscious as well and even directly at odds with one's conscious beliefs. The profound influence of such unconscious or masked emotions on the state of the body may be the single most important determinant of our health, much of our behavior, and indeed the whole course of our lives.

"Because of these factors, the body and its musculature are often fixed into unconscious patterns of holding and protecting. These unconscious patterns, which originate in the mind and are demonstrated in the body, keep the body from functioning in a fluid and pleasurable manner. The body is certainly rational enough to prefer pleasure to pain, but because of this early conditioning, the body's *right* to pleasure must be sanctioned and reaffirmed, in most cases repeatedly."

In order to work on many levels while educating me in the techniques of this powerful healing modality and help me to release these early imprints, Dr. Masters designed a program of psychophysical exercises to assist me in arriving at a more heightened sense of clarity, freedom, and relaxation. The exercises began with of a series of gentle repetitive motions designed to bring new awareness and mobility to specific areas of my body that needed nurturing and release. While performing these exercises I tuned into the area being worked in order to sense restrictions, release tensions (whether physical or emotional), and discover more relaxed and pleasurable ways of moving. As I worked with these exercises I discovered that, like so many Americans influenced by outdated Puritanical beliefs, even though I had struggled so hard to alter my mental and emotional patterns I still retained confusing imprints about my body, sensuality, and the experience of pleasure.

In order to gain greater awareness of the nature of these imprints Dr. Masters and I went deeper into my psyche. Using the healing practices of Sekhmet to engage all five of my bodies, we examined the recurring signs and symbols of my visionary states, dream states, and my waking life. Through this process I was able to identify the specific patterns of energy, emotion, action, and reaction that pervaded my life. I began to distinguish more clearly between my imprinted, ego-centered personality—the part of me that bears witness to its thoughts and actions—and the sacred current of spiritual awareness that runs through it all.[4]

As a result of our work together, I gained greater insight into the relationships between the physical and subtle bodies. I was also given direct knowledge of a powerful system of healing that had been utilized by the priestesses and priests in the temples of ancient Egypt. This made me able to assist my own students in their healing processes; for I knew from experience that it was better to turn and face one's demons and anxieties then let them continue to haunt the mind and spirit. As I watched my students discover, work with, and release their imprints; as I gave them techniques for bringing the powerful light of the divine Shakti into their lives; as I saw them transforming before my eyes into more conscious, courageous, graceful, sensuous, and loving women; and as I watched their luminous bodies begin to shine with a new radiance, my heart was filled with joy.

I love this realm of healing. To this day, I feel that it offers me the cleanest, clearest way to integrate all areas of my training in the sacred arts in order to assist other human beings. It gives me a means by which I can call on all my innate feminine gifts and continue the loving, selfless work of the priestesses, healers, and wise women of old.

During the year in which I worked with Dr. Masters, as we went deeper into the sacred mysteries of the goddess Sekhmet, a clear sense of openness and trust developed between us. I found a place of safety in which old wounds from distorted or inappropriate interactions with men could be recognized and released. As friends working together within clear and appropriate boundaries, we were able to link our minds and direct our energies toward growth and healing. The natural energy that flows between female and male, priestess and priest, yogini and yogi, was channeled in the most loving and supportive manner.

I believe that this interaction made it possible for me to enter the next stage of my mystic quest, one that would not only help me discover the power and potential of female and male union, but would also lead me to discover that the teachings about the luminous body and the power of the Divine Feminine existed deep within the heart of the Judeo-Christian tradition of my birth. Like Dorothy in *The Wizard of Oz*, who traveled over the rainbow only to realize that there was no place like home, I too was on a magical journey that would lead me back to the very place from which I had started.

4

The Keepers of the Light

*I know myself, that the Goddess Isis is the mother of
all things, that she bears them all in her womb and
that she alone can bestow Revelation and Initiation.
You unbelievers, who have eyes that you may not see
and ears that you may not hear, to whom do you
address your prayers? Do you not know that you
can reach Jesus only through the intercession of his
Mother; Sancta Maria, ora pro nobis?*
—FULCANELLI, THE MYSTERY OF THE CATHEDRALS

*hum dhum taka tak, dhum taka tak, taka dhum dhum taka tak,
dhum taka tak.*

The sultry rhythms of sensuality were calling. I had entered
the magical world of ancient Egypt through the doorway of the
healer and the temple priestess. My years of training in the spiritual teachings and practices of Tantra, Dzogchen, and the healing arts
of ancient Egypt helped me travel the physical and psychic-energetic landscapes to
explore the magical domains of the temple dancer, priestess, yogini, and healer. Like
a serpent shedding its skin, I had cast off yet another layer of conditioned responses,
fears, assumptions, and compulsive emotional cravings that had haunted me. With
every passing day I could see with greater clarity the divine light and energy of the
Goddess as it flowed into, through, and between all beings. It was time to take the
next step on my lifelong search to remember the signs, symbols, and teachings that
formed the heart of the sacred feminine mysteries. I was refreshed and revitalized
from my recent work with Dr. Masters and the goddess Sekhmet, and the drums were

calling to me, inviting me to once again take up my lifelong passion and enter the dance.

In search of another essential key to the mysteries of ancient Egypt, I entered the sensuous, exotic, and initiatory realm of Middle Eastern dance. As I stood in the crowded Manhattan dance studio filled with women of all ages, shapes, and sizes, all of whom were doing their best to follow the sensuous movements of our beautiful Gypsy teacher, I wished that I could share with them the rich and subtle teachings of my guruji Sitara, Norbu Rinpoche, or Dr. Masters. The women, dressed in glittering bras, coin-draped hip belts, and colorful transparent skirts, were receiving training in what I knew to be the last surviving remnants of a once sacred art form. For hidden in the movements, postures, expressions, and gestures taught to us by this graceful instructor in her early sixties, I could see a rich and compelling language deeply connected to goddess worship and the feminine mysteries.

Casting aside the veil of the contemporary, secular, and titillating manifestation of cabaret belly dance, I sought out the subtle energetics and teachings intrinsic to the movements of the dance. Trained as I was in the art of the temple priestess and healer, from my perspective these movements had not been originally designed as ways to entice or mesmerize a man sitting in the audience, as we were being taught, but the physical expression of primal patterns of feminine energy. To me these were movements that demonstrated the fertile, fluid, initiatory power and vibration of the divine Shakti herself.[1]

I could feel that what my exotic brown-eyed belly dance instructor called a shimmy was not a lurid shaking of the hips but a trembling or quickening that resounded throughout the sacred vessel of my body. These rapid, ever-so-subtle motions of the shoulders, hips, heels, and entire body recalled the fertilizing and rejuvenating power of the rain as it falls in varying tempos and quantities on the earth and seas. Depending on the force and cadence of the movements, they evoked the fiery thundering force of the wrathful goddess, the shimmering, ecstatic bliss of the sensuous goddess, or the soft and delicate effulgence of the peaceful goddess. The spiraling and circular movements of the chest, hips, arms, and hands we performed were not some lascivious exhibition but a clear demonstration of the spiraling patterns of feminine energy swirling into and out of the chakras of our luminous bodies and the primordial heart of creation. I did not consider the serpentine, figure-eight undulations so unique to this ancient art form as ways to ensnare a mate and demonstrate my flexibility as a sex partner, but as a symbolic expression of the vital force of the Kundalini Shakti, or female serpent power, making her way up the central channel of my body. I was also aware that these supple figure-eight patterns could be read as a glyph representing infinity, harmony, balance, and the nourishing aspect of the Great Goddess herself.[2] In addition, I knew that the number eight was associated in Tibetan Tantra with the number of petals or spokes emerging from the lotus, or whirling energetic wheel of the heart chakra.

As we danced together to the powerful rhythms of the drum, I was fully aware of the energetic and symbolic significance of each of these movements. With each rippling wave of energy, I felt the awakening, regeneration, and purification of both my physical and subtle bodies. From this place of outer fluidity and inner luminosity, with each inhalation I opened my heart to receive this delicious energetic nourishment. Allowing my whole being to ingest this divine energy, with each exhalation I sent divine radiance out into the world, imbuing the psychic-energetic landscape with the fluid wavelike patterns of life and light so natural to the Goddess and her female counterparts. I was filled with the magnetic power and playfulness of the sensuous goddess, and every so often I would feel the touch of an accent, a change of pace, a syncopation, and send a flash of her joyous feminine energy outward from my eyes, hips, shoulders, or hands.

In one of these Middle Eastern dance classes I met Ramzi El Edlibi, a drummer, choreographer, and dancer whose fascination with the movements, rhythms, and symbolic expressions of world cultures paralleled my own. Over the next five years Ramzi and I worked together as partners. Interweaving our knowledge of the physical and psychic landscapes with our choreographic creations, he mapped out the outer patterns and composition of the dance. I added the inner teachings—the myth or story and its spiritual or cultural connotation—as well as the energetic nuances, symbols, and mudras. Like the Kathakas of old we traveled throughout the country embodying the myths, teachings, rhythms, and expressions of cultures from around the world. From the temples of India and Egypt to the villages of Africa and Hawaii and the streets of Spain and South America we took our inspiration, transforming into queens and kings, heroines and heroes, goddesses and gods, for the schoolchildren, college students, and members of cultural organizations who came to witness our magical display.

But it was ancient Egypt, the birthplace of Western civilization, that brought us our greatest inspiration. Ramzi, a man of Lebanese birth who had the heart of a Sufi, became the great god Osiris. I, Sharron, the Jewish princess from Baltimore, became the great goddess Isis. In this sophisticated realm of the arts there was no anger, hatred, or resentment between Muslim and Jew, but only a beautiful blending of art and creativity that focused on the richness of mutual understanding that could be gained from this interaction.

I assumed the task of embodying this great goddess, who was at one time

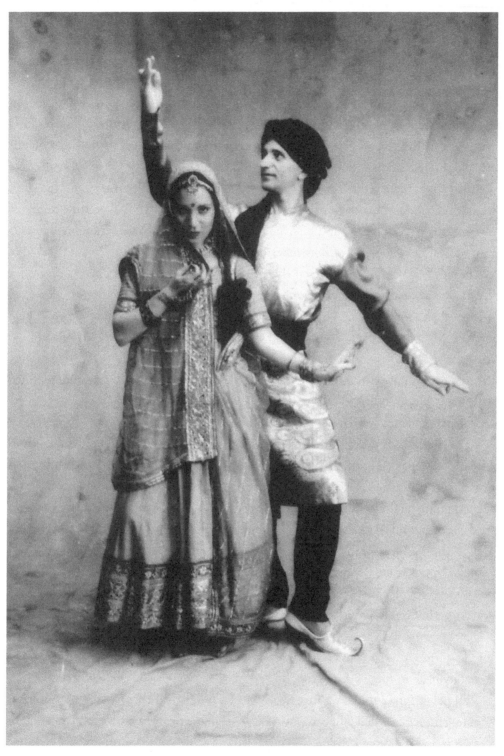

The author and Ramzi. Photograph by Ken Kobé.

worshipped throughout the Western world with the same fervor I approached all the deities I had previously encountered. This time, however, there was no living teacher of the lineage to transmit her essence to me. To fill this void I read everything I could find about the mysteries of Isis. I was assisted by the work of Dr. Houston, whose book *The Passion of Isis and Osiris*, had filled me with inspiration. This is also when I began my study of Egyptian art and hieroglyphs, seeking the sacred gestures, postures, and symbols within them. To my delight, I discovered that encoded in the hieroglyphs and paintings of ancient Egypt were numerous representations of universal symbols of manifestation, such as the lotus flower, the risen serpent, the sun, the moon, the stars, water, and fire. In these ancient works of art I also discovered ritual gestures and postures of invocation, praise, and offering. Ramzi and I incorporated these movements into our dance, the dance of remembering.

From my research I discovered that Isis and Osiris were the archetypal form for the Tantric couple of the West: woman/man, sister/brother, queen/king, goddess/god. Within their story was the key to the ancient Western mysteries that flowed like a river of light out of Egypt. Their legend was the story of birth and rebirth, death and resurrection, darkness and illumination. Isis and Osiris were credited with bringing the arts of civilization to humanity. They were perceived as the divine couple, filled with love for each other and for their people, whose stories and deeds provided inspiration and guidance for humanity.

The dance of Isis and Osiris that Ramzi and I created was based on the myth in which Set, their evil brother, overwhelmed by jealousy of the divine couple, murders Osiris, cuts him into fourteen pieces, and scatters the pieces throughout Egypt and the adjoining lands. In her overwhelming grief at the loss of her consort, Isis wanders through the world to recover these dismembered pieces. She finds all but his phallus, and so she fashions one out of gold. The dance Ramzi and I choreographed was inspired by a passage written by Normandi Ellis that is included in *The Passion of Isis and Osiris*. It depicts the scene in which Isis, through the medium of a magical ritual, performs what is referred to in the medieval alchemical literature as the mystical marriage, or *conjunctio*. Through the power of her magic she impregnates herself with the divine spirit of Osiris's son, Horus, who goes on to avenge his father's death and bring harmony back to the world.

I'll never forget the day I first heard Dr. Houston read this passage to me. I was standing in her crowded office taking a break from my healing work with Dr. Masters. In her rich and dramatic voice, she provided me with the story that would help me fashion the movements, mudras, and expressions of Isis and Osiris at the foundation of this dance.

In her sorrow she began to dance, to weep, to spin, her feet raising great clouds of dust. She spun round and round. She keened. She sighed. Her arms became great feathered wings. Kitelike she fluttered above the corpse of Osiris, chanting, singing, crying, as she had done in Byblos. Mad with the grief of separation even now as he lay in her arms, enchanted by the power and hunger of her love . . . It was as if she were making life anew. A god blinked in the darkness. A god rose up, bright fire from the watery abyss. He and She. She and He. In the beginning the one became two, the self and the other, the selfsame self. Now, she cried, "Merge and merge and merge again. In the flesh the two are made one."

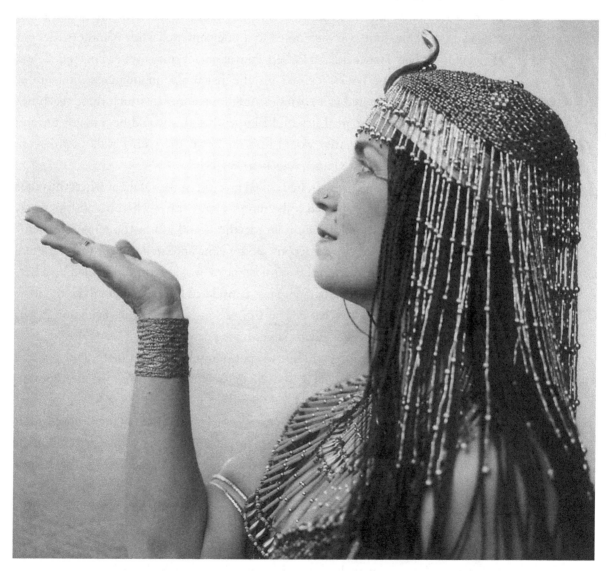

The author as Isis. Photograph by Tom Lounsbury.

As I traced the glyphs and figures so essential to Isis's teachings, as I placed them within the sacred vessel of my body, as I read the texts devoted to her worship, Isis—like Tara, Durga, Saraswati, Mandarava, Sekhmet, and all the other goddesses I have had the privilege to embody—began to silently reveal herself. As I consciously moved through the postures and gestures of Isis, they wove themselves into a fluid dance of invocation, praise, and worship. The dance grew and changed each day, inspired by each new connection, each new insight into her mysteries. The dance was a prayer, an offering, a simple display of divine feminine energy in which radiant patterns of light poured out of my heart like a healing balm to ease the pain of living amid the chaos and ignorance of the Kali Yuga.

Because Ramzi and I possessed the ability to translate this compelling myth into visual and symbolic form, we were asked to accompany well-known authors Richard Hoagland, Graham Hancock, and Robert Bauval on a lecture tour of England. These authors—whose latest books focused on the teachings, monuments, and art of ancient Egypt—had invited us to demonstrate the manner in which these teachings had been encoded in the art. Little did I know that this would be a major turning point in my life, an event that would lead me down the path I walk at this very moment, where I put pen to paper, fingers to keyboard.

Isis, goddess of the alchemists, had called me. Just at the moment when the outer circumstances of my life appeared to be running smoothly—when friendship, work, art, and remuneration flowed beautifully together—and just at the moment when I had let go of desire, of longing for a consort, someone appeared and my world shifted.

While preparing for the tour I was told that we would be accompanied by a hermetic scholar named Jay Weidner, who was considered by the authors to be the foremost authority on Isis. After our arrival in London I noticed that everyone in our group was drawn to Jay, a charismatic silver-haired man. Filled with a wealth of information on sacred geometry, world history, politics, religion, and more, Jay appeared to possess in-depth knowledge of the inner symbolic teachings of the Western alchemical tradition, which he told me originated in ancient Egypt. Over the next few days we became constant companions. I was so taken with Jay that I phoned Ari in New York to tell him about this highly intelligent man I had met. Ari was then sixteen years old and had become engrossed in the study of Medieval history; he was especially interested in the tales of the Knights Templars and the Freemasons. He was pleased to hear that I had met someone who could give him greater insight into this subject matter.

From the moment that Jay and I began to speak it was as if two scholars and practitioners of the ancient traditions of Tantra and alchemy had been brought together to discover their common ground. Over the course of the tour that led us from London through the ancient Celtic ruins of Stonehenge and Avebury to Leeds, Jay and I began a deep and intimate conversation and quest for the sacred that has continued to this very day.

For years I had hungered for a true consort with whom I could share and expand on my knowledge of the sacred sexual mysteries that were vital to the training and initiatory practices of the temple priestesses and yoginis of India and Tibet. Perhaps the depth of the work I had done with Dr. Masters to uncover and release my confusing imprints about men had opened a new doorway for me, or perhaps it was just another magical coincidence, but here I was, being inexorably drawn to Jay. From the moment of our first kiss under the shadow of Stonehenge, we were inseparable.

It was that very evening in the ancient city of Avebury that I began to share with him my knowledge of the sexual teachings of Tantra. I sent him out to buy some wine, and I took a shower, massaged my body with the oils of sandalwood and amber, and wrapped a red sari around me. While chanting special mantras of purification I prepared a bath for Jay, lit candles and incense, and tossed red rose petals across the clean white sheets that covered the bed. When Jay returned, like the temple priestesses of old I bathed him, wiped his body dry, and led him to the bed. Placing my hands underneath his head, I tuned in to the flow of his cranial rhythms and gently coaxed his nervous system toward a place of quietude and relaxation. At this point I began my teaching on the Kundalini Shakti. Before his eyes I filled my body with this sacred feminine current and transformed into the sensuous goddess, all the time explaining to him every aspect of this potent energetic process. (For "The Energy Field of the Sensuous Goddess," see chapter 8.)

I told Jay about the training of the temple priestesses and yoginis, explaining their knowledge of how the passion and power of the sex drive could, when properly harnessed, become extraordinary fuel for enlightenment. He told me that the alchemists and their consorts, known as *soror mysticas* or mystical sisters, were also schooled in the ancient art of lovemaking. They too believed that the most powerful physical, psychological, and energetic experience that could take place between a man and woman was that of sexual intercourse.

As we sat together in union I guided Jay through the breathing techniques and visualizations I had learned for awakening the radiant light and energy of Shakti and bringing it slowly up the central channel of the body. From the base chakra we visualized this light rising through and permeating the seven subtle lotuses of our luminous energy bodies. We did this by alternately generating and building the sensation of pleasure and then relaxing and allowing it to flood each successive chakra. Finally it felt as if there was one great current of liquid light streaming up and around our conjoined bodies. The sense of I and other began to melt away as our physical and subtle bodies were flooded with bliss. Bathed in the ecstatic experience of female-male union, we sent streams of love and radiance outward from our hearts to infuse the energetic landscape with the sweet nectar of our sacred union.

In the years since this first powerful experience of union, Jay and I—as lovers, researchers, tantric consorts, alchemist and soror mystica, husband and wife—have journeyed through the visible and invisible realms, seeking the cultural correspondences inherent in the universal language of the spirit. This intermingling of knowledge, experience, and energy has given us a great deal of fuel for inner purification and spiritual growth. Our commitment to a true tantric-alchemical relationship has provided us with the opportunity to experience times of deep communion and connection, as well as times of severe testing and confrontation. As sounding boards and mirrors, as friends and companions, we have worked to assist each other in becoming aware of and releasing the false projections and negative imprints embedded in our psyches. In this way the relationship itself has become the holy alchemical crucible in which all impurities, even those carried down through generations, are surrendered, heated up, and melted away in the blazing fire of love. Through the darkest nights and the brightest days, through felicity and adversity, we have worked hard to never lose sight of the immense beauty and power of the flickering flame of spiritual light that burns between us.

In those early days of our relationship I constantly questioned Jay about his upbringing and his own mystic quest for knowledge of the Western alchemical tradition. He told me that he was born in the heartland of America to a Roman Catholic family of Celtic origin. Therefore, deeply ingrained in his bloodline was a familiarity and resonance with the sacred traditions of the Celtic people that were forced to go underground with the coming of the Inquisition and the suppression of the feminine principle throughout Europe. Jay's grandmother's name was Mary Magdalene, and his genealogy contains numerous other female ancestors named Mary Magdalene. In fact, he was amazed to discover that his ancestors had built many churches throughout the world dedicated to this foremost disciple of Christ, who was disparagingly referred to in the literature as a reformed "prostitute." Clearly this gave Jay pause for reflection on the contradictions and inconsistencies inherent in Church doctrine.

A sensitive, inquisitive, and intellectually gifted child, from his early days Jay was moved by the majestic nature, beauty, and spiritual power of the cathedrals. As an avid reader always in search of rare and odd volumes, particularly those relating to history and mysticism, Jay visited a garage sale in North Hollywood at which he came across a book titled *Les Mysteres des Cathedrales* by a mysterious French alchemist called Fulcanelli. This was a turning point in his life.

Jay took the book home and attempted to read it, but had difficulty understanding its strange allusions and allegorical references, as well as the author's constant darting back and forth between myth, legend, and established fact. But intuitively Jay knew that there was something truly profound in this book, and over the years he kept referring back to it, perusing its pages over and over until he had uncovered its mysteries.

One evening as we sat together by the fire in our home high up in the Colorado Rockies, Jay told me that, essentially, Fulcanelli believed that everything we in the West think we are, all that our historians and scientists have been telling us about the nature of who we are, is wrong. "In fact," he said, his sky-blue eyes twinkling with an inner light, "prior to the Inquisition in Europe the West held a great and glorious spiritual current, a living lineage of transmission dating back to ancient Egypt, a tradition of

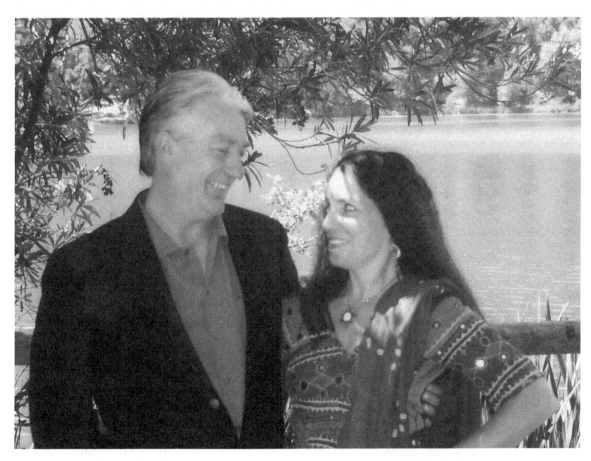

Sharron Rose with her husband and hermetic scholar, Jay Weidner.

devotion to the feminine in both her earthly and divine forms. While most histories of the initiatory traditions in the West go as far back as the 1500s with the creation of the Rosecrucians, Fulcanelli proves that this tradition, which included light body practices similar to the ones you have learned from your teachers, was evident in Europe at the time of the construction of the Cathedrals in the 1100s. You, who have brought my beloved goddess Isis to life before my eyes, will be pleased to know that this lineage, like Tantra and Dzogchen, is an initiatory tradition that is said to have begun with Isis herself and her interaction with an angelic being."

Jay pulled out notes he had taken on the hermetic text *Isis the Prophetess to Her Son Horus* and continued.[3] "It was during a unique alchemical moment when the stars and planets were in perfect astrological alignment that Isis begins her tale: 'It happened that one of the angels who dwelt in the first firmament saw me from above and came towards me desiring to unite with me sexually.' You see," Jay explained in his inimitable way, "in her role as prophetess and liaison between the luminous and corporeal realms, Isis is keenly aware that she has a great opportunity to receive sacred knowledge. So she strikes a bargain with the angel. She tells him that she will only perform this sacred act if he first agrees to present her with the keys to the great alchemical mysteries. To this offer he replies that he will return the next day with another angel named Amnael, who she will recognize by the sign of a ceramic vessel full of shining water on his head.

"From a symbolic perspective," Jay said, "this sign is extremely significant. It reveals that Amnael held what is known in the alchemical lore as the hermetic vessel, vase, or crucible, which houses the 'vital spark,' or 'universal solvent containing all the virtues of heaven and earth'—what you would call the essential light of Shakti. Knowledge of this secret metaphysical fire of the wise is at the root of what is known as the Great Work of alchemy. By reading this glyph, one can see that Amnael possessed the very secrets of illumination itself."

Jay continued, "As promised, the next day Amnael appears. Upon seeing the beauty, charm, and magical allure of Isis, he too is filled with sexual desire for her. In the text Isis describes their interaction: 'When he stayed with me, I did not give myself to him. I resisted him and overcame his desire till he showed me the sign on his head, and gave me the tradition of the mysteries without keeping anything back, but in the full truth.'

"Amnael then reveals to Isis the great alchemical secrets, including the mystery of the *prima materia,* or first substance from which all others are formed, and a number of alchemical recipes such as the elixir of life. After this Isis takes an oath never to reveal what the angel has told her to anyone except her son, who is her closest friend. She never even reveals whether or not she has performed the sacred act of sexual union with Amnael."

I interrupted, "Coming from the Tantric and Dzogchen lineages, which are passed along from master to student through a chain of direct transmission, I can easily perceive the basic theme inherent in this text. There is the acquisition of what the Tibetans would call a terma, or treasure text, via an interaction or initiation with an angelic messenger from the luminous realms. This initiation most likely included the mystic act of tantric union between female and male, and the taking of a solemn oath to protect its secret and lineage. In this traditional manner Isis as prophetess becomes the lineage holder and Great Mother Goddess of alchemy who receives, reveals, and transmits the sacred teachings to her progeny.

"I must admit," I said to Jay, "that I find this to be surprising. From all of the tales I heard before I met you I thought that alchemy was some obscure 'magical' practice of attempting to turn lead into gold, and that it was exclusively performed by men in Europe during the sixteenth and seventeenth centuries. I had also heard that these men, the predecessors of our modern day chemists, were supported by kings and noblemen, to whom they had made claims of being able to perform this physical transmutation of metals and also synthesize an illusive substance called the philosopher's stone. This exceedingly coveted substance was purported to have the power to bestow immortality on the owner. From these tales it seemed to me that this art was merely concerned with making strides on the material plane."

Jay commented, "I must say, Sharron, your presumptions about alchemy are very wrong. In fact, the stories you have heard are just the outer trappings of a deeply spiritual tradition—a tradition that, like Tantra and Dzogchen, transmitted its mysteries through myth, symbol, metaphor, allegory, and parable.

"According to Fulcanelli the mystical science of alchemy, like that of Tantra, works backward from the belief in a divine source. For these alchemists who traced their lineage back to Al Khem, or ancient Egypt, every physical process had a metaphysical correspondence. Therefore intimate knowledge of every minute aspect of physical reality was vital, for it was the means by which they could discover the Divine. To seek the Divine within all things, to search for the spark of light that resides in all life, to perceive the interconnectedness and interdependence of all living things: This was the quest of these ancient scientists."

Jay added, "Because they knew that each living thing holds a vital spark of divine energy, the alchemists created experiments to reveal and liberate this light from matter. The alchemists were obsessed with the prima materia; they called it the black virgin, for its color was black, the root of all colors, and it was a virgin in the sense that no alchemical transmutation had yet been performed on it. This original substance from which all alchemical transmutation manifested, the base matter from which life arose, was known to contain the secrets of life, death, and resurrection. The alchemist's task was to investigate, reveal, and reflect on the elemental components of the prima materia, and through this process gain a profound knowledge of the very secrets of life itself."

I responded, "So what you are telling me is that the alchemists of the West, like the Tantrics of the East, understood that all reality is essentially made up of light, and they were actually seeking to discover the essence of this light or the nature of Shakti herself."

Jay affirmed, "That's right, but this purification and liberation of light and energy from the heart of matter was only one aspect of the art and science of alchemy, or the Great Work. On a deeper level, these alchemical teachings, like the teachings of Tantra and Dzogchen that you have shared with me, were merely an outer display of the level of gnosis, or direct experiential knowledge, the adept had attained through his or her private metaphysical practices. For unbeknownst to most, the primary focus of these adepts was attainment of the fully illumined state, and its most secret practices were created to enable the adepts to transform all aspects of their beings.

"The alchemists studied the movement of the stars in the heavens and their relationship to human events, seeking out the most favorable times and circumstances for their magical experiments. Then at the most auspicious moment, in their secret laboratories, in their crucibles and alembics, the alchemists and their soror mysticas would endeavor to generate the philosopher's stone, or key to the secret of eternal life. By performing specific practices that gave them the ability to unite their energy, they were able to directly influence both the physical and psychic landscapes. The myths say that through the knowledge they obtained on an exoteric level, they gained the ability to turn lead into gold. And on an esoteric level they gained the ability to transform themselves into fully realized beings of light."

Jay pulled a book from the shelf and showed me pages of alchemical drawings. They depicted many of the essential themes found in Tantra: the elements—earth, air, fire, and water—portrayed both as feminine figures and geometric shapes, as well as female and male joined together as a hermaphrodite, which was reminiscent of the images of Shiva and Shakti as one. There were also images of both women and men together and separately performing alchemical experiments, clear evidence of the important role women played in the alchemical arts. And there were images of queen and king, moon and sun, performing the sacred act of sexual union. These drawings, like those from the tantric tradition, were filled with symbolic representations that were part of a sacred initiatory language that clearly transcended culture and therefore could be read and interpreted by those who had been trained to perceive them.

Later that evening Jay and I lay in bed perusing the books. "You see," he said, "medieval Europe had a different culture from that of the East, and so they spoke a different metaphorical language. What you would call a tantric union they called the conjunctio, or mystic marriage. What you call rainbow body they called resurrection, transfiguration, or body of glory. European village life was built around the knowledge of various crafts. Every village had its blacksmith, carpenter, healer, and chemist. So when these alchemists spoke of the light body practice, they used terms that were guided by the same imagery that was used in these crafts. Just as today we use computer terms such as *download* or *up to speed* to explain a particular process or activity, the alchemists used terms from their crafts to explain these processes. So the alchemical phrase *lead into gold* is merely the physical vernacular used to explain this metaphysical process.

"Evidence of this alchemical focus on the attainment of the light body can be found in an early Hellenistic text known as the *Book of Comarios*," Jay reported. "The primary character in the book, you will be happy to discover, is a woman named Kleopatra, who is a disciple of the alchemical arts. In this text she speaks about the underlying relationships between the physical and metaphysical procedures, which form the base of the Great Work. For example, she describes the metaphorical correspondences between the development of an embryo in the crucible of the mother's womb and a metal being transmuted in the alchemist's crucible of glass. She also speaks of the purification and liberation of light from matter, or the soul from the confines of the material world. She describes the use of sexual symbolism that is inherent in the art and imagery of alchemy, and the intimate relationship between material and spiritual alchemy."

According to Kleopatra, who should not be mistaken for Cleopatra the Egyptian queen and wife of Ceasar, after having been regenerated by a process of psychophysical purification and distillation known as the *pharmakon,* or medicine of life, the adept regains the luminous state of spiritual perfection enjoyed by humanity in the Golden Age. In other words, through this process, the adept attains the glorious body of light.[4] Kleopatra noted, "When the spirit of darkness and unsavory odor has been cast out the body is filled with light. Soul and spirit rejoice."[5]

"To me," I told Jay, "this text contains evidence that the fundamental goals of Tantra and alchemy are the same, and that their inner teachings were designed to assist practitioners in the process of 'resurrection,' spiritual purification, attainment of the body of light, and subsequent reintegration with the original primordial state."

Over the next few days Jay continued to reveal the history of the great Western alchemical tradition to me. "It was during the Hellenistic period, in the time of hermeticism," he shared as we walked along one of the many hiking trails that led through the snow-covered mountains surrounding our home, "that the great symbols, myths, and sacred knowledge of Egypt were transmitted from the temples to the mystery schools of Greece and Rome. The essential metaphysical teachings of the Egyptians were also retained and transmitted through the inner circles of the Islamic, Hebrew, and early Christian traditions. At the heart of the alchemical transmission was an extraordinary spiritual and secret teaching known as gnosticism. This teaching is believed to be the spiritual base of Christ's essential message to humanity. Gnosticism valued the feminine qualities of receptivity, intuitive perception, and visionary experience. It was a teaching of love, selflessness, harmony, and communion.

"The mystic experience of and communion with the essential grace and majesty of divinity lay at the heart of the gnostic current. The clear and immediate experience of this awakening was known as *gnosis*, or wisdom. Often translated from its Greek root as 'knowledge,' gnosticism goes much deeper than merely intellectual understanding. Like a brilliant flash of light emerging from the darkness, this understanding arises in the individual as a bright lucid awareness—an intuitive realization of the pure essence, nature, and energy of divinity as it flows through oneself and all creation.

"From the gnostic viewpoint the answers to all of life's questions can only be found when one opens oneself to this divine current, to 'allow oneself to be penetrated by it to the point where one is possessed and transformed by it,' as described by Giovanni Filoramo, a great alchemical scholar." I was amazed to receive this teaching, for I now realized that even though they used different terms, these Medieval women and men were attuning themselves to the divine current of Shakti.

We stood atop the mountain, looking out at the pristine beauty of the environment. Jay said, "Gnosticism, like the Sufi and bhakti movements you have told me about, was revolutionary because it revealed the process by which any individual—female or male, rich or poor, Jew or gentile—could travel beyond the veils of the material world into the luminous energetic realms, where one could directly experience the pure light of God. Gnosticism enabled one to experience this direct communion with divinity without the intercession of a priest or rabbi ordained by the church or temple. In this way it was a clear break from the fixed dogmatic and authoritarian view that prevailed over many religious systems.

"Two thousand years ago, after the death and resurrection of Christ, which was considered by some to be a clear demonstration of the great alchemical transmutation from physicality into the illuminated body of glory, the secret teachings of gnosticism and hermeticism made their way to southern Europe, particularly the area around southern France and northern Spain. Besides the already established Celts, many Greeks, Jews, Arabs, and other peoples came to this area. In the midst of this cosmopolitan confluence many spiritual, philosophical, and symbolic links were discovered between these peoples and their traditional belief systems.

"For the next twelve hundred years the people of southern France were at the forefront of a revival of spiritual awareness and feminine values that wove itself into the fabric of the psychic landscape of Europe. It was a period of love and romance, of the Knights Templars, the Cathari, and the troubadors, the era in which the Jewish mystics recorded their secret oral tradition in the form of the Kabbalah. At the heart of this mystic reunion was a desire to reinvigorate Europe with the ancient alchemical knowledge of the path to liberation and enlightenment."

Jay proceeded, "But this last flicker of grace, beauty, and renewed respect for the feminine mysteries was overtaken by the horrifying surge of tyranny and repression that has been the signature of the Age of Iron. From the rise of the Roman Catholic Church around A.D. 300 until the Renaissance, there was a gradual destruction of these ancient sacred belief systems. The mystical and scientific insights from these great traditions were denigrated and called 'magic' by the hierarchy of the Roman Catholic Church. The great teachings of alchemy that had been gathered over thousands of years were nearly lost in this holocaust of ancient pagan Europe. The discarded teachings included the use of herbs for medicinal purposes; the awareness of the sacred relationship between man, woman, and the Divine; the mysteries of nature; and the physical and astronomical teachings, including the secrets of Isis.

"But the hidden masters—the great alchemists—had foreseen this era of fear and ignorance. Fully aware of the alchemy of time, they knew that the shadowy tentacles of the Iron Age were reaching out to grasp hold of both the physical and psychic landscapes. They realized that they must find a covert means through which to preserve their metaphysical teachings for future generations. And so, like their Egyptian ancestors, the alchemists encoded their sacred mysteries in the art and architecture of their temples: the Gothic cathedrals. The cathedrals were sacred hermetic 'books' carved in stone, for they held within them the secrets and symbolic transmission of the Western tradition that had flowed out of ancient Egypt."

As we made our way down the mountain Jay finished his tale of this secret history of the West. "It turned out that the building of the Gothic cathedrals was the final display of this ancient alchemical tradition," he said, stopping for a moment to help me cross a swiftly running stream. "After the destruction of the Cathari in A.D. 1210, the alchemists sensed danger and began to move underground. As the Iron Age grew to ripeness, these men and women withdrew from history. This does not mean that they stopped helping seekers to find their way; it merely means that as part of a hidden group I call the Keepers of the Light, they chose more subtle methods of communication. I believe that Fulcanelli was one of these hidden masters, and that is why he had to remain anonymous."

Having been made aware of this hidden history of the West and filled with the desire to have firsthand knowledge of the places that still retained the mystic teachings of Isis, alchemy, and gnosticism, Jay and I embarked on a series of journeys to France. With Fulcanelli's *Les Mysteres des Cathedrales* as our guidebook we began our quest in Paris, the City of Light whose name etymologically can be linked to the pre-Celtic *Par-Isis*, the grove of Isis. As Jay and I stood hand in hand before the facade of the Western porch of Notre Dame de Paris, Jay began to explain the symbolic meaning of the architecture. Surprisingly, this journey was about to lead me into some of the deepest secrets of the Goddess herself—and also into the Hebrew tradition of my birth.

Jay began, "At the heart of the mystic tradition of Judaism known as the Kabbalah lies a symbolic glyph known as the tree of life. Encoded in its design is the key to the secret mysteries of divine manifestation. It contains three pillars joined by a latticework of twenty-two paths, and it describes the unfolding of light and energy from the primordial source through a series of ten sephiroth, or divine potencies, represented by circles. As one meditates on this sacred glyph and its symbols, both the mysteries of emanation from God—the divine source, beyond male or female characteristics—and the knowledge of the path of reunion and reintegration with this source is revealed."

Jay had just revealed that, unbeknownst to all but a few, encoded in the architecture of this façade of the Notre Dame Cathedral and of numerous other Gothic cathedrals throughout the world is the symbolic map of manifestation as perceived by the Jewish mystics. Jay pointed out the relationship of the architecture to the sacred Hebrew glyph and said, "On the two sides we see the right and left pillars of duality, of male and female, of the divine potencies or sephiroth of wisdom and understanding, severity and mercy, splendor and victory."

I remarked, "From my perspective, these correspond to the right and left channels of the subtle energy body known to tantric practitioners."

"Rising between these two pillars is the central pillar of union," he continued.

"This could be seen as the Shushumna, or central channel from the tantric perspective," I chimed in.

Jay replied, "This is the sacred pillar of initiation—what the Egyptians referred to as the djed pillar—representing what you might call the middle way or path of resolution of opposites. Many layers of physical and metaphysical teachings are encoded in it. The hidden crypt, which lies below the cathedral, represents our earthly kingdom, physical reality, and the prima materia of alchemy designated at the base of the tree of life by the sephirah or divine potency known as Malkuth. The front door signifies Yesod, the moon, the energetic realm of emotions and sexuality. The beautiful rose window signifies Tiphareth, the sun, or heart center, the mediator and point of equilibrium

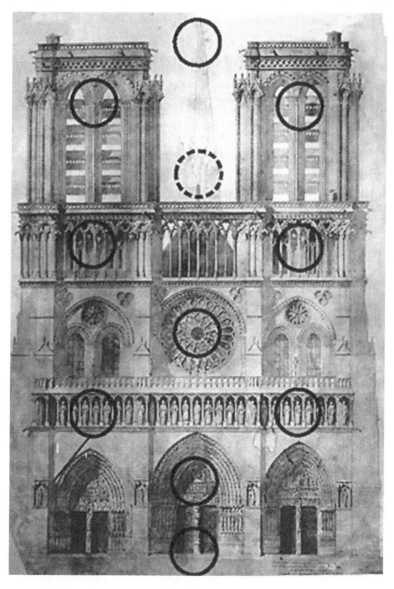

The tree of life superimposed on the façade of the Cathedral of Notre Dame.

between heaven and earth, spirit and matter, from which love and compassion is born. The empty space above that symbolizes Daat, the secret hidden sephirah, the abyss, void, or gateway to the inner planes. And the crucifix that sits atop the spire is Kether, symbolizing the crown of creation or primordial source, where all opposing forces are reconciled in the one Supreme Being."

This was an intriguing introduction to the teachings encoded in the tree of life, teachings that, as a Jewish female, had been closed to me. To discover them imprinted on the very entrance to this refuge of the Catholic faith was astonishing. But this was only the first part of the secret teaching that Jay presented, for according to his research the origins of this sacred Hebrew glyph could be traced back to ancient Egypt.

"This same archetypal pattern of the tree of life can be found in the ankh, which, as my beautiful Isis, you hold in your hand," Jay said, lightly tracing out the symbol on the palm of my hand. "Furthermore, as you will see when we enter Notre Dame, or any of the Gothic cathedrals, the entire ground plan of the building is laid out in the shape of the ankh, the ancient Egyptian key of life."

From reading Fulcanelli, I had learned that to the ancient initiate the ankh, or its later manifestation in Christianity as the cross, is the alchemical symbol for the crucible in which the spiritual transmutation takes place. It is in the crucible that the first matter (prima materia) dies to be revived, purified, spiritualized, and transformed. This is why the ankh is called the key to the mysteries.[6] Jay told me that he believed that Christianity was essentially a recast version of the myth of Isis, Osiris, and Horus, with God as Osiris, Mary as Isis, Jesus as Horus, and Satan taking over the role of Set, the evil and jealous brother.

Jay explained, "The ankh also reveals another essential teaching about the mysteries of Isis. The ancient Egyptians believed that Isis, as the Great Mother, was the womb of all creation, which on a physical level corresponded to the center of the galaxy itself. In the view of the ancients, the center of the galaxy was the prima materia and the source of all becoming. In fact, for the Egyptians, who sought out the correspondences in all things, the act of Isis giving birth to her son, Horus, was perceived as a metaphorical reflection of the mother galaxy giving birth to our sun—the Great Mother giving birth to the child of light. Indeed it can be said that everything that is—all of nature, human beings, even human consciousness—originally comes from the womb of Isis, which is represented by the empty space within the upper portion of the ankh."

As we walked through the giant oak doors of the cathedral, I was deeply moved by its regal splendor. I realized that we were now standing in the building that was a centerpiece of French history; since the day of the trial of Jacques de Molay, the proud leader of the Knights Templars, to its near destruction during the French Revolution and the coming of Napoleon, many historic events had occurred within these hallowed walls.

Slowly and reverently Jay and I walked down the central aisle. I became keenly aware of the patterns of multicolored light that filtered down through the hall. Looking up to discover their source, I was struck by the beauty and power of the stained-glass windows. Depicted in the design of the windows themselves I recognized a symbolic manifestation of the higher dimensional realms of the Divine. Here were depictions of Jesus, or the Virgin Mary and child, surrounded by saints and angelic presences that, from my Eastern indoctrination, resembled the circular, mandalic depictions of the realms of the buddhas and bodhisattvas that were so essential to the symbolic art of Tibet. Intuitively I felt that these windows must have been created to give the parishioners a personal glimpse of the subtle realms of light.

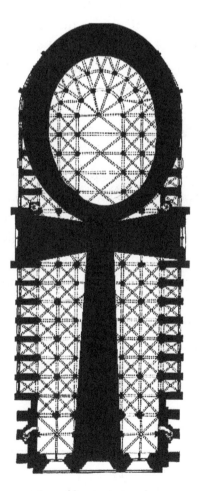

An ankh superimposed on
the floor plan of the Cathedral of Notre Dame.

We stood in front of the altar at the heart of the cathedral, which was positioned at the center of the cross, or ankh. Before us stood a remarkable statue of Isis in what I came to know as her later incarnation as the Virgin Mary. There she was, as a full-bodied woman, filled with life and light, the body of her crucified son splayed across her lap. This powerful statue, commissioned in 1630 by Louis XIII as a gift to Notre Dame, symbolized for me Christ's birth out of the crucible of his mother's womb into this earthly realm and his subsequent sacrifice and return to the kingdom of divinity via the crucible of the cross.

Moving from the intellectual to the intuitive, I sat down before this living goddess of the West to contemplate her teaching of the ankh, the tree, the cross, and the crucible. I wanted to feel her teaching within the cathedral of my physical body and open my heart to its message. As a healer, at the beginning of every session I would feel the essential shape of the cross in my body as I aligned myself with earth and sky. This allowed the light of spirit to flow from the central point in my heart down through my arms and out through my hands. Now I was to perceive the cross on yet another level. For as I closed my eyes and traveled into the visionary landscape to sense the energy of this essential symbol, another image juxtaposed itself upon it.

From the space between my eyebrows I suddenly beheld images of stars pouring out from what resembled the dark core of the galaxy in a burst of shimmering sparks. The sparks radiated outward from the heart of emptiness, the womb of the Goddess. The sparks then formed into the oval-shaped outline of the ankh, glowing like a nimbus, or aura, around my head. As I let myself relax and melt into the experience, images of saints and bodhisattvas, deities and healers, from many sacred traditions began to flow through my mindstream. This same halo of light, the visible expression of their luminous spiritual awareness, surrounded each figure. They seemed to superimpose themselves upon each other, until they dissolved into one distinct image: that of Isis herself as the Universal Mother. I was taken by the beauty and radiance of this image, and in homage to her I whispered her Egyptian name, *Auset*. A wave of warm and soothing energy streamed out of my heart and flowed through my body as I felt myself magically transform into the Great Goddess. No longer was I merely seeing her in the mirror of my mind, but I was feeling her divine healing presence flowing through me, enlivening my tissues.

The lotus flower of my heart spun open. My breasts began to tingle as I sensed her sweet nectar of compassion pouring through them and into the hungry mouth of the child who magically suckled at my breast. I was the loving mother of the universe nourishing her children. I was Isis nursing her son, Horus; Mary nursing her son, Jesus; Sharron nursing her son, Ari. I was simultaneously the image and the sensation, the symbol and the metaphor. As I was overwhelmed by the power of this experience, tears of gratitude welled up in my eyes, and from the heart of this sacred abode I offered up a silent prayer. It floated skyward from my heart through my eyes, now wide open and gazing upward toward the heavenly realms of light. To my astonishment and delight, adorning the very top of the nave was the image of the Blessed Virgin herself, riding across the ocean of existence on a crescent moon, waiting to receive my prayer and guide me toward true liberation.

Jay and I left Paris and continued on our pilgrimage to the places sacred to the alchemists and gnostics, the places that silently whispered of the beauty and power of the sacred union of earth and sky, feminine and masculine. It was in the heart of Chartres Cathedral, considered by many to be the most beautiful of the Gothic cathedrals, that I first encountered another living representative of the lineage of Isis, one that I would encounter over and over throughout the course of our travels: the Black Madonna.[7] In preparation for this journey, this pilgrimage, I had read the few books I could find that spoke of her mysteries.

In Ean Begg's *The Cult of the Black Madonna* I discovered that throughout the former Celtic lands of Europe, and especially in France, statues of the Black Madonna appeared spontaneously in this earthly dimension. These statues were discovered in the depths of the forest, in streambeds, on the shore of the sea, or emerging from the earth where a farmer plowed his field. Time after time these statues were taken to the local church only to magically reappear in the place of their discovery, upon which a chapel was then constructed for the Black Madonna's worship and adoration. Tales also exist of how these statues of the dark goddess were brought to Europe by pilgrims and knights who had traveled throughout the Holy Land. Legends told of the magical healing powers of these representations of the Divine Mother.[8] Most often the Black Madonna was placed near the well that lies at the crypt of each cathedral. Once upon a time these wells were sacred to the Celtic people and their druid priesthood. The wells, which were fed by underground streams, symbolized a magical space that was feminine in nature, a space in which the subtle energies of the earthly and supernatural realms converge, a portal between the numinous and the corporeal.

In *Les Mysteres des Cathedrales* Fulcanelli explicitly states that the symbols of the Madonna and child, as well as other characteristics of the Black Madonna, are based on those of the goddess Isis and her son, Horus. He also informs us that the cathedrals were built over former Greco-Roman temples dedicated to the mysteries of Isis. "Formerly the subterranean chambers of the temples served as abodes for the statues of *Isis*," Fulcanelli states, "which, at the time of the introduction of Christianity into Gaul, became those *black Virgins*, which the people in our day surround with a quite special veneration." He went on to say that for the alchemists the Black Virgins represented Isis before conception; the attribute of the virgin that symbolizes the "earth before its fecundation and which the rays of the sun are soon to bring to life. . . . They represent in hermetic symbolism the *virgin earth*, which the artist must choose as the subject of the Great Work."[9]

Chartres Cathedral is unique in that it contains two statues of the Black

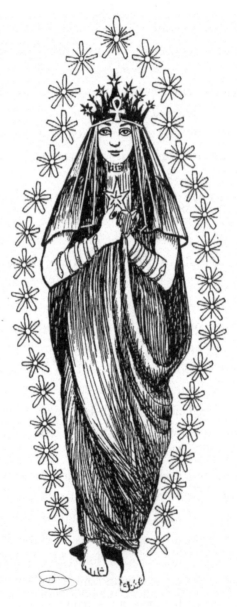

A circle of Nuit stars surround the Black Madonna, honoring her ties to ancient Egypt.
Black Madonna statuary was kept deep within the secret crypts of some
French Gothic cathedrals. Illustration by DARLENE.

Madonna: one in the nave and one in the crypt. It was in this church, where the statue of the Black Madonna has remained since the thirteenth century, that I first had the opportunity to greet her, place my heart in her hands, and ponder her mysteries. I knelt down before her, my palms gently held together in the universal mudra of prayer, and contemplated her image.

She was as black as night, as the prima materia, as the virgin earth; black as the void, the source, and matrix of all becoming. Was this the embodiment of both Isis and the Virgin Mary I beheld, or was this Kali, tantric goddess of this dark Age of Iron? From my perspective as a yogini the Black Madonna appeared to be the Primordial Mother herself, the creator, protector, and destroyer who dissolves all illusions and machinations of the mind. Or Kali Ma, the fearless warrior of truth and integrity whose immaculate heart is a cremation ground on which all egotistical cravings are offered, purified, and transmuted.

As I placed my head at the base of the Black Madonna's pedestal to ask for her blessing, I felt the presence of the multitudes of worshippers who have opened their hearts and placed before her their every longing, every dream, every prayer. I heard them weeping, chanting, crying out to this exquisite embodiment of the secret mysteries of life, death, and regeneration. Going deeper and tuning into the power of the place, I felt rushes of energy course through me as shivers raced up my spine. Light suffused my body, spiraling up through my central channel and engulfing my energy field until I was magically transformed into a radiant ball of light.

In the blink of an eye I found myself traveling through a long, dark winding tunnel from which I was promptly expelled into a silent space of emptiness, of nothingness. There I rested—floating, relaxing—into this vast expanse of empty space. I felt as though I was being absorbed into the very heart of the Mother herself, dissolving into her soothing blackness.

At the moment of my deepest rest I was suddenly propelled outward. I felt myself spinning, spiraling, dancing through the darkness. All around me I saw a host of glowing balls or sparks of light, each shining with its own radiance. We moved together on a vast plane of energies, with stars being birthed out of the heart of the galaxy. I was one of millions of stars that glittered and danced and wove themselves together to form the great spiraling arms of the Milky Way.

I opened my eyes to see the Black Madonna, the Primordial Mother, standing silently before me, waiting patiently to take me in her arms and listen to my prayer. Like those who had come before me, I opened my heart to her. I asked for her assistance in my personal quest for gnosis and illumination. I spoke to her of my longing for grace, beauty, and truth to return to this world. And I prayed that all humans would turn their hearts toward her once again, so that every being could feel the primal power of her loving presence—the vast healing and transformative power of the Divine Feminine.

From Chartres, Jay and I traveled south to Provence to follow in the footsteps of the gnostics, my ancestors Mary Magdalene and the Hebrews, and all the other refugees from the far reaches of the Roman Empire. Jay and I were intrigued by speculation about the intimate relationship between Jesus and Mary Magdalene and the infusion of their bloodline into the heart of France (as first documented in *Holy Blood, Holy Grail*), so we began this new part of our pilgrimage on the shores of the Mediterranean Sea outside Marseilles at Les Saintes Marie de la Mere. In a small chapel dedicated to Mary Magdalene that had been consecrated by Archbishop Roncalli (who later became Pope John XXIII) were paintings of her arrival from Palestine on these shores in a small rudderless boat.

According to legend, soon after the crucifixion and resurrection Mary and her family were expelled from the Holy Land and set adrift on the waters of the Mediterranean Sea. Following the family's arrival in France, Mary was said to have traveled the land preaching the authentic gnostic gospel of Jesus, which had been revealed to her through her personal interaction with him during his mission on earth and in mystic visions after his return to the subtle realms of light.[10]

According to the gnostic gospels that were discovered in 1945 in a cave in upper Egypt near the village of Nag Hammadi, Mary Magdalene was said to be an inspired prophetess who, like Mirabai of India, continuously experienced the living presence of her Lord within her. In addition, French religious literature of the Middle Ages abounds with legends of the life of Mary Magdalene. Tales of her miraculous healings, her aid in fertility and childbearing, and even her ability to "raise the dead" are told.[11] Reportedly there is a secret tradition of the healing arts alive in France today that traces its roots back to Mary Magdalene.[12]

After her prophetic mission was completed, Mary, like many of the yoginis of India and Tibet, is said to have withdrawn to a cave in Saint Baum, where she spent the remainder of her days in prayer and solitude. She is believed to have been buried at Saint Maximin, where from the fifth century until the Saracen invasion her remains were guarded by Cassianite monks.[13] In 1058 a papal bull by Pope Stephen acknowledged the existence of her relics in the church of Vezelay. Consequently it became one of the major places of pilgrimages during the Middle Ages.

This story gave Jay and me much fuel for contemplation. Did Mary Magdalene really carry the thread of the mystical teachings of Egypt to France? I found evidence of this in an early gnostic text titled *Pistis Sophia*. This mystical text relates an extraordinary view of cosmic unfolding. It claims to reveal the secret teachings of

Jesus delivered to his disciples from the shining realms of light thirteen years after his resurrection. These teachings symbolically "connect directly with beliefs and rituals found in the Egyptian *Book of the Dead*."[14] It also recognizes Mary Magdalene's essential role as seer and prophetess in this transmission. In the *Pistis Sophia,* after Jesus presents the first part of the mystical teachings concerning the aeons, orders, and regions of the "Great Invisible," he recognizes Mary Magdalene's superior capacity for contemplation, insight, and revelation:

> It came to pass then, when Mary had heard the Savior say these words, that she gazed fixedly into the air for the space of an hour. She said: "My Lord, give commandment to me to speak in openness." And Jesus, the compassionate, answered and said unto Mary: "Mary, thou blessed one, whom I will perfect in all mysteries, of those of the height, discourse in openness, thou, whose heart is raised to the Kingdom of Heaven more than all thy brethren."

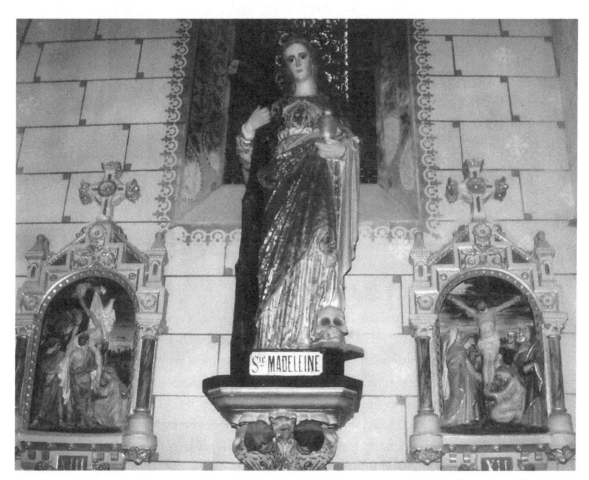

Devotional statue of Mary Magdalene from Rennes Le Chateau, France. Photograph by Jay Weidner.

After listening to her interpretation of his teaching, Jesus again acknowledges her perceptive abilities:

> "Well said, Mary, for thou art blessed before all women on the earth, because thou shalt be the fullness of all fullness and the perfection of all perfections."[15]

But this is only one of a number of early gnostic texts that speak of both Mary's gifts and the enigmatic relationship between her and Jesus. In the Gospel of Mary, from the Nag Hammadi collection, Mary Magdalene the seer relates to other disciples teachings that were revealed to her through prophetic vision. Mary is perceived to fully understand the power of silence, a power or attribute that the gnostics describe as feminine. After revealing to the male disciples Jesus's mystic teaching on the ascent of the soul as it returns to the light, Mary concludes with a description of the final act:

> "I left the world with the aid of another world; a design was erased, by virtue of a higher design. Henceforth I travel towards Repose, where time rests in the Eternity of Time; I go now into Silence." Having said all this, Mary became silent, for it was in silence that the teacher spoke.[16]

In the Gospel of Phillip, from the same collection, the disciples appear to be jealous of the intimate connection between the teacher and his talented female disciple:

> The companion of the savior is Mary Magdalene. But Christ loved her more than all the disciples and used to kiss her often on the mouth. The rest of the disciples were offended by it and expressed disapproval. They said to him, "Why do you love her more than all of us?" The Savior answered and said to them, "Why do I not love you like her? When a blind man and one who sees are both together in darkness, they are no different from one another. When the light comes then he who sees will see the light, and he who is blind will remain in darkness."[17]

This text is often used as evidence by those who speculate on whether Jesus and Mary had a physical relationship. Some modern researchers conjecture that Jesus and Mary had a tantric relationship, a "sacred alchemical marriage" uniting both flesh and spirit. In fact, in recent years there has been much speculation about whether or not Mary arrived in France pregnant with Jesus's child, who gave rise to the royal Merovingian bloodline of the early mystical kings of France.[18]

As a tantric practitioner I found all this information fascinating. The intimate relationship between Jesus and Mary Magdalene as described in these texts finds its parallel in that of Padmasambhava and his consorts Yeshe Tsogyel of Tibet and

Mandarava of India. From this perspective, the male teacher and enlightened emissary who is born miraculously into the patriarchal world of the Kali Yuga transmits the sacred teachings of the way of light to his female disciple, who, following his departure from the material realm, goes on to become both transmitter and caretaker of the lineage. In addition, both Padmasambhava and Jesus clearly acknowledge the intuitive capacities of their female disciples.

According to Church doctrine Mary was a penitent whore from whom Jesus had cast out seven demons. She was also the one to care for him and anoint him before the Crucifixion. In the Gospel of Luke, Mary is described as the one who "bathes his feet with her tears, dried them with her hair, and then anointed them with her oils."

To me this role seems similar to that of the priestess in the funerary rites of ancient Egypt. I wondered, *Could Mary Magdalene have been trained in these ancient feminine arts?* Such training would have prepared her for her mission. The rigorous and extensive schooling for this exalted position would have allowed her to be privy to knowledge of the sacred symbols and mysteries of this ancient tradition of the Goddess. This sacred training, which included travel into the mystical world of vision, certainly would have prepared her to become a fitting companion for Christ and a ripe vessel for his teachings.[19]

And what of the casting out of the seven demons? Was this merely a metaphor for Jesus's assistance in the purification of the seven centers of her luminous body, which are known in the East as chakras? I knew that this type of cleansing is essential to the tantric process of transformation. It seemed to me that the expulsion of demons from Mary's body, mind, and energy field corresponded to this essential aspect of Tantra, in which the student uses specific practices to become aware of, work with, and release negative thoughts and their resulting actions.

But as I was a Jewish woman and a devotee of the Goddess, and now actively in search of my sacred heritage, this was only one of the teachings on the power of the Divine Feminine that I was to uncover in the Western spiritual transmission. For as Jay and I continued our travels I was thrilled to walk through the regions of Provence and Languedoc, where the Goddess as an invisible force or "indwelling presence of God," the Shekhina, had been integrated into Judaism. Here, at the end of the twelfth century, the oral tradition of the Kabbalah (which literally translates as "received") was encoded in mystical books such as the *Bahir* (Illumination). In the Kabbalah, the Shekhina, like Shakti of the Hindus, is seen as the "principle and essence of this world," and "the brilliance taken from God's primal light which is the good light stored away for the righteous."[20] She, like the divine Shakti, is also viewed as "that aspect of Deity that can be apprehended by the senses."[21]

As the feminine potency of God, the Shekhina, like the Great Goddess herself, is alternately referred to as Mother, Daughter, and Bride throughout Kabbalistic works. The *Zahor*, another important Kabbalistic text that is said to have emerged from neighboring Spain during the same period, describes the Shekhina as the "Woman of Light, in whose mystery are rooted all the females of the earthly world."[22] In the gnostic Hebrew mythos she is even spoken of as the soul itself, and her exile from her original home with God into the material world was seen as a metaphor for the exile of the Jewish people from the Holy Land.[23]

For the Kabbalists, this exile or separation of the feminine and masculine aspects of divinity was brought about by the sins of Adam and Eve, who before the fall from paradise were purely spiritual beings clothed in bodies of light. Since that moment, sparks of the Shekhina have been scattered throughout both the physical and psychic-energetic landscapes. It follows, then, that the primary role of every Jew is to travel the path of redemption in which these sparks are gathered in one's being and the pristine state of primordial bliss is restored. This is accomplished through living a life of righteousness and honor in keeping with the laws of the tradition. The great Kabbalistic scholar Gershom Scholem writes:

> In redemption everything is restored to its place by the secret magic of human acts, things are freed from their mixture and consequently, in the realms of both man and of nature, from their servitude to the demonic powers, which, once the light is removed from them are reduced to deathly passivity.

Therefore the Kabbalists believed that "every religious act should be accompanied by the formula: this is done for the sake of the reunion of God and His Shekhina."[24]

That evening, as I sat gazing up at the stars from the window of our hotel room in the beautiful Medieval city Carcassonne, contemplating this mystic teaching of my ancestors, a memory of the precious days I spent with my guruji, Sitara, floated into my consciousness. She was in the midst of demonstrating a karana of the goddess Durga for me. As she assumed this beautiful and wild posture, she seemed to grow in stature. "I am Shakti, the great light and the sacred syllable," she said as her eyes shone with the inner radiance of the Goddess. I am the eternal fire, the holy flame burning in the space in the heart. Although I have innumerable incarnations, essentially I am one. I am the sacred light of divinity that illuminates the world." With those powerful words my guruji magically vanished from my inner vision.

Shakti, Shekhina, Shakti, Shekhina. The names, which sounded so similar to me, resounded over and over in my mind. I wondered, *Were these two manifestations of the Divine Feminine essentially one and the same?*

Later that evening I was overjoyed to discover that sexual union between hus-band and wife was considered a holy act and means of divine meditation by the Kabbalah. In their writings Hebrew scholars Raphael Patai and Gershom Scholem reveal that sex played a central role in Kabbalistic rites.[25] In his thought-provoking book *The Hebrew Goddess* Patai beautifully describes this sexual relationship, which mirrors both the sacred alchemical marriage of the king and queen and the mystic copulation of yogi and yogini in the tantric rites:

> The union of man and wife was considered by the Zahor to be a replica of the union between God and the Shekhina, and at the same time the fulfillment of one of the greatest sacred commandments, because it mystically promoted that divine union and thus contributed to the oneness and wholeness of the deity.[26]

Every Friday evening at the beginning of the Sabbath, or day of rest, which was to be fully devoted to the contemplation of God, Jewish husbands and wives were required to partake in sexual intercourse. This sacred act was preceded by the decla-ration "I fulfill the commandment of copulation for the unification of the Holy One, blessed be He, and the Shekhina."[27]

My childhood Hebrew-school training ran counter to these teachings on the power of both the feminine principle and the act of sexual union. I wondered if I had found a vital link between the mystical teachings of Tantra and Judaism. Had there once been a place for the worship of the Goddess in the Hebrew tradition? Had the patriarchal forces that have so dominated the Kali Yuga forced this knowledge to go underground? In *The Hebrew Goddess* Patai reveals that for 236 years statues of the Canaanite Mother Goddess, Ashera, were present in the Temple of Solomon. The author states, "In Jerusalem, the statue of the Ashera was present in the Temple, and her worship was a part of the legitimate religion approved and led by the King, the court, and the priesthood, and opposed by only a few prophetic voices crying out against it at relatively long intervals."[28]

After the destruction of the Temple of Solomon exoteric Judaism returned to its monotheistic roots. But esoterically, did it retain a sacred spark of the alchemical-gnostic transmission from Egypt? This is very likely. Did this current then flow through Jesus and Mary Magdalene to southern France, or did it merely arise in this magical time and place from the confluence of cultures? It is even possible that there was direct influence from India and the legendary land of Oddiyana, where Padmasambhava spent many years of his life. In this flourishing center of medieval French culture commercial ties to these Eastern lands had been developed. This must have created an atmosphere conducive to the exchange of ideas and material goods.

It was obvious to me that in the same manner that the cult of the Virgin Mary, the Black Madonna, and Mary Magdalene had entered the heart of Christianity, these Kabbalistic teachings must have arisen out of a longing for the return of a loving, nurturing, passionate, and compassionate feminine figure to grace what had become a distinctly patriarchal religion. This longing is mirrored today in the hearts of so many of us Jewish women.

Finally Jay and I traveled to Montsegur, the most holy site and the final stronghold of the Cathari, the last group of Christian gnostics who openly transmitted their sacred teachings before the Catholic Church systematically eliminated them. Labeled as heretics by the Church of Rome, the Cathari were hunted, tortured, and burned at the stake for their beliefs. Jay was very passionate about this act, which he called the "first Inquisition." He explained, "The Cathari were a selfless, altruistic, and compassionate people who, like your saddhus and wandering mendicants of India and Tibet, renounced all worldly possessions and fully committed themselves to the path of spirit. The [word] *Cathari* is translated from the Greek *Katharos*, meaning 'pure ones,' and they claimed they were inheritors of the true teachings of Jesus. These were secret teachings that came from a tradition believed to be much older than that claimed by the Church of Rome. Like Jesus before them, they rebelled against what they considered to be the excesses of the priestly hierarchy. They felt that the Church of the Romans, with its grandiose pageants, expensive vestments, loose morality, and intolerant views, was exactly the opposite of what a true Christian believed and practiced. But that is not all. To the Cathari, the very tenets of Catholic doctrine were seen as blasphemy.

"The doctrine of the Cathari, like those of all gnostics, delineated the dualistic nature of the world we live in, the eternal struggle between good and evil," Jay said as he looked out over the quiet countryside that surrounded us. "According to these teachings, Jehovah, the wrathful god of the Old Testament, was seen as a false god and an expression of what they referred to as the *demiurge*. For how could a truly enlightened divinity contain within him negative human emotions such as anger, jealousy, or vengeance? In their view, the real God was a loving deity equally and directly accessible to all. This God taught that compassion and the true sacrifice and transformation of the self, or ego, was the highest spiritual path.

"The Cathari, like all gnostics, believed that the plan of this demiurge, or Satan, was to trap spirit in matter, and that the earth itself was a prison in which souls were exiled from the divine source. The real world for them was the nonmaterial world of spirit, and all their rituals and practices were designed to prepare them to enter this divine realm. Therefore, they felt that anyone who claimed authority in this world had to be evil, hence their disdain for the Church of Rome."

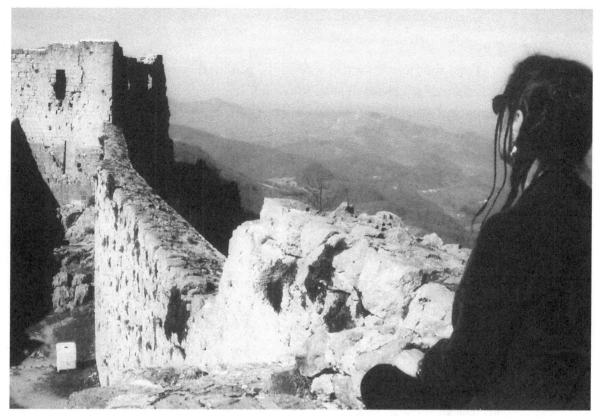

The author meditating at Montsegur. Photograph by Jay Weichner.

That evening as I conducted further research I discovered that for the Cathari, Jesus was perceived as a direct emanation from God. Jesus was a divine messenger or the son "born of the Father before time began," who had come to show the Cathari the means by which they could find their way out of this impure world of matter, darkness, and suffering and return to their true home in the light.[29] The Cathari ardently believed that they were the true heirs of Jesus's secret teaching, a direct energetic transmission of the pure and radiant light of God's Holy Spirit. From the perspective of many gnostic communities, this divine current was, like the Shekhina of the Jews, perceived as the feminine, nurturing energy of God.[30]

The transmission of this feminine energy was the center of the Cathari's most sacred ritual, the *consolamentum*. The ritual was performed by the physical laying on of hands by one who had experienced the power of the transmission. In *Massacre at Montsegur*, an excellent book on the Cathari, Zoe Oldenbourg states:

> There is no doubt that this rite, the consolamentum, contained genuine supra-
> natural virtues for the Cathars. In their eyes, it actually brought down the Holy

Spirit upon its beneficiary . . . This act formed the keystone of the central truth of the Catharist Church."[31]

Once the Holy Spirit had entered the person, they became known as a *perfecti*, or perfected one. He or she had to commit himself or herself to follow the selfless, caring, and moral lifestyle of the Catharist Church or the divine spirit could be lost. This was a lifestyle of constant generosity, prayer, and communion. The most pious of the Cathari were known to never raise their voices or utter an offensive word. Mild-mannered and known for their charitable works and skill in the healing arts, the perfecti provided spiritual and physical strength to noble and peasant alike.

Women were particularly drawn to the tenets and practice of Catharism, a faith that encouraged their natural gifts of vision and intuitive perception. Like Machig Lapdron and the chod practitioners of Tibet, these Cathari women traveled about healing the sick, educating the masses, and even assisting workers in the fields. It is no wonder that the simplicity, generosity, and faith of the Cathari women and men inspired both peasant and aristocrat.

As Jay and I sat together atop Montsegur, he spoke of the horrors that Pope Innocent III had perpetrated against these humble adepts. "In his overwhelming lust to regain both physical and spiritual control over this wealthy region of southern Europe," Jay related, "Pope Innocent issued a proclamation, calling upon his fellow countrymen to rise up in a Holy Crusade against these subversive men and women. Methodically, relentlessly, with great malice, his armies marched through the towns, villages, and citadels of Languedoc, attempting to root out what he called the Cathar heresy.

"The pope's general, knowing that throughout the area Catholics, Cathari, Jews, and pagans lived in harmony, complained to Pope Innocent that he did not know how to tell the difference between them. It is from this horrific crusade that the famous dictum, 'Kill them all; God knows his own' has been handed down through the annals of French history. It is estimated that more than sixty thousand people died in this holocaust. In the end, some two hundred Cathari were trapped here at the castle at Montsegur, where on March 14, 1244, the last refugees of this powerful spiritual tradition slowly descended the steep path you see before you. Down there in the field that even today is referred to as 'the field of the burnt ones,' the Catholic army had built a huge bonfire that they planned to use to slowly torture and kill the Cathari. Instead the Cathari deeply disappointed the army of Rome by suddenly running into the fire en masse."

In my mind's eye I could see the Cathari, these noble women and men who constantly felt the living presence of the Holy Spirit within them, whose hearts were filled with goodness and compassion. I felt the fleeting shadows of their presence around us, watched them as they moved throughout the land, teaching by example and silently imbuing the physical and psychic landscapes with their transformative current of love, grace, and compassion. And I felt the extraordinary power of their faith, a faith so strong that they were willing to face the intense physical agony of the flames rather than deny it.

We sat together in this holy place nestled in the Pyrenees Mountains, and Jay offered his understanding of the core of our Western lineage of transmission. He began, "Hermeticists do not seek credit for their actions. Silently, from a place of deep serenity, they move among the people of the earth, ceaselessly working to alter the psychic landscape of our reality and lead us toward spiritual enlightenment. These humble, generous, and gracious Keepers of the Light, who have not only existed in the West but in cultures across the planet, are the ones who have, through their selfless activities, saved us from ourselves countless times in our history. To do what is right, to simply open one's heart to the beauty and wonder of the world, to live together in peace and quiet contemplation aligned with the path of spirit: This is the way of hermeticism. This is the true way toward the light. The human race owes everything to this secret society, these Keepers of the Light, for without them we would be left floundering in the darkness. You see, my love," Jay said with a warm smile, "we are all members of this group. We just have to decide to join. And then we have to live in the light."

I thought about the courage and foresight with which our sacred ancestors—the teachers, adepts, healers, yoginis, yogis, priestesses, priests, wise women and men—had for so many centuries kept the bright lamp of spirit burning in the darkness. An intense wave of gratitude swept over me, filling my eyes with tears. And in that moment, at that holy place now bathed in the golden light of the setting sun, I took a vow to hold the teachings in my heart. I promised to continue to seek, contemplate, and integrate their teachings within the sacred alchemical vessel of my being, so that one day I might have the honor of telling their story to all who would listen. As Jay and I sat together hand in hand, I gently relaxed into the silent place of bliss and emptiness that resides in the core of my being. Gazing out into space I saw the luminous currents of the divine Shakti/Shekhina calling me home.

5

History and the Feminine Mysteries: Reflections on the Cycle of the Great Yuga

*If one does not understand how the fire came to be,
he will burn in it, because he does not know his root.
If one does not first understand the water, he does
not know anything. . . . If one does not understand
how the wind that blows came to be, he will run
with it. If one does not understand how the body
that he wears came to be, he will perish with it. . . .
Whoever does not understand how he came will not
understand how he will go.*

—"Dialogue of the Savior" from the Nag
Hammadi Library

*Myth is the history of the soul; the memory of our
greater Being; ritual and sacrament are the reminders.
In the continuing Fall the part breaks away from the
Whole; to make something sacred, one must
reconnect the part to the universal Whole.*

—William Irwin Thompson, The Time Falling
Bodies Take to Light

From the time I was first introduced to the teachings on the yugas, or cyclic ages of humanity, by my guruji, Sitara Devi, I was fascinated by this ancient view of history in which the Goddess plays such a dominant role. Over the ensuing years, as I continued my quest to uncover both the sacred mysteries of the goddess and the feminine experience, I began to discover that there were teachings comparable to these in the mystic traditions of many of the world's great religions. These teachings bring to light a very different view of history than the one we have been presented in our schools and universities. It is this alternative view of history that I present to you in this chapter, which I offer as a conclusion to Part I of *The Path of the Priestess*. Based on my years of research and experience in these sacred traditions, it is designed to provoke contemplation about who we really are by opening your eyes to an extraordinary metaphysical perspective on history, spirituality, and the power of the feminine principle that has been handed down to us through the ages.

As you become acquainted with this traditional perspective on the perpetual stream of human events please keep in mind that they unfold over vast expanses of time, and that from our current location in this unfolding the veils between the spiritual and the material worlds have become so thick that unless we have had the great fortune to be initiated into the mystic teachings, we can only speculate on what has transpired. Clearly these teachings counter our modern-day view of the evolution of humanity.

Prior to the art of writing, the history of humanity was passed down through oral tradition from mother to daughter, father to son, elders to community members. Today the only remnants we have of these early events are the myths and legends that have survived through time. The imparting and recording of events is and has always been a relative activity based on the social imprinting and unique perspective of the person witnessing the events. Every culture has its own special view and agenda. When we look back into what we know as documented history, we can see that stories were often written and rewritten, and tales were told, altered, or suppressed according to the worldview of the dominant civilization. Many believe that beneath the linear history of our material world lies another story: the story of the sacred mysteries, the hidden history of the human race. Our ancient ancestors from civilizations the world over postulated that all life flows in great transformative cycles, from the seasons of nature to the phases of the moon and the birth, growth, maturation, and death of all living creatures. They explained that just as we individuals experience the ebb and flow of these smaller cycles, humanity as a whole experiences the rise and fall of a larger cycle. In the Indo-Tibetan, Bon, Zoroastrian, Greek, and alchemical traditions, this great cycle was said to be composed of four yugas, or ages of humanity.[1]

According to the ancient texts the cycle of the ages begins with a Golden Age of beauty, harmony, and grace, an age in which both female and male are fundamentally connected with their own divinity and living lives of truth, fully aligned with the universal spirit.[2] But as the ages progress metaphorically from gold to silver, bronze, and iron, humanity draws farther away from the radiant light of spirit. We move toward an age of total materialization and concretization, a time of ignorance and delusion, a time in which the bright light of spirit is all but extinguished. The ancients called this age the Kali Yuga, the Age of Iron.

This is the age in which we now reside, and in keeping with the teachings of a number of current spiritual groups, it is the age from which we are now emerging.[3] It is the age in which the tantric texts foretold that the great goddess Kali would rise up and perform her powerful dance of destruction and transformation. Through this transformative dance she will draw all the dark and destructive energy of this yuga into the secret core of her being. Then from the depths of her heart, the source of infinite wisdom and compassion, she will absorb and transmute this energy, cleansing and purifying earth and mankind alike. Through this primordial dance, the veils that have blinded us to our own radiance will be lifted. Humanity will then awaken to its immortality and enter a new Golden Age of divine insight and luminosity.

The texts tell us that as each of the four ages arises and ripens, faith, integrity, and allegiance to spiritual values are decreased by one-fourth. A symbolic image that is often given to illustrate the increasing loss of spirit and its resulting acceleration of weakness and infirmity in humanity is that of a cow who in the first age, or Satya Yuga, is standing boldly and resolutely upon its four legs. With the passing of each of the yugas the noble cow forfeits the use of one of its legs, as one-fourth of human virtue is lost. Therefore, in the Silver Age, or Treta Yuga, the cow stands on three legs. With the arrival of the Bronze Age, or Dvapara Yuga, the troubled cow stands on only two legs, as virtue and spiritual essence are now depleted by half. By the appearance of the Kali Yuga, or Age of Iron, the barren, tormented cow has only one leg left to stand on. Humanity, shrouded in the increasing darkness of depravity and corruption, retains only one-fourth of the original light of spirit.[4]

The cow is a symbol that can be found in cultures throughout the world. Feminine in form, she stands for fertility, nourishment, support, and preservation. She represents the Mother, our first teacher, and our eternal patroness of righteousness and integrity. She is the strong and solid foundation upon which the spiritual sustenance of humanity rests. Isn't it fascinating that a feminine symbol should be used to transmit these teachings of the cyclic destruction of humankind? Could this mean that, contrary to our contemporary Western indoctrination of the spiritual power of women, it is women who hold the primary responsibility for maintaining spiritual and moral alignment? Could this also mean that as the light of spirit diminishes and as women increasingly turn away from their true spiritual natures and primary roles as teachers and nurturers, all of us—both female and male—degenerate?

As the ages unfold, not only do we lose our spiritual luminosity but also we become densified, more material and corporeal. We are born fresh, pure, and newly formed, projected from the formless heart of the Divine. In the beginning, at the instant of creation, the moment that the divine androgyne reflects on itself and divides into essence and energy, when Shiva sends out his Shakti and the Lord God sends out his Shekhina, we emerge from the heart of emptiness in an exquisite display of vibration, sound, and light.[5] Radiating with the pure light of spirit, filled with endless vitality, we are in tune with every subtle nuance of universal expression. But according to this view, in this cyclic dance of creation the time of harmony must end. From the exquisite radiance of the first moment of creation the process of entropy ensues.

Entropy is the second law of thermodynamics, and it states that everything in the universe is slowly disintegrating. While it is true that matter cannot be destroyed, as time passes it does move into a more ineffectual state. In our reality all systems are prone to eventual breakdown, death, or transformation to another mode of being. This is true of the human body, the trees and plants, and the stars and planets. For example, even though the matter that makes up a log is not destroyed by a fire, it is reduced to ashes, which are a disintegrated form of the wood. The key word here is *disintegration*—the movement away from the integrated or unified state. As this happens there is an incremental increase in the number of souls born; a decrease in strength and longevity; and a proliferation of disease, suffering, and madness.[6]

Through this entropic process of descent from the primordial unity into separation and densification, spiritual authority is traded for secular domination, quality is exchanged for quantity, and the sacred vanishes into the profane. In fact, the end of a cycle appears to be the inversion of the beginning, and the world's values are turned upside down.[7] As a parallel to the fast-paced times in which we live, it is also interesting to note that during the progression of the cycle time literally speeds up, with life passing by at an increasing velocity until time itself ends and the present manifestation is dissolved and a new *mahayuga*, or great cycle, begins.[8]

How does this view of the development of the ages—with its emphasis on the increasing loss of spiritual union, intimacy, beauty, and truth—apply to our quest for understanding of the feminine experience? Recently many scholars have postulated that there was a time in which our current male and female roles were reversed, a time in which women held dominion. However, when one looks back in time from the perspective of the continuous cycles of the ages, or yugas, new insights into the relationship between woman and man and humanity and divinity begin to emerge.

The Golden Age: The Age of Divinity

*O people of the earth, born and made of the
elements, but with the spirit of Divinity within you,
rise from your sleep of ignorance! Be sober and
thoughtful. Realize that your home is not on the earth
but in the Light. Why have you delivered yourselves
over unto death, having power to partake of
immortality? Repent and change your minds. Depart
from the dark light and forsake corruption forever.
Prepare yourselves to climb through the Seven Rings
and to blend your souls with the eternal light.*
    —HERMES MERCURIUS TRISMEGISTUS, *THE DIVINE
    PYMANDER OF HERMES MERCURIUS TRISMEGISTUS*

*There is in everyone [divine power] existing in a
latent condition. . . . This is one power divided
above and below; generating itself, making itself
grow, seeking itself, finding itself, being mother of
itself, father of itself, sister of itself, spouse of itself,
daughter of itself, son of itself—mother, father,
unity, being a source of the entire circle of existence.*
    —HIPPOLYTUS, *REFUTATION OF ALL HERESIES*

According to the ancient texts human beings did not evolve from some inanimate and simplistic form, as our modern scientists would have us believe. Rather, we emerged fully realized at the start of the Golden Age. Every spiritual tradition speaks of this time, whether it is known as the primordial paradise, the Garden of Eden, the first world, the Dreamtime, or the Satya Yuga. In fact, teachings from spiritual traditions around the world describe this as an age of primal perfection in which humanity was one with nature and spiritual order prevailed.[9]

During this idyllic age the world and all its components—from human beings to plants and minerals—were seen and experienced as the immense manifest body of the formless. We were part of the dance of divinity unfolding itself. Therefore we had no need of outward images, rites, and rituals to help us maintain our link with divinity. According to the great French alchemist Fulcanelli, we experienced total balance and alignment with the universe. Female and male lived together in a state of continual bliss. Fulcanelli states, "Living a contemplative existence, in harmony with a fertile, rejuvenated earth; our blessed ancestors were unacquainted with desire, pain or suffering." In this luminous garden of delight we were at peace with ourselves, each other, and the world we inhabited.

In the Golden Age, which is extremely difficult for us to even imagine, let alone articulate, because of our current position in the cycle, our reality was not as solid as it appears to our modern earthbound senses, but rather an exquisitely subtle vibratory reality composed of light and sound. This was the period of new beginnings, when the divine intelligence manifested itself in the wealth of forms that make up our world and the spiritual realm became conscious of itself as the manifest world and as the divine power governing it.[10] In this remarkable age all beings, knowing themselves to be the energy of divinity fashioned into a luminous form, were naturally conscious of the world of spirit, and their external reality reflected this spiritual consciousness. This was the mythic age of goddesses and gods, the age of the immortals. There was no veil separating life and death, and our innate consciousness was free to fly between the spiritual and material realms.

In the myths and legends of many civilizations we discover these goddesses and gods, our divine progenitors. In their shimmering, translucent world of light, which existed prior to the formation of the veils of linear time, the process of entropy had not yet begun.[11] The laws of physics and the forces of gravity of the later ages did not constrain these suprahuman beings. Therefore, in their deeds and demeanor they demonstrated abilities that appear extraordinary to our modern sensitivities.

This was an epoch of purity, innocence, beauty, and truth, the era that the Australian Aborigines refer to as the eternal Dreamtime that occurred before time began. In this first age of the Dreaming, it is said that the vast expanse of primordial space was infused with the power and intensity of great mythical energies and beings who realized their dreams and visions without the limitations of embodied existence.[12] As vital forms of fluid, divine energy joyously weaving, playing, and manifesting their inner light as external reality, they planted the essential seed emerging from the residue of the former mahayuga. From this perspective our original ancestors were not primitive apes but a magical display of the very essence, nature, and energy of the primordial source of all creation fashioned into a luminous form.

One of the most insightful explanations of the beings of the Satya Yuga can be found in the Tibetan Buddhist teachings. These teachings describe a subtle dimension of light known as the Sambhogakaya, or wealth dimension.[13] It is a magical realm composed of the luminous essence of the elements that make up our concrete physical world. As we have seen in chapter 2, to the initiate these essential energies appear as multiple symbolic forms or realized beings known as dakinis, dakas, bodhisattvas, herukas, and so forth. Each of these forms is perceived by the initiate as the personification of a principle of pure wisdom, and each serves as an inspirational role model whose qualities are in perfect alignment with the highest spiritual values. But this is not the only ancient tradition in which the sacred beings of light appear and interact with the awakened practitioner. The angels of the Judeo-Christian and Zoroastrian traditions, the kachinas of the Hopis, and the neters of the Egyptian tradition can all be considered present-day links to this extraordinary age. For this was a time in which dynamic archetypal energies radiated like shimmering rays of light from the primordial source of all becoming. How would it affect our perception of ourselves as human beings if we were to imagine that these radiant beings were our ancestors?

The Silver Age: The Age of Ritual

In the ancient way of being, the earth not only
creates, feeds, and protects life but, like a mother,
whispers through natural signs and images the secret
knowledge of how body, mind, emotions and spirit
work upon each other in an intricate, invisible
weaving.

—JOHANNA LAMBERT, WISE WOMEN OF THE
DREAMTIME

Ritual fuses in simultaneity the seed and the tree, the
potential and the actual, the dreaming and the reality.
—ROBERT LAWLOR, VOICES OF THE FIRST DAY

As the periodic cycle of the ages unfolded, most of humanity drifted farther away from this paradisiacal state, traveling on a course that led downward from the subtle light of spirit into the darkness and densification of matter. As the process of entropy ensued we slipped away from this pure awareness of our own divinity. Our essential light became shrouded by the veils of corporeal existence. We descended from a state of divine union and bliss into a state of separation, of other and I, subject and object, light and dark. With this new era of human experience came the laws and experience of duality. No longer did we innately recognize our connection with our divine progenitor, but we instead saw it as something independent. No longer did we rest completely in the light of divine love. With this sudden fall of consciousness into matter, many of us began to identify ourselves with the physical body and could no longer see beyond death. This was the beginning of our collective amnesia, the first days of our sad journey of forgetfulness. Perhaps this is the fall from grace that is spoken of in so many ancient texts.

Isolated, confused, and living in this dual reality separated from divinity yet longing to remember who we were, we humans endeavored to hold on to the radiant threads of our spiritual light. At this time we began to create what is called ritual. In order to retain and transmit the celestial beauty and rapture of what we remembered from our previous idyllic existence, oral tradition and symbolic expression were born. Our sacred memories, visions, and heavenly aspirations were communicated through stories, which we now call myths and legends, and through mantras (sounds that carry the vibrations of divine energy) and mudras (hand gestures used for the worship of and communication with the Divine).

Our ancestors were at first a nomadic people, still awed by the power and potency of nature and the cosmos. They worshipped the elements, the weather, and the principles of the natural world. From their dual perspective the masculine was seen as the static, inert principle (the source of divinity) and the feminine was seen as the kinetic principle (the energy of divinity). The female was the voice of divinity, expressing herself through the countless forms and forces of our physical world. With this recognition of our fundamental divinity, our ancestors embarked on a sacred journey of self-discovery. Their newly formed material vessels and the radiant manifest world around them fascinated these spiritually attuned beings. And so nature, the human body, and the vast cosmos that unveiled itself every evening became the people's medium for exploration and understanding. So closely aligned with nature and living in a world where time had a very different flow and meaning than in the mechanized corporate world of today, the women and men of these ancient civilizations would spend entire lifetimes observing, meditating on, and documenting all the facts of their three-dimensional reality. The forms and cycles of the natural world; the development of the human body, mind, and spirit; the paths of the stars and the precession of the equinoxes were all sacred mysteries to be acknowledged, reflected on, and revealed.

Since the veils between the physical and subtle energetic dimensions were still porous, these ancestors still retained the ability to perceive and travel the mystic roads between them. From their visionary perspective all the manifest world appeared to be surrounded, penetrated, and interconnected by a great web or network of light that constantly flowed out from the primordial heart of creation. As a result of this enhanced perceptive ability they understood that the patterns and systems manifesting in the larger universe mirrored those within the earth itself and within the inner realms of the physical body. Like a great interwoven matrix of light these systems were perceived to nest together like boxes within boxes. The patterns governing reality were considered to have the same essential geometric structure, no matter how infinitesimal or infinite in their scope. Each system held the key to the entire structure of universal manifestation.

Therefore, on both a physical and subtle level, the human body, its organs, systems, movements, rhythms, and cycles were believed to have a direct relationship to the cycles of the earth, planets, stars, and universe. For example, the human body, like the Earth itself, was believed to be made up of the elements earth, air, fire, and water. The element of earth was equated with our bones and tissues, as well as the rocks and minerals that make up the solid body of the planet. The element of air was equated with the winds that sweep across the Earth and the breath that flows through our bodies. The element of water was equated with both our bloodstreams and the rivers and streams that run through the Earth; the element of fire was equated with the electromagnetic currents of energy that flow through the energetic body of the earth, as well as through our nervous systems.

In addition, these highly attuned women and men were also able to perceive the more subtle geometric shapes and currents of energy that flow through the great luminous web of creation. They perceived that just as the human body contains a radiant network known to mystics today as channels, chakras, nadis, and meridians, so too does the earth contain subtle energetic pathways known to shamans as ley lines and spirit paths. As we have seen throughout this book, these channels are conduits for the flow of the serpent power, or Kundalini Shakti, the vital, creative feminine force that is constantly pouring out of the still source of creation. This divine cosmic energy, continuously weaving and flowing throughout the universal matrix, was perceived to vivify, sustain, and enlighten all manifest existence.

During this magical Silver Age, not only was phenomenal reality divided into female and male principles but also each manifestation, force, or expression of nature—such as heaven, earth, sun, moon, rivers, mountains, wind, fire, dawn, and dusk—was recognized and detached from the others. Every aspect of the natural world was transfigured into a distinctive entity that commanded reverence.[14] All were seen as separate aspects of the consummate mystical powers of divinity, which, according to the setting and situation, could be invoked, venerated, and petitioned.

Perceiving the land as the sacred body of the Great Goddess, our ancestors, who are known to modern-day scholars as hunter-gatherers, freely wandered from holy place to holy place performing their practices and rituals. Effortlessly perceiving and interacting with the subtle forces that wove the luminous web of life, these women and men were fully in touch with the psychic-energetic-emotional landscape of reality. Day after day they journeyed on their sacred walkabouts, traversing the vibratory song lines or flowing streams of vital energy that arise from the earth.[15] These subtle lines of force mirrored not only the physical positions of the stars but also the subtle pathways of the eternal realms of spirit. In his superb book *Voices of the First Day*, which documents the ancient teachings of the Australian Aborigines, author Robert Lawlor describes these magnetic currents as "an invisible web extending throughout the universe on every level, from atom to galaxy." According to Lawlor's research these people who trace their lineage back to the first days of creation knew that "magnetic fields of influence integrate the universe, earth and every living creature so that each communicates its rhythmic resonance with all the others."

At first our ancestors were connected to the movements of spirit, and they possessed capacities that are today the subject of lore in some cultures and secret practices in others. These include abilities derived from intimate communion with the elements, such as nourishing themselves with ingested light, keeping themselves warm by raising their inner metaphysical fires, or journeying in dream and vision to the stars and beyond.[16] The nomads traveled without possessions, naked at first, and as time progressed and they lost some of these capacities they clothed themselves with simple garments, communing with the earth and mystic world of the ancestors.

Humanity's creation of religion was a direct result of the turn of the seasons from the end of the Golden Age to the beginning of the Silver. The practitioners of this new religion performed their acts of worship—the prototypes of our sacred rituals, songs, and dances—in the midst of nature, in the woods, along the banks of the river, and on mountaintops. In resonance with their natural environment, they embraced Mother Nature in all her beauty and might. Even today shamanic societies that still adhere to these ancient principles teach that we can commune with our ancestors through our contact with the elements. In the words of Adelina Avla Padilla, spiritual leader of the Chumash tribe of Santa Ynez, California, "In the whisper of the wind one can hear the voices of the ancestors and feel their gentle touch; in the warmth and flicker of the fire and the rays of shining light of the rising and setting sun they are present, waiting for us to recognize and commune with them."[17]

In the ancient hunter-gatherer societies daily tasks that were essential to survival and deep and intimate rituals involving sexuality, social conditioning, and initiation were divided equally between the genders. Females performed their essential roles as childbearers, instructors, healers, and nurturers, while males performed their roles as providers, mentors, and protectors. Creation was believed to be the result of a cosmic relationship between the receptive and nurturing feminine body of the earth that opened herself to receive the indispensable seed of her divine consort, the masculine sky.

During this age of balance women's bodies were seen as magical vessels. Like the process that brings forth the riches of the earth, from deep within the confines of the woman's body new life would miraculously spring. Women, who have the extraordinary capacity to experience a new human life take root, grow in, and emerge from their wombs and into the world, were seen to be intrinsically connected to the great mysteries of manifestation.[18]

The process of pregnancy and giving birth was seen as an extremely sensual and life-altering experience. It was recognized that throughout pregnancy the mother's body was suffused with vital energy. This energy gave her increased attunement with every sensation within her physical body, and it seemed to heighten her ability to travel in the etheric and energetic realms as well. To these simple and wise people it was only natural that women going through this profound experience, which mimicked the very act of creation itself, would innately comprehend the essential dynamics of the heart —of love, tenderness, compassion, selflessness, and protection.

The woman's work had only begun at birth. For it was the mother's role to not only nurture and maintain the physical health and vitality of her child but also to nurture and maintain its spiritual growth as well. This work was given the highest priority in these ancient societies. As mothers, women were the first teachers and guides. They were the healers, nursemaids, and custodians of the spirit; the acknowledged weavers and keepers of the psychic-energetic-emotional landscape. Fully aligned with the truth, women understood and transmitted the spiritual and moral values of the clan or society to their children. Numerous rituals existed in which women were the spiritual guides, and they assumed the roles of priestess, educator, and initiator into the sacred mysteries of sexuality and spiritual transformation.[19]

Through continuous interaction with each other, their children, their mates, and the environment, as well as through intuition and trial and error, women were able to accumulate a highly specialized body of knowledge and expertise. Today we call this body of knowledge women's mysteries. These mysteries included comprehension of the underlying principles, cycles, and flow of nature and the cosmos; the hidden secrets of life, death, fertility, and sexuality; the arts of healing, such as the magic of plants and herbs; insight into the nature of the psychic-energetic-emotional patterns flowing between the physical body and the luminous energy field; and receiving, transmitting, and interpreting messages from both the physical and visionary realms.

Although many aspects of this knowledge were shared and discussed with men, it was more often than not considered the intrinsic realm of the feminine. It was preserved and handed down through oral tradition and direct energetic transmission from mother to daughter, woman to woman. This fertile period of human history is often spoken of as the time of the matriarchy, a time in which women were fully empowered. During this era men had equally essential roles to play, and there have been many volumes written about their ways and practices throughout history. In this story, however, we will focus primarily on how the flow of the ages shaped feminine lives and experiences.

The Bronze Age: The Age of Doubt

> *The arts are not for our instruction, but for our delight, and this delight is something more than pleasure, it is the godlike ecstasy of liberation from the restless activity of the mind and the senses, which are the veils of all reality, transparent only when we are at peace with ourselves. From the love of many things we are led to the experience of Union. The secret of all art is self-forgetfulness.*
> —ANANDA COOMARSWAMY, THE DANCE OF SHIVA

> *By definition the Symbol is magic; it evokes the form bound in the spell of matter. To evoke is not to imagine. It is to live; it is to live the form.*
> —R. A. SCHWALLER DE LUBICZ, THE TEMPLE OF MAN

As time inevitably marched on, the downward spiral of the great yuga unfolded and the pure light of spirit diminished once again. Only half the initial light of creation remained. According to numerous texts, this was the crucial period when the balance of power, of light and darkness, shifted. It was a catastrophic time compared to the earlier idyllic existence, which was dominated by feminine values and the collective experience. One could speculate that until this moment in time we retained a strong telepathic connection with each other and the animals, and forces of the natural world. Intimate with the elements and the subtle vibrations of a larger reality, we could perform what we today consider extraordinary feats of extrasensory perception such as clairvoyance, telekinesis, and astral projection.

This was the legendary time of the Tower of Babel, a time in which great catastrophes such as floods, earthquakes, storms, and fires ravaged the land. Communities were torn apart and the natural fertility of the planet began to be compromised. This was an age of material and spiritual separation, a time of confusion and disorientation in which we lost the ability to speak to each other in the same language.[20]

We then moved into an era of increasing materialization in which we began to identify ourselves with our physical bodies and the ever-densifying material world. In this second half of the mahayuga, which was dominated by the fundamental forces and energy of the male principle, inherent trust for the nurturing and sustaining qualities of the earth had clearly diminished. We humans began to limit the scope of our vision and to attempt to control Mother Nature and each other. With the discovery of agriculture as a way to provide for ourselves and prove our dominion over natural forces, our contemplative nomadic existence, with its wide-open spaces and panoramic views, was traded for the agrarian, pastoral life. The hunter-gatherer tribes moved into the stable, immobile farming communities. Frightened by the powerful forces of nature, we no longer felt free to wander the earth living on nothing but the natural fruit of the land. With the advent of agriculture, civilization—with its settlements, hierarchical power structure, and rules and regulations—slowly became the guiding force.[21]

In the early agrarian civilizations of this period, worship of the Great Mother Goddess, the symbol of fertility, was still performed. The womb was still perceived as the primordial doorway to creation, the holy vessel that brought new life. It was equated with the storehouse, or the place in which the grain was kept. It was seen as a horn of plenty that mirrored the abundant nature of planet Earth herself. As women traveled the inner and outer roads of feminine experience from young girl to mother and fully mature female, they were seen as great repositories of knowledge and wisdom. It was the mother, the priestess, and the wise woman to whom all would come for healing of body, mind, and spirit. Essential to women's roles was the maintenance of the psychic-energetic-emotional landscape of their communities.

But as time went on and farm turned to village, village to town, town to city, and city to nation-state, a new social structure was formed. Society was divided into castes or classes, each individual assuming her or his own distinct role. This was the beginning of the era of the great theocracies. Kings and queens, believed to be the living embodiment of the Divine, ruled these civilizations. Men were especially affected by this alteration. In the new world order the male began to change his responsibilities from those of hunter and provider to that of guardian. At first his responsibilities were that of protector of the land; later they were that of warrior and conqueror. Because the veil of darkness and densification had begun to descend, the average man—immersed in his role as farmer, shepherd, laborer, and warrior—was given little time to contemplate nature and the manifold expressions of divinity. Women, in general, maintained their familial roles.

As the great cycle unfolded, more and more souls were born into the world. Some chose to incarnate throughout the cycle to keep the light of spirit burning, and today they still retain the innate knowledge of truth and virtue and the spiritual vision of our divine beginnings and the primordial paradise. Others who were newly incarnated had only the knowledge of their immediate time and place in the cycle.[22] Working the fields, many times with women and children by their sides, and struggling with the forces of nature and each other in order to protect their land and possessions, the average person had less time and inclination to seek the pathways of spirit and explore the wonders of life.

Because of this constraint and our increasing concern with the conditions of daily life, an intermediary was needed to link most people with the world of spirit and help them remember their divine heritage. A special hierarchy of priestesses and priests arose to traverse the pathways between spirit and matter. Symbolic rites and rituals and artistic expression in the form of dance, music, sculpture, theater, and painting became the vehicles through which our ancient stories, dreams, and memories were transmitted. The myriad aspects and forces of our material world and its dual nature became personified as goddesses and gods, monsters and demons. This anthropomorphization came about as a means by which to transmit the early knowledge of our divine beginnings and the enormous potential of the individual human being. By depicting these powers and forces in sentient form, our spiritual leaders were teaching us that as embodied beings we had a conscious choice whether to rise to the heights of the gods or to sink to the depths of the demons.

Our myths, legends, magic, and mysteries—the vast wealth of human knowledge, which had been passed down through oral tradition—were now encoded in songs, dances, hieroglyphic symbols, and images. This was the beginning of culture and the encoding of the sacred arts. The idols, icons, and images—replete with their symbolic gestures, postures, implements, and attributes—and the mystic rituals and practices of the priesthood became the vehicles through which the average person could perceive and commune with the subtle and sophisticated world of divinity. According to the ancient texts, this is when the sacred remnants of the Golden Age, the high arts of civilization and of refinement and sophistication, were given to humanity. And who was the giver of these heavenly gifts? The Mother herself, the Great Goddess in the form of Inanna in Sumer, Isis in Egypt, and Saraswati in India. As emanations of the Great Goddess, or voice of divinity, goddesses such as these were often associated with the art of weaving; for as embodied manifestations of the Divine Feminine force, it was their role to continuously weave her sacred currents of spiritual light, beauty, truth, and grace into the fabric of our world. These goddesses became the caretakers of the tradition and the vehicles through which divine knowledge was transmitted.

As time went on and the forces of materialization took hold, holy temples were built to house the energy and images of the goddesses and gods. The temples were constructed according to the sacred teachings of the societies. Based on a perception of the divine order of the universe, constructed through the use of sacred mathematical and geometric principles, and filled with exquisite art and sculpture, the temples were designed to provide the multitudes with a personal experience of the celestial realms.

Amid this heavenly atmosphere sacred rituals composed of dance, drama, music, and chanting were performed. These rituals were created not only to further enhance the religious experience but also to convey the basic principles and practices of the culture's faith. In essence, the sacred temples and the ritual activities that took place within them were created to provide the individual with the opportunity to experience the energies (sounds, visions, feelings, and so on) of a larger reality. The buildings became huge womblike generators in which the average human being could be immersed in the power and potential of divine union.[23]

The sacred rituals and works of art that were housed within the temples still held the potential to open the doorway to multiple layers of understanding, even in the average viewer. Through the vehicle of a ritual performance, a statue, a painting, the architectural grandeur of the temple, or a sacred monument, the spectators or participants could be mystically transported from their simple tangible world to a magical display of the celestial realms. In these treasured moments they could experience the beauty and wonder of their divine inheritance. Because of the overwhelming power of this spiritual experience, everyone who participated came away with the feeling that all human beings still possessed the innate capacity for divine insight and inspiration.[24]

According to Hindu beliefs it was at this time that the *Natya Shastra*, the fifth Veda, or sacred text on the science of dramatic art, was revealed. It was brought forth from the great compassion of the Creator for the new souls being born into the Dvapara Yuga, or Bronze Age. These new people's minds were believed to be clouded by the vicissitudes of earthly existence. In the myth the gods saw that most people were now bound by the seduction of the senses and were living under the relentless sway of earthly passions. Knowing that the inherent joy of humanity was constantly mixed with sorrow, the gods asked the Creator to provide a means by which all classes of humanity could contact their divine inheritance. The Creator then fashioned a pastime that would be called theater. He said:

> All the themes of mythology and heroic tradition will be combined. This Veda will lead to Rectitude and Justice (dharma), to Wealth and Plenty (artha). It will bring fame, it will impart learning, it will be adorned with a set of maxims, it will show the future world every possible act or deed, it will contain the meaning and bearing of all sacred knowledge, it will bring to life every facet of the arts and make them prosper.[25]

This was the age of the temple priestess. Young girls whose manner and bearing revealed an innate connection to the Divine were consecrated at the temples and initiated into the feminine mysteries. They were trained in the sixty-four sacred arts, which included religious rites, dance, theater, music, poetry, weaving, adornment, massage, herbal elixirs, the practices of healing and divination, and the secret mysteries of sexual union.[26] As priestesses they mastered ritual practices that enabled them to realize the Goddess within. Through this training their bodies were transformed into holy vessels through which the pure power and energy of the Goddess flowed. Each movement, expression, gesture, and posture was perceived as a blessed act of worship and consecration. Essentially, they became living symbols of divinity: goddesses in the flesh. In many cultures these priestesses were considered emissaries of divine energy and were encouraged to travel the luminous paths of spirit and bring back fresh images and insights from the more subtle energetic dimensions.[27]

Day after day in their exercises and meditations these priestesses explored and became intimate with the subtle interplay of spirit and matter. Sensitive to every nuance of emotion, passion, and vibration, they were masters at perceiving and influencing the powerful energies of the invisible landscape. Knowledge of this art was crucial to their significant roles as initiators, for it was their responsibility to ignite and channel the spiritual fire of the male inward and upward along the sacred path of enlightenment. In this exacting role they would initiate men into the deep and secret mysteries of the heart, awakening them to their true spiritual potential.

Even with the increasing densification of the material world, myth and legend tell us that until the end of the Bronze Age human beings still had the capacity to perceive and interact with the elemental realms. A popular example of a book that describes the shift that happened between the Bronze and Iron Ages is J. R. R. Tolkien's *Lord of the Rings* series. Filled with fairies, elves, orcs, and other magical beings who interact with humans on an equal basis, this popular series provides a glimpse of a time when the veil between the worlds was more transparent. But Tolkien leaves us with no illusions. He makes it clear that the magical world of hobbits, goblins, and magicians is coming to a close. At the end of the tale, all these fairytale creatures vanish into the mist, declaring that their time in the world has come to an end and it is now the time of man.

The Iron Age: The Age of Chaos

Everything that has any kind of existence, even error, has necessarily its reason for existence, and disorder itself must in the end find its place among the elements of universal order. Thus, whereas the modern world considered in itself is an anomaly and even a sort of monstrosity, it is no less true that, when viewed in relation to the whole historical cycle of which it is a part, it corresponds exactly to the conditions pertaining to a certain phase of that cycle, the phase which the Hindu tradition specifies as the final period of the Kali Yuga.

—RÉNÉ GUÉNON, REIGN OF QUANTITY
AND THE SIGNS OF THE TIMES

Beauty naturally belongs to heaven; on the earth it is only reflected; and when the connection with heaven is broken, when the back is turned towards heaven, then the eyes become focused on the earth and slowly and gradually beauty begins to disappear.

—HAZARAT INAYAT KHAN, SUFI MYSTICISM

As time passed and our focus on the material aspects of existence increased, the sacred rituals, with their sounds, movements, symbols, and images, although continuously developed and refined, were only fully comprehended by an elite group of individuals. These were the privileged individuals who were initiated into the mysteries and who helped bring some of their grace, wisdom, and moral inspiration to the masses. However, a hierarchy was slowly developing that was keeping these magical and vital secrets for itself.

As the forces of entropy and materialization took hold, the mystic ceremonies and stylized artistic representations gave way to the authority of a new medium: the written word. The beauty and spontaneity of spiritual expression, the vibratory power of the vocalized word, and the loftiness of the sacred image now began to be restricted.[28] Written language became the dominant vehicle through which our rites and rituals were preserved. But the written word did not transmit the richness of spiritual experience in the same manner as direct personal communication, verbal expression, sacred gesture, and artistic symbols. The book could never replace these more vital mediums. This new art form lacked that essential feeling of spontaneity, immediacy, and dynamism that are unique to the direct energetic experience. It also lacked the vibrant power of the sacred image to evoke within the reader multiple layers of intuitive connection.[29] While the written word helped us keep our memories intact through a graceless age, it provided only a map of reality. After the written word became the dominant medium for expression and transmission we began to mistake this map for reality itself.

Another issue that the increasing dominance of the written word calls forth is that education in this new artistic form was only offered to certain individuals who were, with the very rare exception, men.[30] This exclusive club of men now possessed a new art form that they could claim and control. Some men, such as the mystics and poets, who were still guided by the radiant light of spirit, used this new form of expression to inspire their readers to seek the sacred ideals of truth, virtue, and beauty. Their works were designed to communicate their visions of the artistry and brilliance of the heavenly kingdoms. Their writings, designed to immerse the reader or listener in the dynamic flow of narrative, were filled with nuance, allusion, metaphor, and parable. But with increasing frequency these mystic writings, and particularly any references to the Divine Feminine or women as spiritual guides and mentors, were discouraged and suppressed.

Civilization, a term that actually did not come into existence until the eighteenth century in Europe, once more "advanced." The pure light of spirit had been reduced to one-quarter of its original radiance, and in a devastating wave of fear and repression the Kali Yuga was born. As the light of spirit grew dimmer and the shadow of darkness stretched over the Earth, our minds became haunted by images of evil and depravity. Cities turned into nation-states, individual religions became a cause for separation and subjugation, and the world of politics and religion became indistinguishable. The manifold pathways to spirit were now hunted, seized, and patrolled by cadres of religious and political elite consisting of "pious" priests and "noble" aristocrats. Access to the realm of spirit was increasingly permitted only to men who would tow the party line. Unfortunately for women, not only did these men dominate the pathways to spirit, they also began to hold dominion over all aspects of human life. The events of this era of human civilization—starting from the middle of the Bronze Age, when our oral tradition was encoded in stone, an era dominated by the forces of the masculine—are being taught to us in modern schools and universities as "history." It is a fitting description of this time, for it truly is the time of male dominance—*his story* as opposed to the earlier ages of *miss story*, or mystery.

At this time a new relationship with the earth and the feminine was brought forward. From this moment on, we humans perilously lost touch with each other and the natural world. We increasingly abandoned our spiritual values for supposed security and material gain. Not only did we continue to lose touch with our spiritual essence, but we also lost touch with our own personal magic, our insight, our imagination and creativity. No longer was the earth seen as an expression of the spirit of the Divine Feminine opening and flowing up to embrace and unite with her divine consort, who was flowing down to plant his seed within her. Instead the earth was considered a wild forbidding place to be feared and conquered.

Men, who frequently looked to the outer world of form, became the vehicles through which this new perspective of reality was transmitted and enforced. The written word became one of the greatest tools of this dominant group. By controlling the art of writing and suppressing, dominating, or eliminating the sacred arts of dance, music, and performance they believed they could grasp the psychic-energetic landscape and manipulate the minds and emotions of the people. They knew that readers and listeners, whose minds were now fully focused on the linear visions provided by the priest or writer, could be drawn into the priest or writer's inner world; they could be influenced and directed. History could be altered, books could be written, and tales could be told to cut us off from the sacred knowledge of our own divine beginnings.[31]

Fear and the violence that stems from it became the devices by which we were enslaved. The priests and their hierarchy taught us that we were essentially evil creatures cut off from our maker, a wrathful and jealous God. As opposed to the great majority of gods before him, this formless, all-powerful being stood alone, without a consort. There was no goddess to bring him joy and ease his wrath, no female partner with whom he might experience the sacred bliss of sexual union. According to this new telling of our history, woman was regarded as the evil seductress whose curiosity and desire led humanity to fall from grace and perfection. Humanity as a whole was seen as totally divorced from divinity.[32]

With this new view of the feminine came a bias about our physical bodies. Our bodies were now considered imperfect vehicles, and our innate desire to experience the bliss and connection of sexual union was seen as a dark, animalistic, manipulative urge that should be subdued. The sex act itself was viewed merely as a necessary means of procreation, of bringing more people into the world to provide a greater workforce for the rulers.

Now came the time of the patriarchy, of male dominance, of viewing nature as a force to be mastered. It was a time of isolation, individuation, and egotism, in which both women and children were thought of as mere chattel. Rather than view the world around them from an interconnected, heart-centered perspective, men began to think of themselves as superior "evolving" individuals who must use the power of their intellect to conquer, scrutinize, exploit, and dissect. This was a time of intellectual dominance, of total separation of the heart and mind, of objectification, of ownership and slavery.

Along with this new view of Mother Nature came a different perspective on the principles of human relationship and interaction. Women were seen as sexual objects to be possessed, utilized, scrutinized, and subjugated. In the name of religion, the sacred mysteries and ancient knowledge that had been preserved throughout the ages were for the most part suppressed or appropriated and then distorted by the forces of the patriarchy. The realms of spirit, like the realms of social leadership (now known as government), knowledge of the forces and forms of the natural world (now known as science), and even the domain of health and healing were considered to be male property. Increasingly women were restricted from performing their time-honored roles. As a result women used the only avenue left open to them to gain some semblance of power: their bodies and sexuality. Women, who had been the teachers of the sacred art of sexual union, were now reduced to using their bodies in exchange for preferential treatment from the ruling warrior caste.

A more disturbing outgrowth of this change in consciousness and attitude toward women was the Inquisition that spread throughout Europe beginning in the thirteenth century. It was during this period that women began to be stripped of their last vestiges of self-esteem and power. One of the main reasons for this Inquisition and the destruction of paganism in Europe was to attack the secret women's mysteries. The priests and other leaders of the Inquisition, threatened by the innate wisdom and power of women, devised stories to produce fear of women and their time-honored mysteries. Women's sacred circles were disgracefully referred to as witches' covens, and their mysteries were said to be derived from the members of these covens consorting with the devil. Through the use of torture the men of the Inquisition would extract from their helpless victims whatever deranged nightmares their own warped imaginations could conjure.[33]

By the 1700s in Europe, industrialization and its factories, toxins, pollutants, and inhuman working conditions appeared. With the arrival of the industrial revolution the raping and pillaging of the planet was now in full swing. This was the complete manifestation of the Iron Age. We collectively entered our current age of the machine, of materialist science and intellect, of rationalism and externalization—an age that has been characterized by the destruction and devastation of the feminine and the earth that gave us life.

Some cultures still sustained a connection with the pure light of spirit. As the force of modernization took hold, however, their sacred art and religion were perceived by the increasingly dominant Western culture as superstition. In a vain attempt to right the wrongs of industrial society, Marx and Engels, the "fathers" of Communism, thought that by abolishing private ownership of property and promoting equal distribution of goods they could turn us back toward the same communal lifestyle that was once practiced by preindustrial people. Declaring religion to be the "opiate of the masses," they frowned upon its practice altogether. In the name of the collective, artistic expression, religious practice, and individual brilliance were suppressed. This made matters even worse. In Communism the state became the new father and god. Meanwhile in the West, science, materialism, and the quest for personal power became the guiding force.

Currently, powerful global corporations and their political and media puppets have become our new parents and priests. In this "advanced" society, our minds are increasingly controlled and manipulated by these forces. In the name of egalitarianism there has been a leveling of society toward the lowest common denominator. In our new "hive" mentality, people are regarded as mere objects, living in mass-produced houses and wearing mass-produced clothing, each one looking the same as the next. With the machine as our inspiration, we are turning into object-producing, mechanical beings who constantly repeat mundane tasks that give us little or no pleasure.[34]

Today most humans spend very little time communing with nature, their children, or each other. Hour after hour, day after day, women and men sit in their cubicles, giving their lifeblood to corporations in exchange for money that will buy worldly thrills and conveniences. Or they sit in front of television and computer screens, pacified, hypnotized, and programmed by other people's thoughts and images.

In our current Age of Iron, dominated by the forces of chaos and confusion, entranced by the flickering vibrations and images of our technological wonders, pumped full of pharmaceuticals and food additives to enhance our sensations or ease our pain, we have not only lost our fundamental virtue and integrity, but we have literally lost our minds.

According to the ancient teachings, by the end of the Kali Yuga the majority of humanity is divorced from the world of spirit and totally immersed in the concrete sensory and phenomenal experience. Yet the Tantras, or sacred texts of the Indo-Tibetan tradition that were created specifically to speak to those of us born in this dark age, say that even the intensity of this material focus can be employed in the pursuit of enlightenment. These teachings tell us that we have the ability to heal our confused and unstable way of life, to restore a sense of harmony and balance. Whether we are in the final phase of the dissolution or, as some teachings argue, merely at the beginning of the end, it makes no difference.[35] Regardless of our exact location in the great cycle of time, as luminous spiritual beings in material form, as Keepers of the Light, we must remain true to the divine principles of honesty and righteousness. Our task in this time of darkness and oppression is to journey to the depths of our beings and rediscover the essential light and power that has always been hidden there by the veils of corporeal existence.

The Time of Transition

Form is destructible, but Life is not; it knows
nothing of death. It destroys the mortal mercilessly,
and decomposes the destructible. But the
indestructible remains. Being immortal, it carries
within it the means of regeneration even as the
means of destruction.

—ISCHA SCHWALLER DE LUBICZ,
THE OPENING OF THE WAY

Cum luce salutem; with light, salvation. First source
of all sources . . . perfect my body . . . [so] that I
may participate again in the immortal beginning . . .
that I may be reborn in thought . . . and that the
Holy Spirit may breathe in me.

—FROM THE PARIS PAPYRUS

For those who are firmly attached to their earthly material existence, who can only see within the limits of their own lives, let alone their own cycles, this chaotic time does appear to be the literal end of the world. The signs of the end, as documented in sacred texts from the Revelations of the Bible to the *Corpus Hermeticum* and the Tantras, can be seen throughout the modern world. For the people who cannot see beyond the veil, we are in the metaphoric "winter of our discontent," the season of death and the deepest darkness. But as all these sacred teachings reveal, from the depths of darkness comes the greatest light. And so for others this is the heralded time of the great alchemical transmutation of humanity. It is the time in which the metaphorical black coal, or prima materia, of our being has the greatest possibility of being transmuted into the pure crystalline diamond. When this happens an extraordinary shift occurs, as we are filled once again with the pure light of divinity and become the spiritual seeds of a new Golden Age.

These sacred teachings of East and West have their parallel in those recently brought forward by medical anthropologist Dr. Alberto Villoldo, who has spent many years studying and transmitting the sacred teachings of the Incan shamans of Peru. These shamans have told him that humanity has reached what they refer to as the *pachacuti*, or period of renewal that occurs at the end of time. During this transitional time of upheaval when the world will be "turned right side up again," there will be a "tear in the fabric of time itself, a window into the future through which a new human species will emerge. They call this new species Homo luminous."[36]

According to the Brahma Kumaris, a spiritual group from the north of India that is steeped in the ancient ways of the feminine and the values of nurturing, communion, and grace, humanity has now moved beyond the Kali Yuga into a new transitional age, which they refer to as the Diamond Age or Age of Confluence. This is an age of consciousness that is not manifested in the physical, when those who have the eyes to see and ears to hear become aware of the great call to the light.

At the heart of all the mystic traditions lies the knowledge of this teaching of the call to the light.[37] It arises within us as a longing for truth and clarity; as an overwhelming desire to be free of our sorrow, pain, and suffering; as a deep hunger for beauty, simplicity, rest, and inner peace. Once our ears are opened to this call our eyes turn inward toward the divine light of spirit, the light of the Great Mother Goddess.

As we open ourselves to drink from her fountain of radiance that ceaselessly flows from the supreme primordial source of creation, it kindles our awareness and provides us with the energy to fight the darkness within. Our subtle consciousness awakens and the shadowy veils that have covered our minds begin to lift. Our senses expand to perceive the shining realms of the spirit, the subtle pathways of the psychic-energetic landscape, and the beauty of our essential luminosity. It is no wonder that in these transformative times interest in and knowledge of the Great Goddess is being rekindled throughout the world. For it is she, the divine Shakti/Shekhina as the great warrior of truth and integrity, as the nurturing mother and primal energy of divinity, who provides us with the strength and fortitude to battle our inner and outer demons.

We sit at the juncture of one of the most critical times of this planet. With each and every passing moment we have a conscious choice to continue on this path of destruction and alienation or have the courage to stand up and face our demons. The greatest spiritual traditions of our world teach that the best way to combat these demons, whether they be in material form or in the depths of one's own mind, is not through mimicking their dark methods but through love and compassion. Only when our actions spring from an honest and open heart can we begin to create a world free of the demons of fear, greed, and deception. Only when we have the courage to clearly see ourselves and freely admit how deeply we are entrenched in the darkness—how far we have allowed ourselves to fall from the pure light of truth and integrity—can we begin to dream a new world and give birth to a new shining age of spirit. For out of the ashes of the Kali Yuga the Golden Age is born. Out of the depths of darkness light is born.

PART

2

Awakening the Divine Feminine

6

Lifting the Veil from the Face of Modernity

If one wants to observe the rays of the sun, the clouds which obscure the face of the sun must be removed first. Then the sun will be visible and the qualities of its self-perfectedness will begin to manifest themselves just as they are.

—Chögyal Namkhai Norbu
The Cycle of Day and Night

If you desire the Light, be sure that you will never find it except by begetting it in your own darkness. Do not blaspheme by calling it incompatible with the darkness of matter; for matter would not exist if the Light were not already formed within it.

And this Light, so soon as awakened, will become your Master, full of power, your God dwelling in you, who transforms all efforts into joy, all storms into exaltation, all mysteries and doubts into Knowledge.

—Isha Schwaller de Lubicz, The Opening of the
Way: A Practical Guide to the Wisdom
Teachings of Ancient Egypt

ooking across the landscape of today's culture, one can easily see that the definition of what is feminine is mired in deep confusion. Hollywood and the media provide us with stereotypical seductresses and vixens; gun-toting, muscle-bound women who turn to violent answers; anorexic models who teach us that self-starvation is eminently attractive; hard-edged businesswomen married to their corporations; and women and girls portrayed as victims, prostitutes, and sociopaths. Then, of course, there is always the example of the woman who has totally subordinated herself to her husband, the image that so many of us rebelled against in the 1960s and 1970s. But is commanding military troops or leaving one's children to spend sixty hours a week fulfilling corporate expectations really what women were fighting for all those years?

Many years ago I was perplexed by issues such as these, and inspired by the teachers and teachings I had encountered I began to question the validity of this newly created feminine path. As a naïve young woman of the 1960s and member of the feminist movement, I had been filled with hope for a future in which women would be seen by men as equals and partners. Yet as time went by and my experience in the world grew, it appeared to me that something had gone very wrong in this quest for female equality—that the focus had been watered down from the optimal goal of genuine equality and mutual support and recognition between men and women to merely financial equality for women in the marketplace. It seemed to me that after years of effort women were valued or compensated only to the extent that we could learn to be like men, and that by taking on the male paradigm as our role model we were losing touch with the very essence, beauty, and power of who we were. As I watched women enter and rise in the corporate world, leaving their children at very young ages to be raised by strangers, women so caught up in the lust for power, fame, and fortune that they had no time to fulfill their time-honored and extremely essential roles, as I listened to children who spent more time watching television than interacting with their parents, it struck me that perhaps this new feminist approach was not what I had envisioned.

While some may argue that women presiding in male-dominated professions are bringing their uniquely feminine gifts to those roles, I have noticed that it is usually just the opposite. Because of imprinted male suspicions of the intrinsic fallibility of the female, in order to gain respect in these institutions women in such leadership positions are forced to abandon the receptive, nurturing, integrative aspects of their nature and become harsh and aggressive. In fact, these women most often discover that this newfound toughness and aggression is cheered on and admired by their male colleagues, while their natural feminine qualities are denigrated. Can you imagine what would have happened to Margaret Thatcher if she had dropped her tough masculine facade and revealed her true emotions in public? Would she have then been admiringly referred to as the "Iron Lady"?

Throughout the years of my mystic quest, as I learned to attune myself to the subtle realms of the Goddess, I became more and more cognizant of the high levels of stress, anxiety, suffering, and exhaustion that are the signature of our modern lifestyle. As I listened to my friends and students speak about their hopes, fears, illusions, and disillusions; as I watched young girls being led farther away from any sort of understanding of their true feminine nature; and as I witnessed how the luminous energy fields of those around me were constantly being depleted of life and vitality, it became clear to me that the prevailing vision of the woman being offered to us by the dream merchants of our contemporary Western society was extremely problematic. As I discussed these issues with others they would frequently agree with this analysis. "You clearly embody a grace, refinement, and femininity that is rare in our society," they would say. "Having studied the spiritual teachings of ancient civilizations for so long, would you speak to us about what you have learned? Can you tell us about where we can find adequate role models for girls and women or paths that lead us to our true spiritual heritage?"

At that point I began to offer my friends and students the fruit of the work I had done and the insights I had obtained into the true nature of the feminine experience. I spoke to them about the teachings, rituals, and practices of the rich and fulfilling path of the priestess, yogini, and wise woman. As I did so, my friends and students began to perceive the severe contrasts between this sacred path and the one we as women have been imprinted to follow by modern Western society. This chapter presents a look at the disparity between these two paths and the resulting impact of it on our lives.

Today as the pressures of our modern world lead us away from fundamental spiritual values such as truth, love, and receptivity into those of deception, fear, and domination, I believe that it is extremely important to look at the part that we, as women, play in this current unfolding of the human drama. With the recent destruction of the World Trade Center, with all the acts of terrorism that are taking place around the globe in which innocent women, men, and children are the unwitting victims of the dark forces of our times, it has become increasingly evident that we need to search for alternative solutions to jingoism, hatred, and war. Based on my years of research into and analysis of these issues, as well as numerous healing sessions and discussions with friends, students, and colleagues, I have written this chapter to provoke contemplation about who we were, who we are, and who we might become.

In ancient times there were sacred schools, temples, and traditions that held women and the feminine principle in high esteem. The most important reason for the existence of these schools was to assist women in understanding and aligning themselves with the spiritual nature of the world around them. Having been created by women and for women, the schools were based on a direct transmission of knowledge from generation to generation. An essential part of this knowledge, which we now refer to as women's mysteries, was learning to perceive and maintain the psychic-energetic-emotional landscape of society, the subtle realm of energy, emotion, vibration, and sensation that is recognized by healers and mystics as penetrating all reality and linking the spiritual planes with the material.

To fulfill this crucial function women underwent years of physical, artistic, and intellectual training, as well as intensive personal reflection. They mastered ritual practices that enabled them to purify their bodies and minds and transform into the Great Goddess, the most profound role model that shaped and preserved culture and society. As the earthly personification of the Goddess, they displayed her divine qualities for their students, communities, and devotees. In this way they provided an archetype for a more refined way of being human. These priestesses, temple dancers, yoginis, wise women, and visionaries would perform a crucial role in society by constantly elevating the human condition to one of grace and aligning it with the essential feminine qualities of courage, elegance, refinement, joy, and receptivity. As teachers, guides, healers, mediators, consorts, and initiators into the sacred mysteries of sexuality and spiritual transformation, they transmitted the spiritual light that sustained civilization.[1]

In these ancient societies, which were fully attuned to the ways of spirit, it was perceived that in the ultimate sense, beyond the laws of physical form and the dual nature of our reality, there is no essential distinction between women and men. From this metaphysical perspective, each human being was seen as an expression of the light and energy of the fundamental unity and one divine source of existence. According to this view, each human being ultimately contains both female and male aspects. At the same time great differences between female and male were recognized. In the ancient world the beauty and wonder of these differences was celebrated. The intrinsic powers and capacities unique to female or male embodiment were understood and channeled in ways most suitable to the health and welfare of the community. Through gender-specific rites of passage the fundamental energies of each community member would be aligned with her or his essential nature. Once this was achieved each could begin to experience and appreciate the energetic qualities of the other. In this way each being could have a direct personal experience of the ultimate union of goddess and god, female and male, that exists beyond all forms.[2]

These civilizations believed that there were at least as many manifestations of the Goddess as there are women on the planet, and even more existed in the subtle realms of light. All women were perceived to be emanations of the Great Goddess, and all men were emanations of the Great God.[3] Like the myriad rays that shoot forth from the light of the sun, the divine effulgence was believed to manifest as the wealth of forms that make up both the physical and subtle dimensions. Each woman, man, animal, plant, and mineral was regarded as a visible expression of that essential spiritual current, or Shakti, emerging from the primordial source of all creation. By their very nature men were believed to be focused primarily on the physical experience of existence. This innate attunement made them most adept at creating the external material landscape of our reality. Women, on the other hand, were perceived as having a natural affinity for the more subtle realms of energy, emotion, and vibration. Therefore they were instrumental in creating and maintaining the inner psychic landscape or equilibrium of the society. Here the word *psychic* is used not in the profane sense of the word that our modern-day "psychics" and purveyors of all things supernatural would have us believe, but as a derivative of its original Greek root *psyche*, meaning "soul." In fact, in the Kabbalistic and gnostic traditions the female principle in humanity was considered an expression of the soul itself.[4]

Since earthly manifestation was perceived to filter down from the divine source into the subtle realms of light and energy and then to the concrete world of matter and form, women held positions of great responsibility in these sacred societies. As they attuned themselves to these energetic realms, it was the women's task to maintain an atmosphere of emotional harmony and balance within the community. Over the centuries, teachings and practices were developed that trained young women to focus and enhance these abilities so that they could maintain the psychic-energetic-emotional equilibrium. In particular they were taught to perceive, understand, and work within the realms of emotion, sensation, and feeling. They learned how to call on and cultivate the feminine gift of second sense that we now call women's intuition. One of the main elements of this training was how to open and expand the senses to perceive and interpret the signs and symbols that are conveyed during every moment of life. These signs and symbols and their underlying meaning come from every nuance of human appearance, such as facial expression, gesture, movement, vocal tone, smell, skin color, and so forth. But the signs also come from the expressions of the world of nature, inner vision, and the land of dreams. Women spent much of their time learning these subtle languages and discussing their underlying meaning and importance to the community. The shapes of clouds, the stars at night, the passing of an eagle, the look of fear or wonder on a child's face—each was a sign to be interpreted. Each reflected something about the current situation in the life of a society. Therefore one's connection to the Dreamtime, or to the invisible voices of nature, became a large aspect of one's everyday reality.[5]

Even today in the fading beauty of the Australian Aboriginal society, it is the woman's responsibility to monitor psychic-energetic-emotional equilibrium. Aboriginal women, who still preserve their ancient rites, gather together to discuss the emotional milieu of the tribe and what action to take in the case of group disequilibrium. The women find a way to restore a sense of harmony within the group, whether through having sexual intercourse with a specific man to soothe a disturbance in his energy field, working with a child to teach him or her appropriate behavior, or mitigating disruptions that come from the larger world.[6]

In *Wise Women of the Dreamtime*, an excellent collection of myths about the initiations, ceremonies, and practices of women in Aboriginal society, author Johanna Lambert states:

> An important aspect of the initiation of a young Aboriginal girl is to develop the sensibilities and concentration that make her aware of the living and symbolic interrelatedness of the natural world. During her isolation, she is instructed to listen to the first note that any bird sings throughout the day, to which she must respond with a particular ringing sound. The birds are believed to be inhabited by the spirits of her deceased female ancestors, and in this way, a subliminal connection is maintained between generations.[7]

Evidence of this innate affinity of women with the subtle energetic realms can also be found in the work of Swiss anthropologist Jeremy Narby, who has focused much of his research on the shamans of the Amazonian rainforest. At a conference in London in 1996, he discussed how chosen women sit with the male shamans, or *ayahuasqueros*, as the men journey into the subtle realms under the influence of the powerful drug ayahuasca. Narby reports that these women, who have not taken the plant themselves, actually travel with the shamans into other dimensions and share in their experiences. At the conclusion of this powerful journey, when the men have returned to a normal state of consciousness, the women assist them in recalling what they have experienced.[8]

In the sacred rituals of the Hebrew tradition one can discover a clear acknowledgment of the importance of these innate feminine capacities to the community.

Every Friday evening at sunset it is the responsibility of the woman of the house to usher in the Shabbat, the holy day of devotion and rest. To begin the ceremony, the woman lights candles and calls on the spirit of the Matronit-Shekhina-Shabbat, the bride of God, to come and dwell within her home. As we have seen in chapter 5, the Kabbalistic teachings document that during the course of this holy night a man and his wife were required to perform the sacred act of sexual union, thus replicating in human form the mystic union of God and his Bride.[9]

According to the Kabbalistic sages it is the wife—naturally endowed with the quality of *binah*, or understanding—who has the innate capacity to sense the deeply spiritual nature of life. This capacity gives her the power to shape the spiritual foundation of the home from a place of profound vision; she is the one who "enlightens the eyes" of her husband and family, and who, as the "guardian of truth," brings joy, love, and honor to them.[10]

In fact, because of this capacity, over the past centuries orthodox Jewish women have taken up the task of maintaining the social and material foundation of the home so that the men would be free to spend their days in prayer. This is contrary to our current perception of the importance of the woman's role in the Hebrew tradition. Could this example be evidence of the fact that since women were naturally aligned with the values of love, devotion, and understanding they took on these worldly tasks so that their husbands could learn to attune themselves to the subtle ways of spirit?

In the tantric teaching of Tibet, women's natural receptivity and affinity for the inner realms of spirit and their extraordinary capacity to experience and express profound feelings are seen as fuel for enlightenment. As the embodiment of wisdom, women's innate receptivity and intuition make them ripe for the subtle teachings. As disciples on the path they are shown to possess strong spiritual resilience, overcoming great hardships to support and maintain their practice.[11] It is for this very reason that the great Tibetan sage Padmasambhava told his consort Yeshe Tsogyel:

> *Wonderful yogini, practitioner of the secret teachings!*
> *The basis for realizing enlightenment is a human body.*
> *Male or female—there is no great difference.*
> *But if she develops the mind bent on enlightenment, the*
>   *woman's body is better.*[12]

There is evidence in the early gnostic tradition of Christianity of this same idea. Mary Magdalene, whom the gnostics considered the foremost disciple of Christ, was known to have abilities that transcended those of Jesus's male disciples. The gnostics— who depicted the eternal principles of wisdom, truth, thought, grace, faith, silence, intelligence, foresight, and direct experiential knowledge (or gnosis) as aspects of the feminine—revered Mary Magdalene as the favorite disciple of Christ.[13] She was the one who realized his highest wisdom. In the gnostic Gospel of Mary she is depicted as being in intimate communion with the risen Christ. In this text she confesses that she is still in communication with her Lord through the means of her inner vision.[14] Her knowledge, wisdom, and insight were said to be far superior to that of the male disciples.

Even though remnants of these ancient women's mysteries can still be found in some of the surviving shamanic and initiatory societies that have survived in remote areas of the world, the images of our Western industrial society dominate today's growing world culture. Throughout the past centuries the minds of women and men have been increasingly indoctrinated toward a secular, consumer-oriented lifestyle that places its highest value on achievement and progress in the material domain. During this time the sacred rites of women—so essential to the maintenance of a truly spiritually oriented society—have been all but eliminated. Not only has this happened, but also our very capacity for working with the energetic realms has been toyed with and turned against us.

In today's materialistic society the sacred paths of the priestess, the wise woman, and the healer are all but forgotten. As the values and seductions of our media-dominated culture consume us, we women have increasingly turned away from our ancient feminine roles—with often alarming results. As many women attempt to redefine themselves by male standards, with no time-honored training or true role models to support their essential feminine spirit and moral values, and as they are separated from their children by their growing need for worldly power and prestige, they have become lost and confused. As a result all of humanity is suffering.

Stop and think about it for a moment. Do you remember any truly powerful female role models presented to you when you were a child? Do you remember any stories in which the dominant theme was what could be accomplished through the mutual support, companionship, insight, and imagination of women working together, uniting their energy and vitality? How many stories do you remember that explored the lives, values, and innate capacities of women? The stories we were told were almost exclusively focused on glorifying the achievements and attributes of the male. In these stories the female was almost always portrayed as being of lesser intellectual and physical capacity and clearly subservient to the male. She was given the role of assistant, the silent force who sacrificed her own dreams for his success. Of course, it is natural for the female to nurture, protect, and support the male, just as it is natural for the male to nurture, protect, and support the female. This is the proper balance and alignment of natural forces—female and male working together in harmony.

However, in today's unbalanced society women have been undervalued and treated as subordinate for so long that they have actually come to believe that their knowledge and abilities are of lesser value. Why is it that women tend to be suspicious, jealous, and judgmental of each other to a degree that they would never be toward men? How many women when meeting another woman for the first time automatically size up the other woman to see if she could be a threat to her job, social position, or relationship?

Over the years I have often heard horror stories about female executives being harsher on their female employees than on the males. It is as if these women, imprinted by the male paradigm, become its most loyal soldiers and henchmen. They dress in female versions of men's corporate attire and surround themselves with male trappings of power. Perceiving themselves as being watched for signs of "feminine weakness" by the men who surround them, they overcompensate by becoming more dominating and more demanding of their employees than any male executive.

What has this kind of thinking produced? A society in which women tend to underrate, discredit, and demean each other; a society in which children are left without nurturing and spiritual guidance; a society of self-centered women motivated by the need to prove themselves in a male world; a society of women who trade in the essential roles of mother, teacher, and spiritual guide for worldly power, fame, and fortune.

With the rise of the patriarchy and disappearance of women's rites women were left floundering in a man's world with no one to help them understand their true natures, capacities, and purposes in life. Separated from their ancient female heritage and living lives dominated by fear and repression, women no longer even knew that it was their task to create and maintain the psychic-energetic landscape in a positive, harmonious way. The result has been increasing disorder and chaos.

The Feminist Rebellion, Mind Control, and the Cult of Consumerism

If women's needs for identity, for self-esteem, for achievement and finally for expression of her unique human individuality are not recognized by herself or others in our culture, she is forced to seek identity and self-esteem in the only channels open to her; the pursuit of sexual fulfillment, motherhood, and the possession of material things. And chained to these

pursuits, she is stunted at a lower level of living,
blocked from the realization of her higher human
needs.

—BETTY FRIEDAN, *THE FEMININE MYSTIQUE*

Time and again women have attempted to recover their rightful place in society only to be disenfranchised and repressed in a new and more subversive manner. The feminist movement of the late 1960s and early 1970s and its repercussions are recent examples of this type of female insurgence. As documented in Betty Friedan's groundbreaking book *The Feminine Mystique*, women rebelled with great fervor against the limited subservient roles our mothers were induced to play in their shiny suburban homes. We rebelled against the delusion that we were weak, inferior beings whose only purposes in life were to breed, clean, shop, raise our children, and cater to every whim of our husbands. Asked to deny our intellect, insights, and intuition; to succumb to laws in whose creation we had no say, to remain chained to a double standard of morality and a belief that even an aggressive act of rape was somehow our fault, it was no wonder that we were frustrated and angry.

In the same manner that some kidnap victims adopt the views of their captors in order to survive and comprehend the experience, we began to take on the values and desires of men. Like Patty Hearst locked in a closet until she had "changed," we have been held hostage to an idea—to a way of life—that is essentially antithetical to our true feminine nature. Living in a secular world in which the sacred women's rites that connected us with the higher meaning of life had been lost for ages, we modern-day women jumped headlong into the political arena and began to fight like our male role models for whatever worldly rights we could acquire.

The feminist movement of the 1960s and 1970s came as a reaction to what we perceived as the virtual enslavement of our mothers in the home and the seemingly empty and unfulfilled nature of their lives. These were women, like my own mother, who prior to and during World War II had risen to new levels of education and experience. But with the conclusion of the war our fathers, traumatized by the horrors they had experienced, longed for the physical comforts and safety of an idealized home. The increased prosperity of the postwar era enabled them to strive toward this make-believe vision of the American dream that included the perfect job, wife, children, and home.[15]

Many of these men and women were children of immigrants who had come to America to follow the dream of a better life. They tried their best to shed their accents and cultural imprints so they could be accepted into this new, thoroughly progressive society. The psychological atmosphere created by the combination of living through the Great Depression, the tests of the Second World War, and the explosion of the atomic bomb made these people ripe for a different way of life. They dreamed of a life in which they could again feel pleasure and take their minds off of the terrible implications of what they had lived through. In the words of Betty Friedan:

> The American spirit fell into a strange sleep; the whole nation stopped growing up. Women went home again just as men shrugged off the bomb, forgot the concentration camps, condoned corruption, and fell into hopeless conformity. . . . It was easier to look for Freudian sexual roots in man's behavior, his ideas and his wars, than to look critically at his society and act constructively to right its wrongs. There was a kind of personal retreat, even on the part of the most farsighted, the most spirited; we lowered our eyes and contemplated our own navels.[16]

At this point our whole society was reoriented from what little had remained of spiritual values toward material ones. The culture of consumerism, of outward appearance, of a man's worth being measured by how much money he accumulated or a woman's worth being measured by her outer appearance, became the guiding force of our society. Earlier in the century the creation and maintenance of the psychic-energetic-emotional landscape that had been the domain of women had been appropriated and distorted by Freud and his fellow "scientists of the mind." Now a new model for modifying human behavior came to the forefront. Devised by B. F. Skinner, the theory of behaviorism maintained that the desires and actions of human beings could be conditioned, controlled, and altered. Like rats in the laboratory, the behavior patterns of women and men became the subjects of numerous psychological studies. The psychic-energetic-emotional landscape was now completely taken over by psychologists, ad executives, editors of the mass media, and motivational researchers selling us the virtues of this new version of the American dream.[17]

To maintain a strong economy, shopping had to become our number one pastime. With no female guides to lead us, to mold and shape us toward the rightful use of our innate energetic and visionary gifts, we became unsuspecting victims of this new and invasive method of mind control. Even the idea that we were responsible for the sustenance of the psychic-energetic-emotional domain had been lost in the well of history. Manipulation of the human psyche toward self-centered worldly goals, external distractions, and novel sensations became the driving force of our culture. The constant barrage of images displayed by the mass-media merchandising machine directed us all to believe that we could not be happy, healthy, or attractive without the use of their ever more indispensable products.

These purveyors of materialism were not at all concerned with looking at the essentially spiritual problem that confronted human society; this idea did not even enter into the equation. Everything had been turned upside down. The materialistic forces were now finding ways to help human beings "adjust" to the addictive demands of the culture they had created—a culture based on use and abuse, at its root directly opposite of the true spiritual nature of humanity.

Eventually, due to the intrusion of the media upon almost every aspect of our lives, we all fell under its persuasion. These new "overseers" of the invisible landscape worked on us until we were mere clay in their hands. Before long the manner in which we walked, the positions and postures we assumed both physically and psychologically, the tones in our voices, the expressions on our faces, and our secret inner thoughts and desires were all being shaped by the subtle masters of persuasion. These "psychic engineers" used every tactic they could to orient us toward the sensational and superficial. In this new world order, where money ruled and a flourishing economy led by a military-industrial complex became more crucial than the human values of love and compassion, it is no wonder that women, who were the traditional keepers of the light and the ways of spirit, were under constant attack.

A look at the work of a very clever man will prove my point. Edward L. Bernays, nephew of Sigmund Freud and author of the books *Propaganda* and *Crystallizing Public Opinion*, was one of the masterminds behind this devious and deceitful programming of our minds and emotions. Venerated as the Father of Public Relations, he took the theories his uncle had developed on the power of the psychic landscape and applied them to what he referred to as the "social science" of influencing public opinion and behavior. He once said that those who understand the mental processes and social patterns of the masses "pull the wires which control the public mind."[18] Learning his trade as part of the Committee on Public Information, one of Bernays's early assignments was to help sell World War I to the American public in order to help make the world "safe for democracy."[19]

Bernays then turned his attention toward an emerging market: American women. By creating the image of suffragettes parading down Fifth Avenue, puffing away on cigarettes, a symbol of male power, Bernays implanted in the minds of millions of American women an association between cigarette smoking and women's liberation. In this clandestine way he encouraged women toward the harmful path of nicotine addiction and lung cancer. Over the course of a career that spanned nearly eighty years, Bernays initiated such tactics as subliminal message reinforcement, the use of hidden agendas, the use of independent third-party endorsements, the setting up of "independent research institutes" to create scientific studies to support his clients' products, attaching the quotes from famous scientists to research that they had no knowledge of, and buying favorable news reporting with advertising dollars. These tactics were devised to create illusions and program and manipulate members of a democratic society who in Bernays's mind, as well as in those of his fellow enthusiasts, were incapable of knowing what was best for them.[20] In *Propaganda*, Bernays states:

> The conscious and intelligent manipulation of the organized habits and opinions of the masses is an important element in a democratic society. . . . Those who manipulate the unseen mechanism of society constitute an invisible government, which is the true ruling power of our country. We are governed, our minds molded, our tastes formed, our ideas suggested largely by men we have never heard of . . . In almost every act of our lives whether in the sphere of politics or business, in our social conduct or our ethical thinking, we are dominated by a relatively small number of persons who understand the mental processes and social patterns of the masses. It is they who pull the wires and control the public mind.

Raised in this exploitative psychic atmosphere, our minds fully oriented toward outer achievement, we young and modern women raced headlong into the fray. Having been raised by mothers who in many cases inadvertently imprinted us with their unfulfilled desires, we inherited the repressed fears, frustrations, unrealized dreams, and longings of women who had been convinced that obedience, passivity, and self-denial were the only appropriate feminine paths. And so we rebelled. On a physical level we shed our make-up, burned our bras, and raised our voices to cry out for what we perceived as equality. We demanded equal rights politically, economically, and socially. Railing against the traps of materialism, the enslavement of our mothers and our marriages, the virtual isolation of the single-family home, and the military-industrial complex that sent our brothers off to fight what we considered an insane war, some of us at the new radical left began to flirt with the tenets of Communism. After all, it was the only other social system of which we had been given any knowledge.

In seeking alternatives some of us left the cities to return to nature and make an attempt at communal living, only to be persuaded to return to the pleasures and conveniences of the growing consumer culture. Others longing for a deeper connection went in search of the ways of spirit, only to be diverted once again by the media onto the superficial path of spiritual materialism offered to us by New Age prophets and gurus. Others entered and fought their way to the top echelon of the male marketplace. Aping our male role models, we made outward gains. We became what we perceived as fully liberated women, who could take drugs, shed all inhibitions, and have sex for the immediate visceral thrill of it. We fought for and acquired rights to have an equal say in politics and the marketplace.

As strong independent women of the feminist movement, we worked hard to bring to the other women of the world a new level of awareness of our social dilemma and what we rightly perceived as the power of imprinting. We showed great courage and fortitude.

Today, however, thirty-five years later, the underlying problem is still facing us. Yes, we have occupied the conventional male-dominated institutions such as the corporate and political worlds, the military and police, sports, construction, and manual labor. We are better paid and have to deal with less overt sexual harassment. We can get loans and buy our own houses, and we can choose our sexual partners and methods of birth control. But has this really eased the confusion, pain, and frustration that lies at the heart of the women's rights movement? On an outer political and economic level we can rightly sing the praises of our achievements, but at what cost? What of our essential selves have we sacrificed?

Our Modern Cultural Malaise

Perhaps it is only a sick society, unwilling to face its own problems and unable to conceive of goals and purposes equal to the ability and knowledge of its members, that chooses to ignore the strength of women.

—BETTY FRIEDAN, *THE FEMININE MYSTIQUE*

The woman who accepts a way of life which she has not knowingly chosen, acting out a series of contingencies falsely presented as destiny, is truly irresponsible. To abdicate one's own moral understanding, to tolerate crimes against humanity, to leave everything to someone else, the father-ruler-king-computer, is the only irresponsibility. To deny that a mistake has been made when its results are chaos visible and tangible on all sides, that is irresponsibility. What oppression lays upon us is not responsibility but guilt.

—GERMAINE GREER, *THE FEMALE EUNICH*

In the days of the priestess, temple dancer, yogini, and adept, when women still maintained our sacred rites, we were attuned to every nuance of physical, emotional, and spiritual expression. With the enlightened Goddess as our role model, with the blessing and support of our male counterparts, we were trained to channel the natural gifts and tendencies of our beings in ways conducive to both our own spiritual growth and that of the larger society. Training in the art of dreaming gave us the ability to read portents of possible threats to community welfare. Learning to expand our senses to perceive and clear the luminous energy body that surrounds and informs the physical gave us the ability to foresee possible illness and dispel negative imprints or memories embedded in the chakras and surrounding energy field, as well as assist in death rites. Training in the art of temple dance gave us knowledge of yogic disciplines, such as muscular and breath control, visualization and concentration, and techniques for refining, transforming, and physically manifesting emotional states. Through this sacred art we were able to embody and transmit the myths, stories, and teachings that sustained our cultural and spiritual heritage. Education in the power of prayer gave us knowledge of how to focus our thoughts and intentions and attune ourselves to the vibratory realms in order to participate in the rites of healing. Since these rites and rituals were passed along orally and symbolically, it is not easy to find written evidence of them today. However, as documented in part one, there are still initiatory societies throughout the world that hold on to vestiges of these women's rites. Through my experiences in these societies, through my years of training in reading and interpreting symbolic expression, through my research into esoteric traditions, I have woven together a personal vision of what the feminine path may have consisted of. This vision, which is based on the model of the three manifestations of the Divine Feminine known throughout the literature as the Triple Goddess, I will now share with you.

In ancient civilizations around the world young women were trained to uncover and align their natural energetic tendencies with those of a specific goddess whose attributes most resembled their own.[21] Each girl, depending on her temperament, was given meditations, exercises, and practices to align herself with one of the three main manifestations of the Great Goddess: the wrathful goddesses of strength and power; the joyful goddesses of fertility, sensuality, and abundance; or the peaceful goddesses of love and compassion. Since every woman was believed to possess the potential to experience every aspect of womanhood, once this alignment was achieved, a female could deepen her knowledge and experience of femininity by learning to embody the other goddess archetypes. In this way young girls learned how to focus, develop, and utilize their innate energetic capacities for the benefit of the whole society. As they traveled through life's passages from children to adults and then to elderly women,

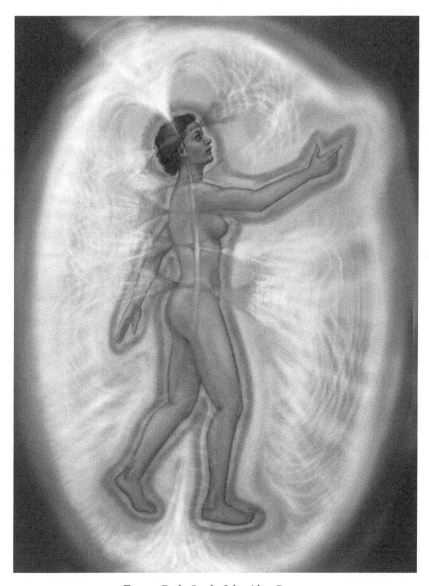

Energy Body Study 2 by Alex Grey.

they were able to fully understand and draw on the richness of their uniquely feminine experience. I believe we can still see these same three feminine archetypes in women's attitudes and behavior in our modern secular society. However, because we lack true spiritual mentors or even acceptable role models, these energies have been confused and distorted.

Just stop for a moment and take a look around. You will find thousands of women working out in gyms, lifting weights, straining their bodies, pushing themselves to be strong and hard. They take courses that teach them how to manipulate, succeed, achieve, and acquire power in a world created for and by men. These are the commanding women who in an earlier time would have been aligned with the divine qualities and energetics of the goddesses of strength and power. These women today push themselves to not just be like men but to be better than men, becoming harder and more cunning and manipulative to meet their goals. These women are constantly measuring themselves by male standards. One does not have to look far to see these highly motivated women struggling in unnatural and inappropriate ways in order to mold themselves into some bizarre image of who they should be and how they should appear—not only physically but also psychologically.

Reflect on it for a moment. How much of their essential feminine natures do these women have to deny to become heads of corporations? How many games do they have to play? How much intellectual and emotional manipulation do they have to practice in order to ascend to a position of power in this controlled and claustrophobic atmosphere? These are intelligent and insightful women who at their core are wounded and hurt and angry. Their once indispensable spiritual and psychological insights have been set adrift in the distorted reality construct of our modern age. Due to a lack of acknowledgment and nurturing of their innate feminine power these women are now attempting to survive and succeed by basically becoming men. With their innate capacity to tap into and guide the psychic-energetic-emotional landscape now twisted by the false prophets of our "advanced" society, these women have traded the perceptiveness of the enlightened feminine for the false security of a masculine corporate identity. Seduced by materialism and worldly authority, women's minds have been manipulated in such a way that they distrust their own innate insight, clarity, and wisdom. Contrary to our modern indoctrination of the "ideal" feminine form, these women of power come in all shapes and sizes. Their initial taste of the supreme energy or essence of Shakti's divine current would have been that of the sacred elixir of truth. As young priestesses, disciples, and initiates, they would have begun their training by becoming acquainted with and participating in the sacred rites of goddesses such as Durga, Kali, Sekhmet, or Simhamukha.

Today we also see women who have at some deep level given up, whose bodies reflect years of surrendering their essential knowledge to a society that still, after all these battles, undervalues them. These are gentle women with big hearts, naturally loving and desiring to be of service, whose overly receptive nervous systems are constantly overwhelmed by the noise pollution, air pollution, water pollution, and the general toxicity of our technological age. Falling for the insistent persuasions of the ever-so-subtle media backlash against the women's movement, fearful of going against the fold, or not wanting to be called a man-eater or an angry feminist bitch, many of these

The dakini Simhamukha.

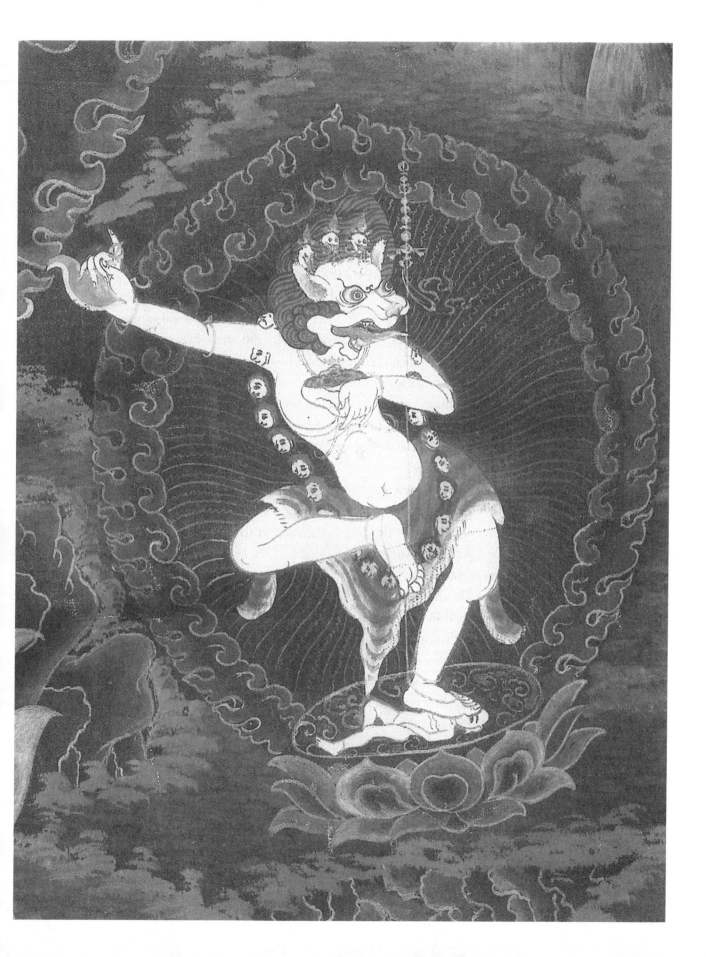

women hold on to the old model of woman as wife, mother, and servant. But like their mothers before them they become wounded from the years of emotional and psychological abuse and the lack of recognition of the bright receptive spirit inside. Since they have been conditioned to believe that they are and always will be sub-servient to men, these women think that they are too emotional and that as women their clarity is naturally obscured by these feelings.

How many times has your honest complaint or opinion been disregarded with "You can't take her seriously, she's just a woman; she probably has PMS"? or "She's just being a bitch"? All around us we see the victims of this type of subtle psycholog-ical abuse. Women's patterns of emotional and psychological rejection of their true feminine natures manifests inwardly as severe depression and low self-esteem and outwardly in weak or unassuming bodies. Heads and eyes lowered, shoulders slouched, pelvises curved under, their minds and bodies numbed by pharmaceuticals but often racked with arthritic pain or the pain of breast or cervical cancer, these women have totally surrendered themselves to the shadowy forces of our age. They are the kindhearted women who would have been aligned with the divine qualities and energetics of the goddesses of love and compassion. They too, like their power-ful sisters, come in all shapes and sizes. Their initial taste of the supreme energy or essence of the Divine Feminine current would have been that of the sacred elixir of love. As young priestesses, disciples, and initiates, they would have begun their train-ing by becoming acquainted with and participating in the sacred rites of goddesses such as Isis, Tara, and Kuan Yin.

In addition, there are women who are naturally endowed with the type of physi-cal beauty admired by the contemporary media and appear to have the world at their fingertips. Generally thin and possessing blond hair, perky breasts, and blue eyes, or else wild and exotic looking, men are drawn to these women like ants to a picnic. Often these women have a zest for life and a sexual magnetism that naturally draws the attention of men and jealousy of other women. They tend to marry attractive men who, often with their support, become wealthy and successful. The women have children. They live in a world of luxury, privilege, and power. They learn every trick offered to them by the media to maintain their imprinted version of sexual attrac-tiveness. And as long as they hold on to their physical beauty this world adores them.

But it is a fast-changing and dangerous world. Time goes by. The successful hus-bands, now middle-aged and prosperous, become bored with the everyday demands of a marriage and family. Lacking the support of a spiritual path to guide them and seduced by the culture of youth and vitality (demonstrated in the supple, wrinkle-free flesh pre-sented everywhere), these once-loving husbands begin to look elsewhere for amusement—no

Tara, by Kay Konrad.

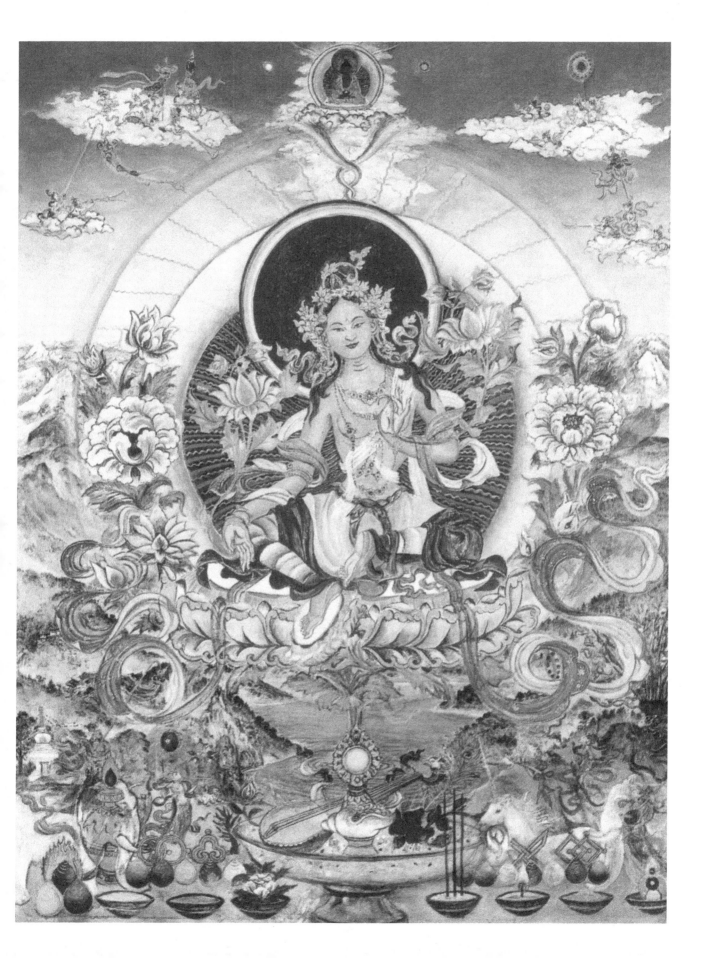

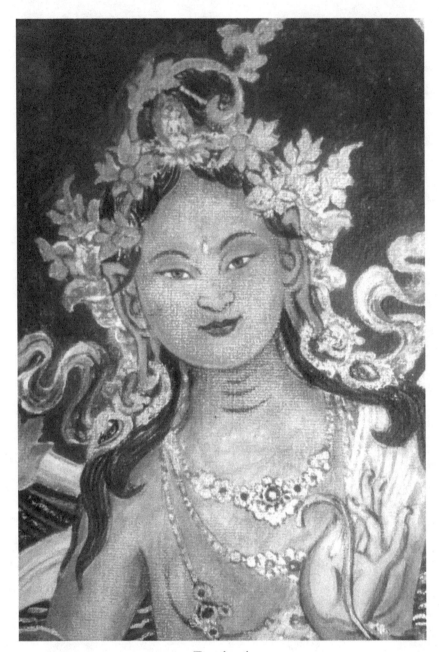

Tara detail

matter that their wives have run to plastic surgeons, attended diet clinics, and tried every new fad that promises a way to retain their youthful splendor. For these women time is a harsh mistress. And so they are left with the house and the kids and the money. In time they start to ache from the faulty breast implants, or their faces begin to take on a strange masklike appearance from the numerous surgeries. These are the captivating women, the natural performers who would have been aligned with the divine qualities and energetics of the goddesses of sensuality. They too, like their powerful and loving sisters, come in all shapes and sizes. Their initial taste of the supreme energy or essence of the Divine Feminine current would have been that of the sacred nectar of bliss. As young priestesses, disciples, and initiates they would have begun their training by becoming acquainted with and participating in the sacred rites of goddesses such as Inanna, Lakshmi, Hathor, and Mandarava.

This realm of sensuality leads us to another significant area of feminine expression that has been distorted and maligned: beauty. In the temples of old, rites of beauty and adornment were part and parcel of the woman's domain. Like the statues and images of the Goddess herself, priestesses wore ornaments, jewelry, and clothing that were designed to symbolize and attune them and their congregations to the spiritual riches of divinity. This focus on the art of adornment was carried over into the daily lives of today's women. Even in modern India one is constantly surrounded by women from every walk of life dressed in the graceful attire of the Goddess. In their positions as shopkeepers, accountants, servants, manual laborers, and so on, they still dress in flowing saris and adorn themselves with jewelry and flowers.

Furthermore, other cultures had views on the outward manifestation of beauty that were very different than those presented to us by our modern American media. For example, when I studied in India I discovered that the slim ballet body I had worked so hard to maintain was not in keeping with the fertile fullness of the classical Indian ideal. "You are just too thin; you look like a boy," my guruji would say. "Eat; enjoy yourself. You are a woman, an emanation of the Goddess. Look at her image, look at her sensuous body. This should be your ideal." At long last I could allow myself to relax a bit and let go of this physical stereotype that had for so long determined my neurotic eating habits.

In the early 1990s Naomi Wolf was disgusted by the media assault on our perception of feminine beauty and so she wrote *The Beauty Myth*. In this eloquent and insightful book she courageously takes on what she calls the "beauty establishment." In doing so she turns our attention toward a new wave of feminine conditioning, one that is even more insidious and insulting to our female sensibilities. In her estimation this new indoctrination arose as a reaction to the growing power and influence of women in Western society. She states, "We are in the midst of a violent backlash against feminism that uses images of female beauty as a political weapon against women's advancement."

Unable to cope with the growing power and independence of women, our masters of manipulation put their heads together and came up with even more devious methods to infiltrate our psyches and turn us into their willing pawns. Suddenly, our natural inclinations toward the art of adornment and rites of beauty were turned into a sick mockery of all that is truly feminine. In Wolf's words, "Somehow, somewhere, someone must have figured out that they [women] will buy more things if they are kept in the self-hating, ever-failing, hungry, and sexually insecure state of being aspiring 'beauties.'" In other words, to keep the economy flourishing, to divert them from their growing recognition of the problems inherent in our society, women and their daughters had to be imprinted with a whole series of new fixations and obsessions.[22]

Today each of us is constantly being assaulted by unhealthy, deprecating images of feminine beauty. Countless newspapers and magazines offer us horrific new pharmaceutical methods and surgical techniques to alter our appearances. Even with the constant revelations about the side effects and suffering that can come from these methods, women spend millions of dollars on diet pills, liposuction, tummy tucks, and breast implants in the hope that the alterations will make them appear more youthful and attractive—and therefore valuable. What kind of diseased culture endorses a cult of self-starvation, self-mutilation, and hysteria in its women?

This is only the tip of the iceberg for us females. Menopause, which was once considered a great rite of passage for women and a time during which we would fully come into our power and wisdom, is now treated as a disease to be resisted and alleviated by costly drugs. Of course, these drugs have side effects, but there is always another pill readily available to relieve the new symptoms. Increasingly, women are told that unless they take these pharmaceuticals they will shrivel up into old, undesirable, dried and wrinkled husks and will be shuttered in some hidden corner of society. Once this natural passage into the wisdom years was treated with reverence. Once our grandmothers were treated with respect. After all, they had a lifetime of experience on which to draw.

According to the research of Johanna Lambert, for the people of the sacred Aboriginal society menopause was considered to be an "initiation into a deeper, more compassionate knowledge. Menopause provided a time for [a] woman to regather, reevaluate, and retrieve the focus of her consciousness from her progeny in preparation for the solitary journey at the end of life. In Aboriginal culture, older women were spiritual authorities and were held in esteem, even by the men."[23] Today these elder women and men, who in a sacred society would have been our sages and teachers, are increasingly isolated from their extended families. What kind of culture is it that thrusts its elderly into "old age" and retirement homes to live out what's left of their lives in front of television sets, their bodies and minds numbed by pharmaceuticals?

After so many years of struggling for freedom, if we take a look around at our modern society, what do we see? We see not only our elders being ignored and pushed aside but also our young girls, our precious daughters, being inundated with the media's versions of femininity. Working hard to live up to this distorted image of feminine beauty, these girls starve themselves, becoming victims of anorexia or bulimia. Or we see teenage girls so lost in the haze of what the media expects of them that they become anxious and depressed. With increasing frequency, girls are given pharmaceuticals such as Prozac and Paxil as a means to alter and numb their troubled minds and emotions. I have seen instances in which girls who are emotionally distraught over the break up of a first love, death in the family, or parental divorce have been automatically prescribed such emotional pacifiers by their doctors so that they will not have to feel the pain of the experience. But since life is filled with both suffering and joy, how can they gain the knowledge of how to cope with these painful life situations if their emotions are masked by these behavior-altering drugs?

Think also of our boys—our sons, active and alive—who have trouble sitting still in the confines of a classroom and are placed on drugs such as Ritalin to turn them into passive, "good" little boys. From youth our children are being conditioned to believe that it is normal to spend one's entire life on medication and that taking a pill will solve every problem. What does this create? A generation of addicts. These are our children.[24]

These precious children, our offering to the future, no longer spend their days communing with us, each other, and the wonders of nature. Instead they sit in front of television sets, mesmerized by other people's versions of reality. Soap operas, "reality TV," and talk shows that pride themselves on parading a never-ending display of the most debased aspects of human behavior now form the moral barometer by which we live. If we continue on our present course the lives of our children will become living nightmares. All of nature for them will become merely a simulated vision that they experience through the technological wonders of virtual reality. Sitting in darkened rooms, their eyes and minds blinded to the miracle of natural life, isolated from the world around them, programmed by dark fantasies, will this be our legacy to our children?

Why is this happening? Why are we forgetting our children and decimating the planet? Because we are living in a society bereft of spiritual values, a society that is increasingly ruled by blatant and unbridled ignorance, lust, jealousy, pride, and most of all *greed*. Nowadays, it is the exceptional person who is honest, forthright and virtuous. It is more important to succeed, to rise to the top of the corporate ladder, no matter who you hurt or what the cost. We are trapped in a nightmare world of our own making. We are so trapped that we do not even know we are in a cage, let alone see its confines. Fighting in a man's world for political and economic equality, molded by forces that seek to blind us to all that is truly just and beautiful, we women have been distracted from the real problem underlying our modern society—a problem that is deeply spiritual.

Spiritual Materialism and the Birth of the New Age

> *The modern mentality itself, in everything that*
> *characterizes it specifically as such, is no more than the*
> *product of a vast collective suggestion which has operated*
> *continuously for several centuries and has determined the*
> *formation and progressive development of the anti-*
> *traditional spirit. The very idea of tradition has been*
> *destroyed to such an extent that those who aspire to*
> *recover it no longer know which way to turn and are only*
> *too ready to accept all the false ideas presented to them in*
> *its place and under its name.*
>
> —RÉNÉ GUÉNON, *REIGN OF QUANTITY AND*
> *THE SIGNS OF THE TIMES*

Some of us are beginning to awaken to the realization that the strides we have made and the goals we have achieved were merely Band-Aids designed to cover wounds that have become so deep and apparent that every living human being feels the pain. As we spiral headlong into the darkness of a technologically dominated world, in which one merely needs to press a button or release a biological weapon to murder millions of human beings, it is essential for us to stop and take a long, hard look at ourselves.

Thirty-five years ago many of us knew that something essential was missing from our lives and that the problem was of a spiritual nature. And so we went in search of spiritual solutions. Conditioned by a mechanistic society in which it was proclaimed that even God was dead (of course, we know that in the "scientifically advanced" Western world, his consort, the Goddess, was killed off centuries ago), we turned our backs on the churches and synagogues that had offered comfort and community to our parents and grandparents. Disillusioned by the ever-increasing materialistic focus of these congregations—in which the chief concern seemed to be how well you were dressed or how much money you could contribute to the new building fund—we went in search of new means for spiritual expression and communion. In a culture where the traditional initiation rituals for coming into adulthood and taking a place of responsibility within the community had all but disappeared, young men and women began to initiate themselves using the mind-altering substances that were readily available to them.[25]

With our senses heightened by the power of psychedelics, some of us began to have glimpses of the subtle highways and byways of a larger reality. In search of the means by which to obtain a deeper understanding of the experiences and insights we had while under the influence of these substances, those who were more scientifically minded began exploring the growing field of psychology, and others—led by the artists, musicians, poets, and dancers—began to look to the East for knowledge and sustenance. Some of us had the courage to leave the comforts of home and immerse ourselves in what remained of the traditional initiatory societies of India, Tibet, the Middle East, and the Americas.

We sat at the feet of gurus, went on mind-altering journeys with the shamans, danced and chanted with the Sufis. Embarrassed by our Western material indoctrination and wanting to reinvent ourselves as what we imagined to be more spiritually aligned human beings, we changed our names and modes of dress. Oriented from childhood toward the outer form rather than direct inner knowledge, we thought that by taking on the outer trappings of a culture we could grasp its inner light. We practiced yoga, the ancient path of union, not for its inner revelations but as a way to keep our material bodies flexible and attractive. We became enamored of Tantra, not in its fullness as a sacred path of inner alignment and transformation but as a method of bringing what we saw as exotic techniques and novel sensations to our sex lives. The few of us who found mentors and who were willing to humble ourselves and do whatever was necessary to purify ourselves, shed our imprints, and walk the timeless path of spirit did our best to keep our eyes and hearts focused on true liberation.

But the shadowy tentacles of our modern masters of manipulation were never far behind. A new movement emerged in America. Fed by early twentieth-century forays into mysticism—such as the Order of the Golden Dawn, Aleister Crowley, séances, scientology, trance channeling, and all things psychic—the movement became a mélange of techniques and practices that prided itself in mixing certain superficial elements and symbols of ancient traditions with a contemporary scientific and medical focus on discovering quick and painless solutions to both inner and outer problems. But this counterfeit New Age movement, with its essentially consumer-oriented, materially based mentality, diverted us even further from understanding our spiritual natures.[26]

Because we were conditioned from childhood to desire instant gratification, the quick fix that would take away all pain and disease, few of us had the inner discipline to walk the difficult path of true initiation and spiritual realization. We wanted instantaneous solutions to our problems. In order to gain courage we walked on fire. We gave money to teachers who taught us to chant mantras in front of strange altars while visualizing the quick attainment of all the material objects we desired. We fasted, consulted astrologers, baked ourselves in sweat lodges, and purchased crystals.

We came in throngs to empowerment workshops and seminars led by military-style teachers who wanted to raise our consciousness by belittling and humiliating us. We screamed and we hugged, experimented with orgies and celibacy, went to therapists and healers. Fueled by Western society's focus on ego gratification we, who were dubbed the Me Generation by the media, kept searching for the ultimate technique that would provide us with the easy yet somehow perfect solution to our problems.

Even today we see people running from guru to guru, longing for the moment when they will receive that special tap on the head that they believe will impart instant enlightenment and with no further work on their part will completely dissolve all their problems. Not wanting to take real responsibility for their own actions, these people are still searching for the elusive father figure who will direct them in every aspect of their lives. Raised in an atmosphere of insecurity, in which their innate perception is given no place of value, many people become almost frozen with fear of the consequences of their actions.

But this is only the beginning of our confusion. Having become oriented toward the external and disconnected from our spiritual inheritance, we were trained to believe that the development of psychic powers was a sign of spiritual development. And so we ran to psychics, channelers, and charismatic "magicians" who we believed could assist us in important decisions, give us insight into our all-consuming problems, and if we were lucky even teach us how to develop and utilize these longed-for powers.

What a travesty! The awakening and development of extrasensory abilities is an experience that often happens along the spiritual path. But from the perspective of true initiatory traditions, it is just a side effect of one's internal meditative practice. In fact, because of the ego's desire to grasp on to these experiences, they are often considered distractions and even obstacles on one's path of realization. Definitely, from the initiatory perspective, the appearance of such capacities is not to be looked upon in an egotistical, self-aggrandizing manner. Like snowflakes melting into the ocean of our awareness, they are looked upon merely as phenomenal experiences to be noticed and released.[27]

In traditional societies it was believed that everyone had the ability to tune in to the luminous energetic world of the Goddess. Understanding the nature and symbology of these realms of vision and dream was integral to the spiritual training that every member of the community underwent. Therefore when they had a vision or interaction with these realms there was a context in which they could place their experience or the message they had received. Those who had a high level of attunement were given more extensive training

Spiritual Energy System by Alex Grey.
This image clearly depicts the toroidal, or cocoonlike, structure of the luminous energy body.

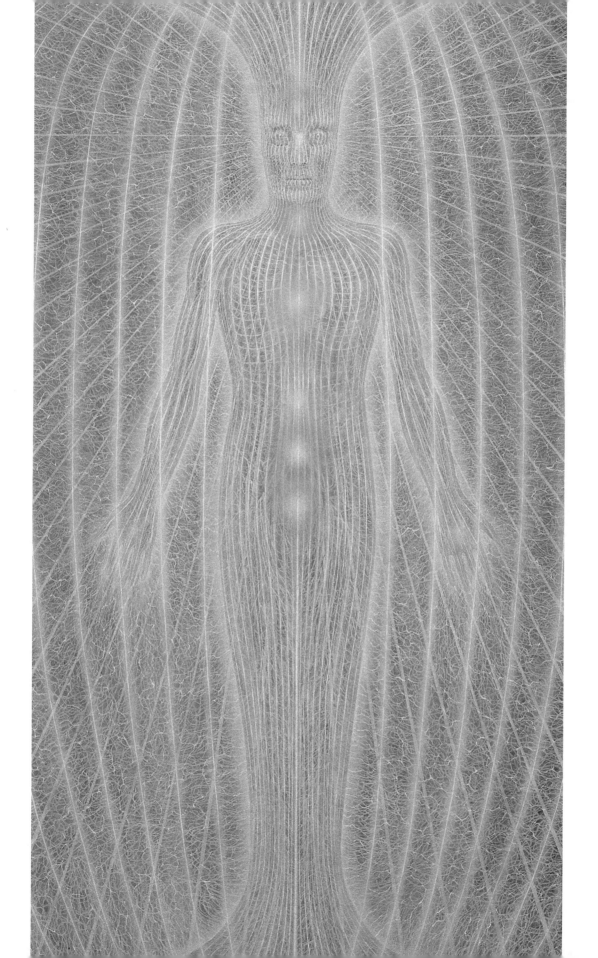

and became the visionaries, shamans, and seers of these communities. This training provided them with the tools to understand the experience or message and its relevance to their lives. In addition, they were taught a system of checks and balances by which they could perceive whether this message was coming from a genuine spiritual source.

Because of the female's natural affinity for these realms, in many societies the woman would take on this spiritual role. For example, the Delphic oracles of Greece, the sibyls of Rome, and other oracles throughout the ancient world were women who had been raised and educated to travel the visionary landscape and bring back insights for those who came to see them.[28] These women were linked to a tradition that helped them clearly perceive the nature of these visions and portents. This tradition remained alive and vital through an initiatic chain of transmission that was passed on through the generations from master to disciple.[29]

In our modern world we still find sensitive individuals who have a natural kinship with these subtle realms, but since they lack the connection with a spiritual tradition and true mentor they have no pure context in which to interpret what they see and no way to perceive the true nature of the source from which they arise. They have no way to know if this source is beneficent or maleficent. With the constant invasion of the psychic-energetic-emotional landscape taking place by forces that increasingly turn us away from honesty, love, and integrity, how are we to discern the false from the true?

In the spiritual supermarket of our modern society much too often we encounter women and men with physical, mental, and emotional wounds engendered through the work of self-styled energy healers, psychics, and channelers of dead or alien beings who have never traveled the traditional path of initiation and apprenticeship.[30] Over the years we have been a great source of profit for many charlatans and false prophets that have increasingly dominated the invisible landscape of our technological age. We have been the unwitting pawns of these masters of collective suggestion whose sole task has been to lead us away from all that is truly spiritual.

This is the nature of our modern age, an age in which our minds have been covered in dark veils of confusion. In order to survive in this age of darkness, during which the rape and destruction of all that is sacred has been the guiding force, we women and men have had to hide the brilliant light of our true essences behind layers of physical, emotional, and intellectual armor. In this appalling age we have relinquished our real power—our vitality and fundamental feelings of beauty, joy, and spontaneity. Because of the increasing levels of deception and discord that have become almost commonplace in the world around us we are out of balance, out of tune. Living lives filled with falsity, our bodies, minds, and spirits have been disturbed and distorted. The psychic-energetic-emotional landscape, once completely attuned to spirit, has been consciously invaded and manipulated for corrupt purposes. Can you even begin to imagine what it would be like to live a life of absolute integrity, totally attuned to the flawless divinity within?

Reclaiming Our Sacred Heritage

The brilliance and clarity of sunlight cannot be dimmed by aeons of darkness; likewise, the radiance of the mind's essential nature cannot be obscured by aeons of delusion.

The empty house that has stood in darkness for millennia is illuminated instantly by a single lamp; likewise, an instant's realization of the mind's clear light eradicates negative propensities and mental obscurations inculcated over countless aeons.

—FROM "THE FLIGHT OF THE GARUDA,"
AN ANCIENT SONG OF DZOGCHEN

If you bring forth what is within you, what you bring forth will save you. If you do not bring forth what is within you, what you do not bring forth will destroy you.

—JESUS, SPEAKING TO HIS DISCIPLES IN
THE GNOSTIC GOSPEL OF THOMAS

We have the ability to heal our confused and unstable way of life, to restore a sense of harmony and balance to ourselves and the world around us. Our task as women in this modern age, in this time of darkness and oppression, is to journey to the depths of our beings and rediscover the essential light and power that has always been there, hidden by the dark veils of confusion and manipulation. We must have the courage to honestly observe ourselves, release our imprints, and discover who we really are.

As women born into this transformative age we must join together to become leaders in the reshaping of our world. Traditional teachers, shamans, and mystics the world over have told me that we actually dream our world; that whatever appears on this earth happens first in what the Australian Aborigines refer to as the Dreamtime, an ever-shifting realm of connections and possibilities. The Dreamtime is created and sustained by the mind. The Tibetan Buddhists and Bon shamans say that manifestation first comes through an imagining in the mind. To them the mind is like a doorway; it receives and projects images. It is a portal to the primordial source—the source of inspiration, creative imagination, and the magical display of divine light and energy that is continuously weaving itself into the forms, feelings, and circumstances of our lives. Its essential nature is pure and untarnished by any experience the ego or personality may have.[31] In his song of introduction to the nature of mind titled "The Flight of the Garuda," Ahakkar Lama Jatang Tsokdruk Rangdrol, a Tibetan tantric yogi of the nineteenth century, relates, "All relative visual and auditory experience is only the natural and spontaneous manifestation of mind itself. . . . The mind is like an artist. The body is created by the mind, as are all the many worlds existing in the three dimensions of microcosmic world systems; all of them are also drawn by the mind."

Once upon a time one of the essential roles of women was maintaining the natural equilibrium of the psychic-energetic-emotional landscape emerging from these projections as the "magical display of mind." Through our sacred rites we learned how to attune ourselves to the radiant light and energy of the spiritual domains and transmit this light to all beings. It is time to reattune ourselves with this inner landscape We have the ability to heal our confused and unstable way of life, to restore a sense of harmony and balance to ourselves and the world around us. Our task as women in this modern age, in this time of darkness and oppression, is to journey to the depths of our beings and rediscover the essential light and power that has always been there, hidden by the dark veils of confusion and manipulation. We must have the courage to honestly observe ourselves, release our imprints, and discover who we really are.

Following this call is the beginning of the destruction of imprints and the beginning of the path to awakening. We must create new standards of feminine expression, seeking as our role models those that offer us the purest and most virtuous goals. As a start we can look back to the wealth of myths, stories, and legends of the Divine Feminine that have survived throughout this dark night of the soul, using them for guidance and inspiration.

Like Mandarava, the princess of India who through her passionate devotion to the dharma realized the luminous rainbow body and became an immortal dakini, no matter what obstacles appear before us we must keep our eyes focused on the pristine path of enlightenment.

Like Inanna, the goddess of ancient Sumer and the queen of Heaven and Earth, on her transformative journey to the underworld, we must not be afraid to relinquish our precious ornaments and implements of worldly power in order to receive the inner treasures of spiritual initiation and rebirth.

Like Kali, the Hindu goddess and Great Mother of time, we must become warriors of truth and integrity, dancing the fearless dance of death that leads to spiritual metamorphosis and transformation.

Like the Blessed Virgin Mary, we must steadfastly hold love and compassion in our hearts, working ceaselessly to liberate all beings from their pain and suffering.

Like Isis, the Egyptian goddess of wisdom and healing, on her long search for the pieces of her dismembered husband, Osiris, we must begin to remember who we really are.

It is time to start a revolution and envision a new society—a sacred society that arises from a real desire for spiritual transformation and the deep stirrings of love and compassion in our hearts. This society would consist of sisters and brothers, sisters and sisters, and brothers and brothers working side by side in grace and harmony.

We have the potential to reshape our reality and change our world. If our reality is manifested in the Dreamtime first, in this fertile womb of vision and imagination that is our natural domain, then perhaps our revolution should begin there. If thought precedes the manifestation of reality then the starting point for the building of a more perfect world is through the creation of a psychic-energetic-emotional landscape that is imprinted with the best intentions.

Womankind, rise up and take hold of your true feminine power! Dare to lift the veils that have obscured your mind and begin to see from deep within your heart. Have the courage to swim against the rising tide of darkness that constantly threatens to overcome you. Do not be afraid to risk all. Do not be afraid to live in truth. Look into the eyes of your children, into the eyes of your mates, parents, sisters, and brothers. See the shining light of spirit trapped within them, imprisoned by the vicissitudes of this Dark Age. Understand that your loved ones are just as confused and afraid as you are. They are waiting for their mothers, teachers, healers, and wise women to wake up from their long, painful sleep and once again guide them toward true liberation.

As we move from this age of male domination and power and of materialism and technology into a new era that promises equality, balance, partnership, and union, it is essential that we women begin to actualize our true wisdom and potential. We must realize the profound significance of our role in this new unfolding of humanity. As intelligent conscientious women who care deeply about the state of the world around us, we must begin to perceive, acknowledge, and take responsibility for our individual and collective roles in creating and shaping the psychic-energetic landscape.

The first step in this process is to learn how to open oneself to the subtle world of light and energy that are the natural domain of the Goddess. The following three chapters will assist you in gaining new levels of knowledge and insight into these mysterious and multifaceted aspects of female embodiment. Based on the main qualities of the Triple Goddess as demonstrated in the myths of numerous ancient cultures, these chapters are designed to lead you into a personal experience of the natural characteristics and manifestations of feminine energy, from the vibrancy and dynamism of strength and power, to the fluidity and bliss of sensuality, to the subtlety and refinement of love and compassion.

Each chapter begins with descriptions of the mythic goddesses themselves, a look into their essential dynamics and symbolic significance, and the myth or story of one of the goddesses of each realm. The myth or story has been included to provide deeper insight into the fundamental nature of the goddesses of this specific realm, whether it be strength and power, sensuality, or love and compassion.

Understanding from an intellectual viewpoint what it means to be a woman is only the beginning of the journey. To walk the path of the priestess, yogini, wise woman, and soror mystica, and the transformative paths of Tantra and alchemy, it is necessary to purify both body and mindstream. Therefore the following chapters are also filled with meditations and visualizations based on my years of research, experience, and teaching in these transformational arts. These exercises are designed to introduce you to the inner landscape of your luminous energy field, help you to become aware of the true nature of your mind and emotions, and teach you how to harness their power and intensity on the sacred path of illumination and integration. As you perform them you will learn how to awaken, channel, and regulate the healing and transformative current of divine light and energy through your chakras, clear away toxic mental and emotional patterns, and fill your luminous energy field with new strength and vitality. You will also learn how to open yourself to the subtle world of feeling and expression that is such an integral part of the feminine experience. As you perform the exercises a subtle reorientation of your luminous energy field will begin to take place, leading you from your habitual imprinted modes of expression to those more in keeping with the enlightened energetic display of the Goddess.

The primary goal of all of these exercises is to offer you the opportunity for insight into the Divine Feminine, an experience that will enable you to do more than just see the Goddess in the inner dimensions of your mind or visualize her standing before you. You will be able to directly experience the extraordinary power of her pure shining presence deep within your own heart. Through this process you will begin to reattune yourself to the radiant light of her divine current and, like the priestesses, yoginis, and wise women of old, once again weave the psychic-energetic-emotional landscape of our world in a truthful and loving manner.

7

Discovering Strength and Power

It of course makes eminent sense that the earliest depiction of divine power in human form should have been female rather than male. When our ancestors began to ask the eternal questions (Where do we come from before we are born? Where do we go after we die?), they must have noted that life emerges from the body of a woman. It would have been natural for them to image the universe as an all-giving Mother from whose womb all life emerges and to which, like the cycles of vegetation, it returns after death to be again reborn.

—RIANE EISLER, *THE CHALICE AND THE BLADE*

What is true feminine power? From where does it arise and how does it manifest? If one contemplates nature in all of her primal power and magnificence, observing her ebb and flow, her cycles of creation, her materialization and dissolution, one may obtain a glimpse of the many facets and expressions of this rich and compelling energetic force. As daughters of the Great Goddess, women possess the essence of nature in all of her beauty, majesty, and horror. We, like the Goddess, are innately wild and passionate, fluid and graceful, strong and resilient. We can be direct and incisive in response to unwarranted provocation, uninhibited and ardent in our lovemaking, and sensitive to our loved ones in times of hardship. As the mothers and caretakers of humanity we possess the intrinsic ability to persevere and guide others through times of sadness, pain, and loss.

The exercises and meditations presented in this chapter are designed to assist you in the process of alignment and embodiment with the powerful Goddess that resides in you. Fashioned in the same experientially based mode of teaching that was utilized in the temples and tantric and gnostic circles, the exercises have been created to provide an immediate perception of this vital, commanding, and resilient mode of being. But before we enter into the richness of this experience let us take a look at the innate qualities and attributes of our divine ancestors and role models, the goddesses of strength and power.

The Goddesses
of Strength and Power

In the sacred texts, paintings, and sculptures of India, Egypt, and Tibet, these powerful female deities—such as Kali, Sekhmet, Simhamukha, and Durga—are known as the strong, fiery, and wrathful goddesses. (They are not wrathful in the sense of anger, but in the sense of movement, energy, and action.) Possessing the fierce and fiery forces of Mother Nature herself, these goddesses are role models of right and appropriate action, who function from a centered and integrated space of wisdom and clarity. Dancing amid flames of wisdom and power, the postures, gestures, and expressions of the goddesses symbolize the playful and passionate outpouring of the enlightened energy of emotion. Holding in their hands sacred implements that assist them in accomplishing their actions, the images of these powerful goddesses inspire us to recognize that true feminine power lies not in anger and destruction but in knowledge, understanding, and transformation.

Kali, the Great Mother of time and the symbol of all the wild and chaotic forces of nature, is the goddess in whom all things are created, preserved, and destroyed. Known as the Black One, Kali symbolizes the essence of darkness, the void, and prima materia from which all of creation arises and into which it dissolves, only to be renewed and reborn. In many of the Hindu Tantras and iconography Kali is the dominant figure, exalted as the most potent of all deities, the essence of the great goddess Mahadevi, and the union of being, consciousness, and bliss.[1] In the *Mahanirvana Tantra* Kali is aptly described as the destroyer of time who dances her transformative dance of dissolution and recreation at the end of the yugic cycle.

Sword in hand, Kali dances naked on the cremation ground, clothed with only her long black hair and garland of skulls. To the uninitiated Kali is the embodiment of terror. Yet when we delve into the meaning of her outward symbolic display, we understand Kali's essential role in the cosmic order. For at her heart she is Ma Kali, the primal current, or Shakti, the mythic embodiment of the great and powerful Universal Mother. As we learn to invoke, embrace, and embody Kali's divine qualities, her potent fiery force provides us with the strength to call up and work with the fundamental energy of fear. In this way she assists us in liberating ourselves from the darkness of our negative thoughts and actions so that we can perceive the beauty of our essential luminous nature.

O Warrior Goddess with streaming
    black hair,
One swing from your sword of wisdom
Will cut every egocentric root
And clarify the heart forever.
I will tame the primal obsessions,

Greed, anger, pride, hatred,
And use them as powerful bullocks
To plow the field of consciousness.
Sowing the seed of Om Kali Ma,
Transmitted to me by a skillful farmer,
I will reap a vast harvest of illumination
    for all living beings.
—RAMPRASAD SEN
(LEX HIXON, TRANSLATOR)

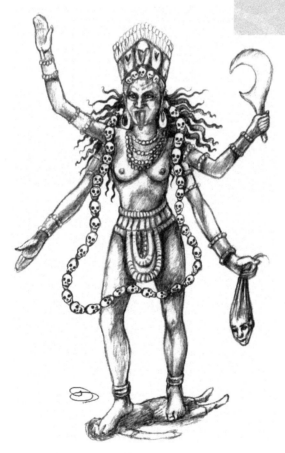

Kali, the great wrathful goddess who with her shining sword destroys egotism and ignorance. Illustration by DARLENE.

Glory and All Praises be Unto Sekhmet,
who burns hot, like the noontime sun
Upon the desert sand
And whose roar echoes
In the caverns of tawny rock.
Mighty Lion-headed One,
Queen of Heaven,
Protectress of truth,
Avenger of Evil,
Guardian of the Kingdom,
Hail to Thee, Unconquered One,
Huntress of Fate who
Commands retribution.
Grant me your courage,
Your strength and fortitude
and Your protection,
so that I, too, may do battle
against the armies of Darkness,
Defending the cause of Righteousness.
AMEN

— "Sekhmet Incantation" by
darlene, Priestess of Sekhmet,
Fifth Way Mystery School

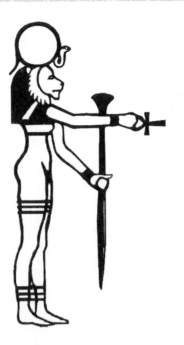

Sekhmet is the wild and passionate lion-headed goddess of Egypt. She symbolizes the blazing, transformative eye of the sun god Ra, the personification of the darkness of chaos from which new light and life emerges. In keeping with the essential role of all of these powerful goddesses, Sekhmet is the protector of the divine order, and as such she protects the gods against evil forces.[2] Stalking the land as the proud lioness, Sekhmet is swift to defend her loved ones. She may strike back with wild and reckless abandon, as she did in the myth of the destruction of humanity, when she was sent out by Ra, the aging sun god, to suppress a rebellion by his subjects. In her frenzy Sekhmet became so intoxicated by the blood of her enemies that she had to be pacified in order to quell her rage.[3] Her attacks, however, only arise when warranted by the malevolence of the situation, and she never strikes out unless exceedingly provoked. Even though the energy of destruction may carry Sekhmet away, she always seeks to restore the sacred principles of righteousness, love, and honor to the world. As we bring the divine energy of Sekhmet into our lives, we begin to acquire the clear perception that leads to the enlightened wisdom of right and appropriate action.

In the ancient Egyptian and alchemical traditions the goddess Sekhmet, like the tantric goddess Kali, is associated with a time of planetary disruption and transformation. If we look beyond the surface we discover that in all the ancient traditions, myths were more than simple morality tales; they were multilayered teachings about the nature of reality, the cosmos, human and divine relationships, and more. The myth of the wrath of

Sekhmet can be seen as a metaphor for the great purification that comes at the end of time. In the myth Sekhmet is the physical embodiment of the blazing eye of Ra and the harbinger of a great catastrophe that occurred thirteen thousand years ago in the former age of Leo, when there was a galactic core explosion that brought about the last ice age.[4] Note that three of these powerful goddesses, like Sekhmet, are lion-headed, or in the case of Durga, riding astride a lion. This symbolically associates them with not only the power and potency of the lioness but also with the destructive age of Leo.

Simhamukha is the Tibetan tantric lion-headed dakini, or sky-dancing goddess, of clear, direct, and active compassion. She is the remover of obstacles who subdues evil spirits and destroys negative thought and delusions of the mind. In the Tibetan tantric tradition, Simhamukha is known as the queen of the dakinis and the goddess of gnosis, and her practice leads to a direct experience of enlightenment.

According to the *Excellent Vase of Precious Jewels*, Simhamukha's principle function as a meditation deity is averting psychic attacks and negative energy and sending them back to their source. One of Simhamukha's primary functions is to protect practitioners against curses and maledictions, and her form and mantra actually repel negative energy and return it to its source. But her rites also include practices for long life, wealth, healing, and magnetizing. In his introduction to the *Excellent Vase of Precious Jewels* translator John Myrdhin Reynolds writes:

> O Jnana Dakini Simhamukha
> You are hereby charged with these
>   actions:
> Pacify all obstacles and adverse
>   conditions
> Afflicting us, both master and disciples.
> And increase our enjoyments,
>   abundance, long life, and
>   harmonious conditions.
> Protect the Doctrine of the Buddha.
> And in order to establish all beings in
>   happiness,
> May you accomplish the realization of
>   all benefits!
> —PADMA GARGYI WANGCHUNG (JOHN
>   MYRDHIN REYNOLDS, TRANSLATOR)

> Even though the Dakini Simhamukha is a wrathful manifestation, she is an expression of enlightened awareness and the compassion of the Buddha. She manifests in her wrathful form only in order to subdue hostile entities, principally evil spirits and demons that oppose the Dharma and attempt to block and impede the course of spiritual evolution. She is like a mother who truly loves her only child,

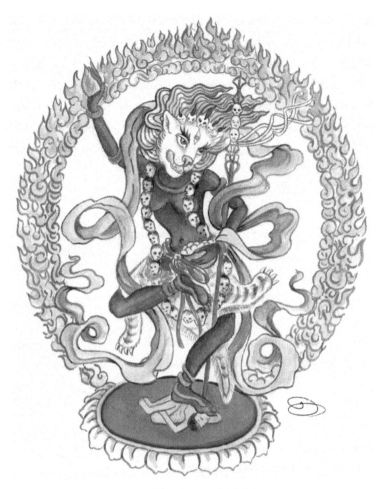

Simhamukha, the wrathful dakini.
Illustration by DARLENE.

but must scold and discipline him because he has done something heedless and dangerous to his own safety and well-being.

Transformation into this powerful queen of the dakinis assists us in removing the inner and outer demons or obstacles we encounter on the spiritual path—such as negative emotions or actual physical or mental disturbances.

Durga, from the Hindu tantric tradition, is the radiant goddess of power and beauty, killer of the horrific buffalo demon, and the destroyer of greed, egotism, and ignorance. Durga is the divine savior, created by the united Shakti, or luminous energy of the gods, who call upon Durga to resolve a cosmic crisis and free humanity and themselves from the dark forces they have helped to engender. Through her power as the feminine principle, the keeper and defender of the light, Durga must arise to rid mankind and the powerful male gods of the evil forces that threaten to overtake the world. As we bring her potent Shakti energy into our lives we are filled with the renewed strength and vitality to stand up and face any situation that may arise before us. Durga's myth is presented here to provide insight into a direct manifestation of the divine Shakti energy from the tantric perspective. In addition, it serves to demonstrate the extraordinary power, majesty, and righteousness of the fiery goddesses of strength and power. It is a story that is very dear to my heart, since it forms the narrative structure on which the dance of Durga, which I first learned from my guruji, Sitara, many years ago is based.

> O Queen of the universe, you protect the universe. As the self of the universe, you support the universe. You are the goddess worthy to be adored by the Lord of the universe. Those who bow in devotion to you themselves become the refuge of the universe.
>
> —FROM THE *DEVI MAHATMYAM*

The Myth of Durga: The Radiant Goddess of Power and Beauty

Adapted from the Hindu twelfth-century text the *Devi Mahatmyam* (Glory of the Divine mother)[5]

Once upon a time, in the first great cycle of existence, there was a terrible war between the gods and the demons. This war raged continuously for hundreds of years. Led by the powerful Mahisha, the demons defeated the gods, expelling them from heaven and forcing them to wander on the earth like mortals.

Mahisha had spent centuries performing ritual practices and austerities. Year after year he stood on one leg in the snow, clad merely in a loincloth, with the raging winter winds chilling him to the bone. Then he sat for an eternity in a meditation box, never moving, never sleeping. He tied ropes around his arms and legs to keep him upright and placed twigs in the corners of his eyes to keep them ever open, never moving except to turn the pages of his precious text. Ever before him was his overwhelming desire to gain enough power to become king of the demons.

The great gods who watch over the earth, seeing Mahisha's one-pointed devotion and determination, rewarded him with extraordinary gifts of strength and power and granted his request that he could not be killed by man or god. But as soon as Mahisha received these powers, rather than use them wisely and compassionately for the benefit

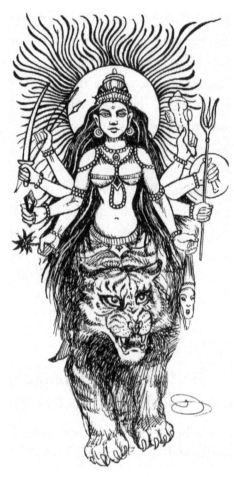

The warrior goddess Durga, emanating protective strength and power,
riding a tiger into battle. Illustration by DARLENE.

of others he and his followers began to seize control of both heaven and earth. Driven by an overwhelming desire for fame and fortune, fueled by his dark hunger for control and domination, Mahisha drove his armies to crush and subjugate both gods and humans. He then placed himself on the throne of Indra, king of heaven.

Defeated, disillusioned, and driven from heaven, the gods, led by Brahma, the great god of creation, sought refuge at the lotus feet of Shiva, the great god of destruction, and Vishnu, the great god of preservation. Upon hearing the gods' tale of Mahisha's uncontrollable greed and abuse of power, Shiva and Vishnu became so angry that fiery rays of light shot forth from the depths of their hearts through their third eyes. This divine Shakti, or luminous energetic force of all the gods, streamed out from them all and united to create a blazing mountain of fire that transformed itself into Durga, the radiant goddess of power and beauty.

From Shiva's Shakti came her luminous face; from Vishnu's Shakti came her exquisite arms. Durga's hair had the scintillating dark of Yama, the god of death. Her breasts were resplendent from the radiant Shakti of the moon. From Brahma's Shakti came her dancing red feet, and from the flames of the fire god her three shining eyes. Blazing out from the hearts of all the other gods came this essential feminine current, which formed her golden body, clothed in the fiery rays of Surya, the sun.

Upon perceiving the immense power and luminosity of this goddess, the gods who had suffered at the hands of Mahisha rejoiced. They knew that Mahisha, even in his wildest musings, could never have envisioned his defeat by a mere woman. Mahisha, in his monumental egotism, had forgotten the great power of the feminine. Desiring to assist the goddess Durga even further, the gods bestowed upon her their magical weapons and implements. Shiva gave her a trident materialized from his own trident; Vishnu, a discus whirling from his own. Vayu, the wind god gave her a bow and quivers filled with arrows, while Indra, the king of heaven gave her a thunderbolt. Kala, the god of time, bequeathed Durga his shining sword and shield.

Armed with these and other sacred weapons, the goddess Durga roared with divine laughter. Again and again she roared, and such was her mystic sound that the sky resounded, the seas trembled, and the earth quaked. The magnificent goddess of power and beauty mounted her valiant lion and descended to earth.

From his very first glance at Durga, Mahisha only had one desire: to have her as his lover. The resourceful goddess demurred. "I am sorry," she said, "a curse has been placed upon me so that I can only perform the sacred act of union with a man who can overpower me in battle." Mahisha, feeling invincible and blinded by his excessive pride, thought that her conquest would be simple. So he sent his demon army to attack her. But each time she easily, playfully defeated them. Soon the battlefield reeked with the odors of the bodies of the dead, and the rivers flowed with blood.

After seeing the utter destruction of his demon army, his commanders, and his attendants, Mahisha took his original demonic asura form—half man, half-buffalo—and in a lone stampede charged the goddess Durga. Mahisha found Durga's unfurled noose closing on him, and so he called upon his shape-shifting powers and slipped into his lion disguise. This was to no avail, for Durga's sword hovered over his mane. Slinking from underneath her sword, he assumed the role of the warrior and advanced toward her, sword in hand. But he was blinded by a shower of arrows, and so he transformed himself into an elephant. Swiftly the great goddess severed his trunk. Finally Mahisha resumed his original buffalo form, horns lowered, hooves stamping, mouth foaming, shaking the three worlds in his rage.

Upon observing this display, Durga laughed with delight and cried, "Roar you fool, roar! Your hour has come!" Then, in one fell swoop, the great goddess severed his head, and his buffalo body sank to the ground, a lifeless hulk.

Suddenly there was light everywhere. The divine Shakti, or vital energy, that Mahisha had stolen from his countless victims was now released from his grasp. The sky was filled with glistening rainbows. Flowers fell spontaneously from the heavens. The gods and sages sang the praises to the goddess Durga, while the heavenly maidens danced for joy.

Jai, Jai Juga Jnanani Devi
Victory, victory to the goddess of wisdom, mother of the world.

The strong and fiery Kali, Sekhmet, Simhamukha, and Durga teach us the true nature of power. They show us that real power is not about control, repression, and domination; it is about flexibility and clarity in the midst of chaos. It is the ability to relax in the face of danger, so that we can perceive the situation and take appropriate action. When we are faced with the abusive situations and demeaning attitudes about women that have become so prevalent in the Kali Yuga, we can take refuge in and sustenance from these strong and powerful goddesses. In these difficult times, we will gain the goddesses' immediate assistance if we have the presence of mind to call out their names, visualize them in our mind's eye, or feel their divine Shakti radiating through us.

The powerful goddesses are our ancestors and role models. They are mythic beings that have traveled the path before us and have transmuted the ordinary human emotions of our day-to-day experience into wisdom—beings that have transcended the relentless grasp of the manipulative ego. Through their myths they demonstrate how to fearlessly face the darkness from within and from without, how to walk toward the shadow, stare fear in the face, be fully present, and feel the ignorance of our habitual tendencies, projections, pride, and egotism. As warriors of truth and integrity, the goddesses of strength and power inspire us to liberate ourselves from the grasp of all the voices of fear and negativity that haunt us. These fiery goddesses also motivate us to dig deep into the dark murky substance of our emotions and experience them for what they are: merely the play of the divine Shakti energy, the subtle dance of vibration.

In the tantric tradition practitioners learn how to work with and transmute anger and fear by transforming into a wrathful deity. For example, students who have a tremendous amount of repressed anger and negativity will imagine themselves as a wrathful deity dancing wildly in the midst of a cremation ground, perceiving their negative emotions as external demons. Transformed into Kali, Durga, or Simhamukha, surrounded by flames of wisdom, eyes blazing with the power of her essential Shakti, imbued with tremendous physical power and mental clarity, the students visualize the act of confronting these inner demons. As they mentally choreograph and participate in this symbolic dance, they see themselves metaphorically chopping off the heads of the demons with the immaculate sword of wisdom, or piercing their hearts with the unswerving arrow of truth, in order to transmute and liberate the energy that has been constricted within their own minds. At the moment of impact, this confused, constricted energy is liberated, converted into radiant light, and joyously released into the universe.

The act of attuning oneself to the powerful and abundant flow of the divine Shakti of Kali, Sekhmet, Simhamukha, and Durga gives you the opportunity to experience the immense power of their potent, invigorating, and cleansing light flowing within the sacred temple of your body. As you learn to awaken the sacred spiritual fire of the Goddess it blazes and fills your luminous energy body with extraordinary strength and vitality. The power of this inner fire of the Divine Feminine is so potent that when it is stimulated and focused correctly it can be of tremendous assistance in your daily life. It will not only help you to melt away impurities embedded in your chakras, but it will also assist you in building a vibrant energetic shield of protection around yourself.

From the visionary perspective of our ancient ancestors, the human body was seen as a sacred alchemical vessel through which we have the potential to discover our true divinity. The body was seen as the gift and blessing of this dimension, a precious medium for growth, experience, and knowledge through which each and every one of us has the capacity to deeply experience all the power, processes, and potentials of life. Encompassing both luminous and physical realities, the human body was recognized as an incredible merging into form of unseen fields and forces. From this perspective, each and every individual was seen not just as a living, breathing body but also as a conscious being animated by the divine light of spirit.

The following exercise is designed to ground and connect you with the earth, acquaint you with the natural upward flow of your sacred inner fire and the basic blueprint of your luminous energy body, and fill you with the vibrant inner sensations of the strong and fiery goddess.

Visualization/Meditation:
The Energy Field of the Strong and Fiery Goddess

Begin by sitting in a comfortable position with your spine straight. Close the outer doors of your perception, release all worldly concerns, and turn your mind inward. As you do, become aware of the responses of your body and breath. Have you ever noticed how the movement of thought through your mind and the flow of breath through your body are completely interconnected? How the ebb and flow of your breath seems to reflect the state of your mind and emotions? How does anger affect its flow? What about fear or bliss or serenity?

Have you ever noticed that no matter how restless and disturbed your state of mind, by slowly taking a deep breath and then fully releasing it your mind and body will begin to relax? And as you focus your awareness on your breath, for that moment your mind will be quiet and the negative thoughts will begin to dissolve. This is probably the origin of the expression "breathing a sigh of relief."

Take a few long, slow, deep breaths in and out. As you do so, travel with me to the land of the eternal feminine, the primordial ground of awareness and holy sanctuary that lies at the *bindu,* or mystic center, of creation. This is a truly sacred space in which all forms appear and disappear; it is the womb of the great and powerful goddess, which exists at the center of our galaxy, our hearts, and the earth. It is the still, silent place of emptiness and serenity, the primal source of life and light.

Breathe slowly and deeply in and out, and as you do so, picture that deep down in the hidden center of the earth upon which you sit is a pool of liquid light, as calm, dark, and placid as a mountain lake surrounded by the blackness of night. Visualize that from the very heart of this blackness a glowing sun begins to emerge, luminous and bright, the secret inner sun of the Divine Feminine, the initiating and nourishing force of life itself. See the primal energy of its shining solar face as a radiant manifestation of the purifying power and wisdom of the wild and fiery goddess.

Now imagine that just like a tree or plant, you have roots at the base of your spine that extend down into this glowing womb of the earth. Through these roots you are able to sense and make a connection with this ancient inner sun. Breathe in. Feel the fiery light rise from the heart of the earth through your roots and into the chakra at the base of your spine. Breathe out. See its cleansing rays stream from this subtle energy center as shimmering particles of light. Relax. Feel the rays radiating out through your thighs, knees, calves, ankles, feet, and toes, clearing away any tension or pain that resides there.

Now picture that running down the center of your body is a subtle, tubelike channel, as strong and supportive as the trunk of a great tree. In the tantric tradition this subtle channel is called the central channel, uma, or Shushumna; in the Kabbalistic tradition, it is known as the central pillar of the tree of life, and in the Egyptian tradition it is known as the djed pillar. According to the mystics this channel begins four fingers below your navel in the area of your cervix, at the base of your womb.

Focus your attention on this area, this vital center of feminine power and creativity. Breathe in as you imagine that through your cervix, or the physical opening to this secret place, you are drawing the magnificent flaming energy of the sun in the form of cleansing terrestrial fire.

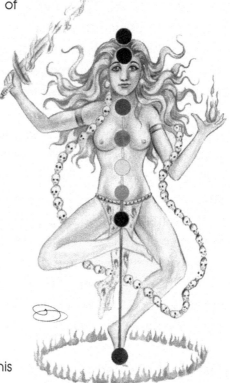

Breathe out. Think of your cervix as a doorway to this subtle central channel. With each inhalation contract your vaginal muscles as you draw the stimulating fire of the Goddess upward into your body. With each exhalation allow these muscles to relax, as your second chakra, which is in the heart of your womb, is overflowing with this enriching light. Feel the glittering rays of the warm solar radiance of the Goddess enter, pervade, and radiate out from this chakra. Feel these rays dissolving any tension, strain, or congestion in your pelvis and reproductive organs. Experience the tension fading away as simply and naturally as the morning dew dissipates when touched by the brilliant rays of the rising sun.

Take a long, slow, deep breath in as you draw this cleansing spiritual fire of the feminine up into your body. Feel the cleansing spiritual fire rise in the form of a bright and shining sun through the central channel of your body, up through your womb, and into your solar plexus, the subtle chakra that corresponds to the powerful physical nerve center located directly below your rib cage.

Breathe out with a soft sigh and relax. Allow the clear lustrous energy of the glistening orb to emanate outward from this subtle center, spreading its cleansing rays of light through your small intestines, stomach, liver, gall bladder, colon, spleen, and kidneys. Feel the energy's deep, liberating power clear away and dissolve any anger, tension, anxiety, and fear in the midsection of your body.

Breathe in. Once again bring the rich and potent energy of the Goddess up through your body in the form of a shining golden sun. Breathe out. Feel the radiant sun passing through each of your body's newly burnished centers until it reaches the still, silent ocean of your heart. Breathe in. See the exquisite beauty and majesty of the Goddess's lustrous face rising from this dark ocean, glowing with the luminous light of her infinite warmth and wisdom. Breathe out. Open your heart to the vast healing power of her divine light and energy.

Relax. Feel the pure, distilled essence of this light streaming through your heart, burning away layer upon layer of the tough protective armor you have created to shield this very sensitive and powerful center. Sense the light absorbing, purifying, and dissolving all the pain and sadness you hold there. Permit yourself to release any sorrow, anguish, grief, or apprehension you may be experiencing.

Feel this sacred spiritual fire of the Goddess kindle the fundamental light of love and wisdom that lies within the depths of your heart. Let this light shine forth from this chakra like a flaming torch, illuminating the darkness of night, awakening you to the immense power and dignity of your own resplendent spirit.

Breathe in, and bring this unwavering flame of feminine wisdom and awareness up from your heart into your throat. Breathe out. Feel the vital energy of the sacred inner fire of the Goddess blaze upward into your throat chakra. With each inhalation and exhalation sense the glimmering warmth of her divine inner sun radiating forth, fully opening this subtle center and encouraging you to release the choked-up feelings and abandoned insights that have been imprisoned by a society that is afraid of the immense power and potency of a woman's emotions.

Imagine that all your speech, all the concepts and words that flow from your mind into the world, are being energized and purified through their contact with this blazing light, until they become a clear reflection of the boundless wisdom, insight, and compassion of the fiery goddess.

Relax deeply and allow your upper body to surrender to this divine purification process. Let the stimulating fire of the Goddess pour from your throat chakra to engulf your shoulders, arms, hands, and fingers. Feel your whole upper body glow with the radiant light of the Goddess's primordial purity and perfection.

With your next slow deep inhale, contract your vaginal muscles as you draw the living flame of Goddess energy into your womb and upward through the subtle chakras of your solar plexus, your heart, and your throat. Allow it to rise into your head until it reaches the psychic center behind your eyes (the pineal center), which is known as the third eye, dakini eye, or eye of gnosis. This is the sacred metaphysical eye that sees in dreams and visions. Breathe out, feeling the bright lustrous energy of the fiery goddess blazing through this chakra, burning away your negative thoughts, judgments, and habits. Let go. Relinquish all the idle chatter that runs through your mind, the incessant flow of thoughts and everyday problems that trouble you.

Breathe in and breathe out. Feel your dakini eye open to reveal the proud dawning of your innate wisdom in the form of a glittering golden sunburst. See its shining rays shoot forth, clearing away the tangled webs of chaos and confusion that surround you and filling your mind with a new clarity and luminosity.

Breathe in, once more contracting your vaginal muscles to draw the sacred inner fire of the Goddess up from its dark depths and through the central channel of your body. Feel its powerful heat rise, permeate, and cleanse your central channel until it is sparkling with the pure fire of divinity. Feel the fire rise even farther, allowing it to make contact with the chakra at the crown of your head—the precious gateway to total illumination. Breathe out, and relax as in a rush of power and sensation you feel this subtle center spin open to allow the pure blazing light of divinity to cascade down and around the entire circumference of your body, until it is fully surrounded by luminous flames of wisdom.

Imagine these flames creating a protective toroidal, or egglike, sphere, sealing and protecting your energy field with flames so powerful that all negativity and provocation are cut off at its boundaries.

As you continue to breathe in and out, feel the extraordinary strength of this sacred inner fire continuously coursing through and around your body, until all your physical, mental, and emotional impurities and obscurations are burned away. Feel its simmering heat melt the dark lead of your being and transmute it into the pure gold of enlightenment. Picture your luminous energy body glowing with this divine radiance.

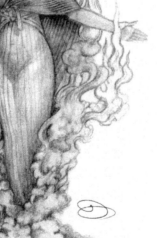

As you feel the pure abundant light of your own essential spirit continue to rise up and blaze within you, visualize yourself as the fierce and fiery goddess exuding luminous flames of clarity, wisdom, and compassion from every cell of your being, dancing with wild abandon the mystic dance of freedom and self-liberation.

The Feminine Art of Emotional Expression

*The eye of the seer becomes like a sword which cuts open all
things, including the hearts of mren, and sees clearly through
all they contain . . . . The glance of the seer is penetrating,
and in this it differs from the glance of the avaerage man. It
has three qualities. The first is that it penetrates through
body, mind, and soul. The second quality of this glance is
that it opens, unlocks, and unfolds things; it also possesses
the power of seeking and finding. The third quality
characteristics of the glance of the seer is more wonderful. It
is this; as it falls upon a thing it makes that thing as it wants
to make it. It is not actually creating, but it is awakening in it
that particular quality, which was perhaps asleep.*

SUFI MASTER HAZARAT INAYAT KHAN,
THE MESSAGE IN OUR TIME

As you have seen throughout this book, the path of the priestess is a path of attunement to the light and energy of Shakti, the Divine Feminine current that resides within us all. This current is particularly evident as it flows from our eyes into the world. It is said that the eyes are the windows of the soul, for it is through our eyes that all our inner feelings are expressed. The eyes can hide or reveal our deepest secrets. They can express power, sensuality, fear, or serenity, for they are linked to the play of the mind. Ancient texts reveal that there are subtle nerves within the luminous body that connect the chakras with the eyes. These subtle nerves channel the energy of emotion upward and outward through the eyes.[6]

In the temples and sacred societies of the ancient world that were dedicated to the worship of the Goddess, an essential part of the training of the priestess, yogini, healer, and soror mystica was the art of emotional expression. Through specialized exercises, practitioners attained the knowledge of and skill for how to discern and personify different aspects of their feminine expression from the enlightened perspective of the Goddess. They would be given specialized instruction that enabled then to understand the essential nature of the energy that emanated from their eyes. By performing these expressive exercises, they were able to directly perceive the difference between the energy of emotions that were based on egotistical cravings and those that arose out of selflessness, wisdom, and compassion. In this way they learned to recognize the intimate relationship between thought, feeling, and action and to refine the manner in which they expressed their feelings to others, and in doing so they gained dominion over the power of their glance. When they had reached the highest level of this training they were able to transmit such clarified energy that they could ignite the spiritual fire within others by merely looking into their eyes.

The emotional expression exercises presented in this and the following chapters are built on the foundation of the ancient teachings of the *Natya Shastra* and the *Abhinaya Darpana* of India, the tantric transformational practices I have learned throughout the years, my work in the healing arts with Dr. Masters, and the writings of the female mystics of early Christianity. The exercises provide a rich vocabulary of expressions based on the many moods, manifestations, and feelings of the enlightened goddesses. Training in these ancient disciplines can bring heightened awareness, sensitivity, and a deep understanding of the drama, energy, and nuance of emotion.

By performing these exercises you will learn to perceive and depict a full range of enlightened feminine expression, from strength and power to sensuality, love, and compassion. You will come to recognize the amazing power and potential of your own emotions and learn to view them not as obstacles or energies to be repressed or endured but as exquisite tools that can assist you on the transformative path of awakening. You will also discover where your own emotional strengths and weaknesses lie by noticing which movements, feelings, and expressions are easy for you and which are embarrassing or difficult. By consciously relaxing, opening up, and allowing yourself to experience the full range of feelings associated with these exercises you will gain increasing insight into your own feminine nature and expressive potential. In addition, you will become aware of the inner dynamics of your own luminous energy body, as well as the energetic displays of those around you. In this way you will develop increasing insight into your own role in shaping the psychic-energetic landscape of our reality.

In my classes and workshops I have found that these exercises are particularly beneficial when performed in groups, with each woman taking a turn reading one exercise to the others. After this I divide the students into two groups, one of which performs the exercise again while the other watches them. Then the groups switch, so that the first group watches while the second performs the exercise. After this we discuss the feelings and insights produced by this experience. I suggest that once you read and perform the exercises by yourself, you then sit together with a group of friends and experience the exercises in a manner similar to that described above.

Expressions of Strength and Power

The following exercises are designed to attune you to the vital, purifying, and transformative energy of the goddesses of strength and power. By attuning yourself to their invincible and authoritative energy you will begin to experience a new sense of your own feminine power. You will also learn how to refine and direct the flow of this powerful energy through your eyes from the place of true inner wisdom, clarity, and perception that is the essential domain of the fiery goddess.

❧ Opening Meditation ❧

Begin by closing the outer doors of your perception and turning your awareness inward. Discover the true space of emptiness and serenity within yourself, as clear, calm, and still as a cloudless sky. Imagine the essential nature of your mind to be like that cloudless sky. Sense the pristine beauty and clarity of your own spiritual essence shining in that empty sky of your being, as luminous and radiant as the sun. See the light of your innate wisdom emanating from you like the glistening rays of the sun.

Now picture your thoughts and their resulting emotions as clouds moving across the sky—sometimes soft and fluffy, sometimes immense and stormy. Sometimes the clouds are so dense that they totally block the light of the sun. Never forget, however, that like the radiant energy of the sun that continuously shines behind those clouds, the crystalline clarity of your inner divinity can always shine forth, undisturbed by whatever manifests before it.

Breathe in slowly and imagine the sacred feminine fire that originates at the center of the earth rising upward. Feel it rising up your spine, filling your body and aligning you with the vital energy of your own divinity. Breathe out and feel it radiate from the top of your head, enveloping your body with its brilliance. With each inhalation and exhalation feel the unwavering light coursing through and around you like a strong cleansing wind, sweeping away all negativity, filling your luminous energy body with its brilliance, and creating a blazing shield of protection.

Now allow yourself to recognize and call on the strongest, clearest, most centered aspect of your being; the part that is pure and true from the beginning of time. Imagine yourself transforming into the Great Goddess in all her divine power and glory. You are strong yet receptive, filled with tremendous vitality, totally awake and alive, and living in the moment. See yourself ablaze with the Goddess's purifying light. Feel her powerful vibration resonating from deep within you.

❧ Self-Confidence ☙

Breathe in, bringing the stimulating fire of the Goddess up through the central pillar of your body. Breathe out. Let this sacred spiritual fire engulf and surround your body with its divine light and energy. Breathe in the sacred fire. Breathe out, feeling it fill your entire energy field with a glowing radiance.

As you breathe in imagine your entire spine is being extended in both directions. As you breathe out feel the back of your neck elongate, relax your jaw, and drop your chin slightly.

Breathe in again, this time feeling the sheer dynamism of this holy inner fire rise into and illuminate your eyes. Breathe out. Let your gaze be firm and your eyes clear, direct, and open. Breathe in slowly and expand your chest as you acknowledge the clear unmitigated power and presence of the divine Shakti within you. Breathe out. Feel your intrinsic energy, creativity, and prowess blaze from your eyes in a magnificent display of strength and proficiency.

Relax and breathe normally. Contract your eyes slightly as you focus inward. Realize that you possess the innate capacity to master any task placed before you. Immerse yourself in the profound experience of faith, constancy, and conviction that comes from being in total alignment with your own essential spirit.

❧ Divine Pride ☙

Now that you have established contact with your pure, essential feminine power, it is time to take pride in that power. Breathe in, feeling the vital energy of the Goddess rising and radiating through your body. Breathe out as it fills you with renewed strength and vitality.

Breathe in and let your spine elongate from head to tailbone. Breathe out, sensing the divine fire of the Goddess engulfing, opening, and elevating your chest. Breathe in. Picture this powerful light helping you to lengthen and elongate your neck as you fearlessly hold your head high. Breathe out. Feel the sacred feminine fire bring a genuine sense of inner warmth and wisdom to your eyes.

Breathe in and out, in and out. Let your gaze be focused and direct, a clear reflection of the splendor of the Goddess. Allow a soft smile of contentment to form on your lips as you experience the pride that arises when every cell of your being is in tune with the pure light of spirit.

Hold your head high. Let your eyes glow with the divine radiance of the Goddess as you survey the world with a feeling of inner accomplishment. Take pride in knowing that as a direct emissary of the Goddess every action flows spontaneously from you and is performed from a place of total harmony, clarity, and boundless compassion.

❧ Glance of Penetration ❧

Relax and close your eyes. Allow yourself to rest in the still, calm place of emptiness and clarity within the core of your being. Breathe in and feel the pure, crystal-clear fire of divinity rising upward. Breathe out. Sense the fire sweeping through your body, cleansing it of all impurities.

Breathe in, allowing your eyes to be drawn slightly inward and upward toward the mysterious third eye of gnosis, which sits midway between your eyebrows. Breathe out and relax. Take a quick breath in and strongly contract your vaginal muscles as you picture the sacred fire flaring upward through the central channel of your body. Breathe out. Feel it entering into, arousing, and opening your powerful dakini eye. Breathe in. Open your eyes as wide as you can and allow the fire to pervade both this mystic center and your eyeballs.

Breathe out. Close your eyes and concentrate your gaze inward. With a quick inhalation open your eyes wide and turn your head sharply to the left as you picture the pure, penetrating light of divine clarity, wisdom, and insight blaze fiercely and directly into and out of your three eyes. Exhale and relax as you continue to gaze outward with this strong, penetrating look.

With a sharp inhale imagine that you are the astute, discerning, and incisive Goddess who with one swift glance is able to cut through and dispel the ignorant, inappropriate, or harmful activity of others. Close your eyes for a moment and rest.

❧ Amusement ☙

Breathe in and visualize the vital effervescent energy of the Goddess rising from the center of the earth through your body like flickering sparks of firelight. Breathe out. Feel the sparks tickling your insides as the light flows up and through your central channel. Breathe in and out. See these animated sparks dancing all around your body like fireworks. Repeat.

Breathe in the light. Breathe it out. Let the light burst from the top of your head and sprinkle your luminous energy body with dazzling flashes of radiant energy as you expand your gaze to the periphery. Breathe in. Feel your eyes twinkle with the sweet brilliance of this radiance. Breathe out. Let the warm pleasurable feeling of the light's sparkling energy percolate through you, causing you to turn both the corners of your eyes and the corners of your mouth upward.

Relax. Allow this gleeful smile of inner amusement to spread over your lips as you look out at the world. Know that as the strong and fiery Goddess your every action is performed from a place of inner joy, clarity, freedom, and spontaneity. From this clear and centered place you will discover that any arrogance, egotism, and pretension on the part of another is both comical and supremely entertaining. Open yourself fully to experience the pure joy, laughter, and delight of the wrathful Goddess.

❧ Majesty ☙

Let yourself rest for a few moments as you take a few soft breaths in and out. On the next inhalation gently contract your vaginal muscles as you sense the warm shining light of the inner sun rise into your body. Breathe out, allowing the radiant beams of this sacred solar fire to spread through you, until every pore is permeated with its divine essence. Repeat.

Breathe in the divine light. Breathe out, letting the powerful Shakti current stimulate, support, and sustain you. Breathe in. Feel this warm inner radiance ascend through your spine and into your eyes as you proudly lift your chest and elongate your neck. Breathe out. Allow both your inner and outer vision to expand to the periphery. Gaze directly forward without blinking. Repeat.

Breathe in, feeling the brilliant beams of luminous sunlight permeating your eyeballs until they are glistening with the powerful transformative light of the sacred inner sun. Breathe out. Feel your senses open and expand as you perceive the clarified light of your own divine radiance emanating out through you luminous energy body like shining golden threads.

With every breath imagine you are growing taller and more magnificent, fully alive, awake, and present in the midst of any situation. Experience the new sense of openness, generosity, and benevolence that comes from knowing that you innately possess the true spiritual strength, dignity, and majesty of the wise and compassionate Goddess.

✲ Deliberation ✲

Now that you have a sense of your own innate strength and majesty, visualize that you are the powerful Goddess immersed in inner meditation, contemplating all sides of a situation prior to taking action.

Breathe in. Look down as you turn your awareness inward toward the sacred feminine flame that rises and dances and swells within you. Breathe out. Feel the flame's strong dynamic energy course through you, creating space between all the vertebrae of your spine. Breathe in as you lengthen your spine and elongate your neck.

Breathe out. Relax your eyelids and focus your thoughts inward in deep contemplation. Breathe in. Contract your eyebrows and turn your eyes slowly to the right. Pause, holding both your gaze and breath still, as if your mind is centered in a moment of clear perception. Breathe out. While maintaining the same inner focus, turn your eyes to the left and hold.

With each inhale and exhale, slowly turn your eyes from side to side, pausing for a moment at each side. Picture yourself as the divine Goddess deliberating on all aspects of a particular problem before making the most positive, compassionate, and lucid response.

✲ Fierceness ✲

The Goddess of strength and power is a fierce protector. Like a wild lioness—alert, aware, senses fully open, living completely in the moment—she is quick to rise up and defend her children from any harmful provocation.

Slowly breathe in her potent stimulating fire. Let it fully empower you,

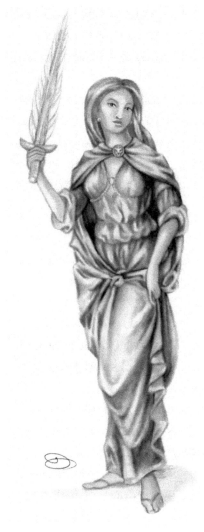

providing a sense of tremendous strength and vitality. Breathe out. Feel the brilliance of this inner conflagration course through your body. Breathe in as you let the sacred fire permeate your eyeballs.

Breathe out. Open your eyes wide. Relax and picture the inner fire fiercely blazing through your eyes, as they are filled to overflowing with its brilliance.

Breathe in. Raise your eyebrows and contract your nostrils as you feel the primal power of the Goddess energy flaring within you. Breathe out. Open your eyes even wider as you feel the boldness, tenacity, and conviction of this fierce protective energy emanating from you as brilliant flames of light.

As you feel this pure flame of the feminine spirit burn within you, imagine yourself as the great fiery Goddess, guardian and protector of universal truth and virtue. Picture yourself transmitting her pure spiritual energy outward from your eyes and body in the form of multicolored flames, creating a powerful and impenetrable shield of protection. Relax.

Pacification

Breathe in. Sense the soothing warmth of the divine solar fire ascending slowly from the center of the earth through your body. Breathe out. Feel the rich sustaining power of this feminine force permeate the marrow of your bones, purifying and relaxing your every muscle and sinew.

Relax. As you feel the warmth of the sacred fire rise and flow through you, experience the quiet pride and fortitude of the enlightened Goddess growing within your heart. Allow the clear warm energy of her limitless wisdom and compassion to expand from your body in the same manner that light is generated from a candle flame.

Breathe in slowly. Open your eyes wide as you use your breath to lift your chest and elongate your spine and neck. With a soft sigh, breathe out slowly, letting your eyelids droop until they are closed. Repeat.

Breathe in. As you open your eyes feel the soft mesmerizing firelight rise, filling you with its radiance. Breathe out. Slowly close your eyes, allowing your whole being to relax into its clear natural state. Breathe in the warm glowing light. Breathe out, and as you gently lower your eyelids send out streams of soft relaxing energy from your eyes.

As you continue to breathe in and out, experience yourself as the Great Goddess, silently pacifying the wrath and aggression of others by revealing to them the still, calm space of clarity and emptiness that lies deep within us all.

✣ Intoxication ✣

Breathe in again, contracting your vaginal muscles as you feel the tremendous potency of the divine fire sweep strongly upward into your womb in the form of millions of charged particles of light. Breathe out and relax. Feel the revitalizing power of this energy spread through your pelvis, hips, legs, and feet. Breathe in. Sense these particles joining together and surging up your central channel as luminous flames of refreshing and purifying light. Breathe out. Feel their intense heat spread out and pervade every cell of your body.

Breathe in and let your head fall back as you feel the overwhelming power of these invigorating flames blaze through you. Breathe out. Feel your eyelids flutter and your eyes sparkle with firelight like two flickering lamps.

With your next few breaths move your head in a circular pattern and flutter your eyelids as you feel yourself becoming intoxicated by the force of this vital fire. Imagine that these flames are streaming outward from your head, forming a glowing corona of light.

Let the divine fire rage upward. As your body is totally filled by its wild stimulating power, allow your head to fall back and a broad, euphoric smile to arise on your lips. Rapidly flutter your eyelids and circle your head as your entire being is filled with the rich, intoxicating power and energy of the wild and wrathful Goddess.

❧ Determination ☙

Slowly take a deep breath. Breathe out with a sigh, allowing your eyes to close and your whole body to soften. Repeat. Slowly breathe in and out, in and out, picturing the fiery pool of liquid light at the mystic center of creation.

Slowly breathe in and contract your vaginal muscles as you draw the unwavering light of the Divine Feminine through the center of your body. Breathe out. Feel this sacred fire release all tension, purifying your body and mind. Breathe in. Drink in the luminous firelight. Feel it rise, filling your body and mind with the renewed strength and conviction to act only from a place of true clarity and wisdom.

Breathe out. Sense your spine elongating and your luminous energy body expanding in all directions. Slowly and steadily breathe in. As the pure power of the Goddess shines from your eyes, contract them a little and focus them directly on an object in front of you. Concentrate on the object with total attention. While maintaining this focus, breathe out. On the next inhalation allow your nostrils to contract slightly as you keep your gaze firm and steady on the object before you. Breathe out. Open your eyes a little more as you display the resolute energy of the strong and powerful Goddess. You are fully awake and aware, your mind clear and incisive.

❧ Playfulness ☙

Maintain your sense of power and intensity of focus for a moment, and then relax. As you breathe, in picture the exhilarating and refreshing light of the Goddess rising in you like a million dancing flames. Breathe out. Imagine these scintillating flames moving through your body with blissful abandon.

Breathe in. Feel the impetuous energy of pure spirit sparkle through you, filling you with such a sense of joy that a smile of sheer delight forms on your mouth. Breathe out as you let yourself fully indulge in these fiery sensations. In rapid succession, let your eyelids move slightly toward each other and then apart, as you send spontaneous bursts of luminous energy outward from your eyes.

As you continue to breathe in and out, let your eyes flash with these rich and spontaneous feelings of pure delight. Visualize yourself as the fiery Goddess, your eyes emitting shimmering flames of energy so tantalizing that they instantly awaken those around you to the immense joy and wonder of life. Revel in the free, playful, openhearted energy of the enlightened Goddess!

❧ Wildness and Passion ❧

Breathe in as you allow these pleasurable feelings to continue to rise within you. Feel the invigorating flames surge upward through the central channel of your body. Breathe out. Let the flames fill you with boundless vitality and inner strength. Breathe in. Open your eyes wide as you feel the brilliant light of the divine fire seeping into every pore. Breathe out. Let your gaze expand as your body, mind, and spirit overflow with the divine ecstasy of the Goddess, filling your luminous energy body with a flaming radiance.

Breathe in. Feel the intense heat of the sacred fire continue to burn through you. Breathe out, allowing a bright spirited smile to form on your lips. With each new inhalation and exhalation, feel the rich purifying flames of the clear elemental energy burning away all impurities and negativity.

As this fresh, untamed energy of the fiery Goddess courses through you, widen your gaze to the periphery, as if you have eyes in the back of your head and are able to see in all directions at once. Shake your head and let a feeling of pure pleasure race through you as you visualize the flames of Shakti's divine fire transmuting your flesh into light. Let the light shine with the brilliance of a million suns from the very center of your being, kindling the innate fire of divinity that lies deep within the heart of every person.

Now that you have explored the wild and sacred domain of the Goddess, let these teachings travel with you. Whenever you are depressed, sad, lacking courage, or in need of strength and stamina, bring the proud spirit of the wrathful Goddess into you. Let her divine power, energy, and lust for life fill your soul and radiate into the world. Let her divine fire nourish and protect you. But always remember that the best protection is to be fully in touch with the pure essential light of divinity that shines deep within your heart.

8

Exploring Sensuality

*The erotic sentiment is the potent "seed" of
mysticism. It is the raw emotion of love, a feeling
that stimulates the passions, "fires" the senses and
awakens the Kundalini-energy at the sexual center.
The erotic sentiment is evoked through the delightful
contact of the senses with the external world. When
refined and channeled, eroticism leads to the
experience of transcendence and ecstasy.*

—Nik Douglas and Penny Slinger,
Sexual Secrets

*I worship in my heart the Devi whose body is moist with
nectar,
Beauteous as the splendour of lightening,
Who, going from Her abode to that of Shiva,
Opens the lotuses on the beautiful way of the shushumna.*
—From the *Bhairavistotra Tantrasara*

ensuality—what a magnificent word. It is a word that is intimately connected to the teachings of our sacred feminine mysteries. Sensuality is a feeling of being totally present in the body, with the senses fully open and expanded, every molecule alive with vital energy. Since we are embodied beings, sensuality is our divine gift. We are embodied so that we can feel, so that we can use our senses to experience the innate beauty and power of our existence. Perceiving the wisdom and power of sensuality is one of the most important steps on the path to self-liberation.

Having been raised in the spiritual traditions of the West, most of us have been imprinted to believe that the path to realization, fulfillment, and enlightenment is about denying the body, senses, and emotions. This imprinting has caused the basic awareness of and respect for the beauty and sensuality of the female body as a receptacle of and transmitter for divine energy to be all but forgotten. Increasingly women have been maligned and criticized for the very aspects of their being that were once considered sacred and magical. From childhood we have been trained to repress the natural feelings of bliss, sensuality, joy, and wonder that are our true birthright as human beings.

Many of us are confused about whether it is socially acceptable to display the intense and abundant energy of our passions. Some of us feel frightened to reveal our sensuous feelings. We find ourselves becoming flushed, uncomfortable, or embarrassed at the thought of outwardly expressing such deep and intimate emotions. Other women have no problem expressing their sensuous feelings in the brassy in-your-face manner that our media mistakes for sensuality. Most of us have little understanding of the essential sweetness, subtlety, receptivity, and refinement that lies at the heart of true feminine bliss.

The fundamental goal of the visualizations and exercises in this chapter is to inspire you to realize the sacred nature of your sensuality. They have been created to take you beyond those familiar imprinted thoughts about your body and sexuality and enable you to begin to experience the passionate dance of your senses, feelings, and emotions from a truly spiritual perspective. As you experience this magical realm of the sensuous Goddess be aware of the feelings and sensations that arise within you. Allow yourself to notice and then release any cynical, judgmental, habituated thoughts about feminine pleasure and sexual satisfaction that have been imposed on you. Understand that they come from a place of fear that is contrary to the loving integrative nature of the feminine. Notice how these negative thoughts disturb the natural flow of your energy, and then let them go. They no longer serve you. Set free your body, mind, and spirit as we enter the playful and passionate world of the sensuous Goddess, a world filled with joy, abundance, and divine bliss.

The Sensuous Goddesses

In the sacred texts, paintings, and sculptures of ancient India, Egypt, Tibet, and the Middle East, the sensuous female deities—such as Lakshmi, Hathor, Inanna, and the sky-dancing dakini Mandarava—are known as the joyful goddesses. They are goddesses of fertility, beauty, and wealth whose postures, gestures, ornaments, and expressions symbolize both spiritual and material abundance. Fully attuned to the rhythms and harmonies of the universe, these goddesses are often pictured dancing sensuously in a lotus field, amid rich vegetation, or in the primordial waters of creation.

The bodies of the sensuous goddesses are ripe and fertile, brimming over with the heat of passion. Full of joy and vitality and thoroughly relaxed, open, and receptive, the goddesses are at the same time totally awake, aware, and responsive. Since their every action comes from clarity, wisdom, and divine rapture, their every sensation, emotion, expression, and movement becomes a spontaneous display of enlightened feminine energy.

The sensuous goddesses are often pictured with their male consorts, symbolizing the harmonious union of the female and male principles. The powerful fructifying energy of this sacred union pours out of this divine couple as a sacred elixir that purifies the hearts and minds of their devotees. As our divine role models these passionate and playful goddesses teach us that true sensuality arises from the bliss of living in total harmony with the vital rhythms of Mother Nature.

Lakshmi of India is the embodiment of the rich nurturing energy of the universe and the inexhaustible source of health, prosperity, and good fortune to all who call on her. Adorned with ornaments of gold and silver, flanked by elephants who shower her with fertilizing waters, and often depicted with gold coins flowing generously from her hands, Lakshmi embodies the beauty and richness of manifest existence.

Lakshmi is also known as Padma or Sri, the lotus goddess who is associated with this mystic flower—a symbol of transformation and enlightenment. She is often depicted standing on a thousand-petaled pink lotus, holding lotus flowers in her hands, and wearing garlands of lotuses.[1] As the radiant consort of Vishnu, the preserver, Lakshmi is the Universal Mother and the caretaker of humanity. Her four graceful hands symbolize her power to grant the four essential aims of Hindu life: *dharma*, or righteousness; *kama*, or love; *artha*, or wealth; and *moksha*, or liberation from the cycle of death and rebirth. In the *Lakshmi Tantra* she describes her role: "Like

> I hereby invoke Sri Lakshmi
> Who is the embodiment of absolute bliss;
> Whose luster is that of burnished gold;
> Who is as wet as it were (from the Milky Ocean)
> Who is blazing with splendour, and is the Embodiment of the fulfillment of all wishes;
> Who satisfies the desires of her devotees;
> Who is seated on the lotus and beautiful like the lotus.
> —FROM THE *SRI SUKTA* (SRI SWAMI KRISHNANANDA, TRANSLATOR)

the fat that keeps a lamp burning, I lubricate the senses of living beings with my own sap of consciousness."[2]

According to the sacred Hindu teachings, Vishnu and Lakshmi represent avatars, or enlightened beings who incarnate throughout the yugas to assist in the preservation of humankind. Through this process, they reveal the path of dharma, or righteousness, as their flawless activities set a perfect example of virtuous and compassionate behavior.

In the iconography, Vishnu and Lakshmi are often pictured together holding hands, embracing, or gazing deeply into each other's eyes. The *Vishnu Purana* beautifully describes their powerful and supportive relationship:

> Where Vishnu is speech, Lakshmi is meaning; where he is understanding, she is intellect; where he is creator, she is the creation; she is the earth, he is the support of the earth; she is a creeping vine, he the tree upon which it clings; as he is one with all males, she is one with all females; as he is love, she is bliss.[3]

In the myth of the alchemical process of the churning of the milky ocean from the ancient Hindu epic the *Ramayana*, Lakshmi makes her appearance when the *devas* (gods), led by Vishnu, and the asuras (demons) agitate the primordial expanse of water to obtain the precious *amrita*, or nectar of immortality. Emerging like a radiant jewel from the distilled essence of these waters, Lakshmi joins her beloved consort:

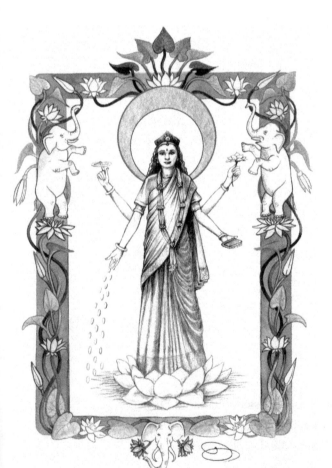

> After a long time appeared the great Goddess, inhabiting the lotus, clothed with superlative beauty, in the first bloom of youth, covered with ornaments, and bearing every auspicious sign; adorned with a crown, with bracelets on her arms, her locks flowing in ringlets, and her body which resembled burning gold, adorned with ornaments of pearl. This great Goddess appeared with four arms, holding a lotus in her hand; her countenance incomparable in beauty. Thus was produced the Goddess Padma or Sri, adored by the whole universe.

Throughout the world the beautiful image of Sri Lakshmi adorns the walls of millions of Hindu homes and places of business, where she is called upon to bring her blessings of wealth and abundance. As we learn to invoke, embrace, and embody her divine qualities we experience a sense of pleasure and contentment that is rare in our modern world. The Shakti energy of Lakshmi is so potent and enriching that our luminous energy bodies begin to shine with greater radiance. In fact, we actually become more physically attractive. Spontaneous feelings of generosity, graciousness, warmth, and affection toward others begin to rise up within us and fill our lives with new experiences of love, caring, and commitment.

Hathor is the beautiful, nurturing, cow-headed goddess of Egypt. She is the goddess of music, dancing, wine, joy, and love, whose devotees celebrate her rich generative powers through song, rhythm, and laughter. As the patron goddess of women and beauty, Hathor presides over the sacred feminine arts of adornment, enchantment, and lovemaking. In the ancient temples of Egypt images can still be seen of Hathor's loving priestesses, their eyes ringed with kohl, their drums, lutes, tambourines, and sistrums infusing the psychic-energetic landscape with the abundant energy of her life-giving power.

Sweet Hathor, queen of beauty,
  protector of the weak.
Shield us against the enemies of light;
Adorn us in the raiment of truth and
  nourish and support us when our
  strength fails.
Guide us in the daily routine of our
  earthly lives.

—MURRAY HOPE,
PRACTICAL EGYPTIAN MAGIC

In her divine role as the goddess of the cycles of life and fertility, Hathor is most associated with the sistrum, a musical instrument similar to a rattle with her face carved on its handle. In ancient times the bells on each of the four bars of the sistrum were tuned to the specific vibration of one of the four elements of nature, and playing the sistrum symbolized both Hathor's generative powers and her ability to keep the world in harmony and balance.[4] As an essential part of the rites of Hathor, her priestesses and devotees would drink wine, sing, and play their sistrums. Moving sensuously to the compelling beat of her vital rhythms, these worshippers would surrender themselves and become lost in the all-consuming bliss of her divine presence as it flowed within them. As these alternating rhythms of the cosmic goddess swelled and abated they generated states of ecstatic frenzy within the priestesses and devotees, which helped them resonate with her universal cycles of nature, birth, growth, death, and regeneration.

Author Jeremy Naydler in *The Temple of the Cosmos* states, "Where there is

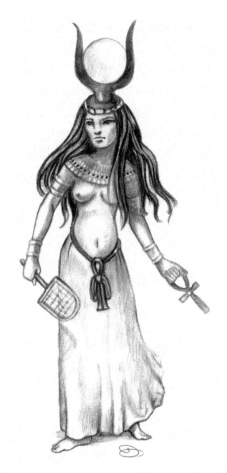

Hathor, the Egyptian Queen of Heaven and goddess
of fertility. Illustration by DARLENE.

lightness of spirit, a benevolent lubrication, then the ancient Egyptians would sense the closeness of Hathor. Celebrants became imbued with her spirit and we may surmise that the individual personality of the celebrant was lifted into a state of consciousness in which he or she felt possessed by the transpersonal energy of the Goddess."

Hathor, in her form as the celestial cow that nourishes all creation, is an ancient goddess who originates in predynastic Egypt. Pictured in this form with stars on her belly, horns of the crescent moon, and a solar disk on her head, Hathor, the mother of the light and the golden one, is the loving consort of the powerful sun god Ra. Throughout the literature she is alternatively referred to as Ra's mother, daughter, and powerful shining eye.[5] According to the eminent scholar of Egyptian studies E. A. Wallis Budge, Hathor was perceived as "the great Mother of the World," and the "power of nature that was perpetually conceiving and bringing forth, rearing and maintaining all things, both great and small." In this role she represented the fullness of the feminine experience. "She was the mother of her father, and the daughter of her son. Heaven, earth and the underworld were under her rule and she was the mother of every god and every Goddess."

In her form as the celestial cow Hathor plays a significant role in the *Papyrus of Ani, the Book of Coming Forth by Day*, known to us as the Egyptian *Book of the Dead*, which was written around 1250 B.C.E. Hathor, as the lady of the underworld, is present to receive the deceased, feed and care for them, watch over them, and assist them in their journey toward illumination.[6] She is present at the critical moment of judgment when the heart of the dead is weighed for its purity, and she brings delight and blessings to those whose hearts have been found pure. In the concluding scene of the *Book of the Dead*, Hathor emerges from the marshes into the light of everlasting life, in conjunction with an epithet:

> Hathor, Lady of the West; She of the West; Lady of the Sacred Land; Eye of Re which is on his forehead; Kindly of countenance in the Bark of Millions of Years; A resting-place for him who has done right with the boat of the blessed; Who built the Great Bark of Osiris in order to cross the Water of Truth.[7]

Transformation into Hathor brings great feelings of joy, eroticism, and ecstasy into our lives. We begin to open ourselves to the sacred feminine arts of adornment, music, and dance and feel the sacred rhythms of life flowing within the temple of our physical bodies. An air of mystery surrounds us and we gain the ability to magnetize and bring into our lives the people and circumstances that will lead us to new experiences of the rich, creative power of the Divine Feminine spirit.

Inanna of ancient Sumer is the glorious queen of heaven and earth and the goddess of the morning star who delights in her sensuality. She is known as the goddess of fertility, bearer of the arts of civilization, and goddess of sensual love. Like an overflowing cornucopia or horn of plenty, Inanna offers her divine gifts of abundance, creativity, passion, inspiration, and contentment to those who worship her. In the book *Inanna, Queen of Heaven and Earth*, storyteller and folklorist Diane Wolkstein describes Inanna's rich and vivifying power as "the cosmic force that descends from heaven to earth. Not only is she a spiritual vision in dreams, she is the awakening force that stirs love in men and ripeness in plants."

In the Sumerian myth "Inanna and the God of Wisdom," Inanna, the queen of heaven, leaves her earthly domain and journeys to the home of her father, Enki, to

The people spend the day in plenty.
The king stands before the assembly in
   great joy.
He hails Inanna with the praises of the
   gods and the assembly;
"Holy Priestess! Created with the
   heavens and earth,
Inanna, first Daughter of the Moon,
   Lady of the Evening!
I sing your praises."
    —FROM *THE JOY OF SUMER*, *THE*
SACRED MARRIAGE RITE (SAMUEL NOAH
   KRAMER AND DIANE WOLKSTEIN,
                        TRANSLATORS)

obtain the sacred *me*, or arts of culture and civilization, to bestow upon her subjects. These arts include ritual, speech, music, architecture, writing, lovemaking, rejoicing, and lamentation, as well as emotions, truth, and procreation.[8] At first Enki and Inanna drink together and enjoy each other's company, and Enki is filled with the warmth of generosity. He freely offers his daughter the precious gifts, which she places on the boat of heaven and then sets sail for home. But as soon as he recovers from his drunkenness he becomes sullen and sends his messengers to retrieve the gifts. But Inanna refuses to give them back. By standing firm she is gifted with these treasures and also magically receives more gifts, including the art of women, allure, drums, tambourines, and the perfect execution of the *me*.[9]

Like Lakshmi and Hathor, Inanna is a goddess of beauty and eros who delights in the rich and luxurious realm of the senses. In "The Courtship of Inanna and Dumuzi," Inanna, as queen of heaven, takes an earthly consort, the virile shepherd Dumuzi, to ensure the fertility and seasonal renewal of the land. Her passionate words of love and longing and the sense of abandon with which she speaks of her body and her desire for the bliss of sexual union provide us with a vision from the era of the temple priestess, when sensory pleasure was still considered sacred and the female body was revered as the holy life-giving vessel. In her song of feminine desire Inanna cries out to Dumuzi:

> My *vulva, the horn,*
> *The Boat of Heaven*
> *Is full of eagerness like the young moon*
> *My untilled land lies fallow.*
> *As for me Inanna,*
>
> *Who will plow my vulva?*
> *Who will plow my high field?*
> *Who will plow my wet ground?*[10]

As the goddess and her shepherd enter the royal bedchamber and consummate their sacred union, they revel in the beauty and power of their lovemaking. Joyously they mix their vital female and male energies, which are poured out for the benefit of the kingdom. In this holy alchemical marriage of the goddess and her consort, of

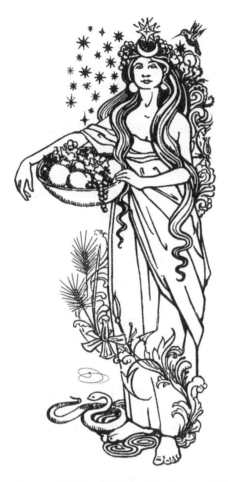

The goddess Inanna holds the bounty of the harvest. Illustration by DARLENE.

heaven and earth, the simple shepherd becomes a king and the fertility and prosperity of the land and their devoted subjects is ensured.

As we bring the sensuous energy of Inanna into our lives, we begin to take pleasure in the fullness and fecundity of our bodies. The immense delight and sense of feminine power she exhibits in each and every aspect of the art of lovemaking inspires us to cast aside our imprinted beliefs and seek out a deeper understanding of the true nature of sexual union. Through this process we can begin to reestablish our fundamental feminine role as teachers and guides in the sacred mysteries of sexuality.

Mandarava is the indestructible dakini of long life from the tantric tradition of Tibet who arises from the great ocean of emptiness and bliss to grant immortality to those who walk in her radiant footsteps. The Indian consort of the great Tibetan master

I pay homage to you O Mandarava,
Radiant Dakini of Immortality
Grant me your blessings,
Fill the sacred vessel of my body with
    the luminous essence of the elements.
Create within me an unwavering pillar
    of strength and vitality.
Eliminate all negative thoughts that are
    obstacles to health and long life.
Increase my knowledge of the true state
    of contemplation.
Bestow upon me your supreme initiation
    of the immortal vajra body.
                —SHARRON ROSE (BASED ON
            THE TEACHINGS OF NAMKHAI
                    NORBU RINPOCHE)

Padmasambhava (like her vajra sister, Yeshe Tsogyel), Mandarava was born on earth in a woman's body and in this form achieved the ultimate state of enlightenment. In the Tibetan tantric tradition, the practice of Mandarava is a long-life practice for increasing one's vital energy. As we feel her divine presence within, our luminous energy bodies begin to glow with the rich restorative energy of the elements. All impurities dissolve, as every poisonous thought and machination of our minds is refined into the rich undiluted nectar of her boundless wisdom. Through her remarkable legend, Mandarava clearly demonstrates that it is possible to purify ourselves to such an extent that even in the darkness of the Kali Yuga, one can achieve the luminous rainbow body

The Legend of Mandarava

Adapted from the Tibetan terma
The Life and Liberation of Mandarava[11]

A long time ago, at the end of the eighth century of our era, in the region of India that is today known as Bengal, there was a marvelous kingdom known as Zahor. This was a rich land of beauty and splendor that was ruled by a generous king and loving queen. One beautiful sunlit day, miraculous signs began to spontaneously occur throughout the kingdom. Rainbows filled the sky and lotus flowers of every conceivable color fell onto the earth like glistening raindrops.

That night at the very instant this royal couple united, a luminous ball of seed essence emerged from the heart of emptiness. Like a glittering star falling through the blackness of the night sky, this essential light of the being that was to manifest on earth as the princess Mandarava joyfully entered her mother's womb. That night the dreams of the king and queen were filled with auspicious signs of dakinis and dakas dancing, singing, and making offerings. As the months went by the queen seemed to grow more beautiful and vibrant. Having been filled with a magical potency, her skin began to glow with light. Wherever she walked the land became lush and bountiful. To all it was evident that she was to bear a very special child.

Then on the tenth day of the tenth month in the year of the male wood horse,

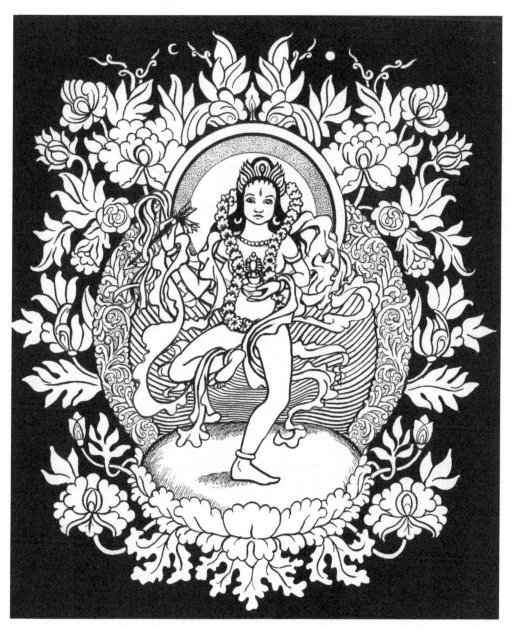

Mandarava, the princess of India who through her passionate devotion to the dharma realized the luminous rainbow body and became an immortal dakini. Illustration by DARLENE.

surrounded by luminous spheres of light, the queen gave birth to her radiant daughter. Endowed with the auspicious signs of a dakini, totally alert and filled with vitality, princess Mandarava immediately stood up and sang praises to her parents. In a sweet and melodious voice she sang of her heartfelt desire to bring bliss, joy, and good fortune to her parents and their kingdom: "As an emanation of the great wisdom dakini, I have been birthed into this world to assist all beings on the path of enlightenment, to tame the hearts and minds of each and every being according to their capacity, and to lead them from the ocean of suffering to the shores of liberation."

Living in this earthly realm as a human being, from her earliest days Princess Mandarava, was inexorably drawn to the path of dharma. Like the Buddha Sakyamuni before her, as Mandarava walked through the world she was constantly touched by the pain and suffering that she witnessed. She knew that human beings were bound by their negative karma and had to endure the endless cycles of birth and death, and so she prayed incessantly for their awakening.

By the age of thirteen Mandarava was fully committed to her spiritual practice. Since she was desirous of a devoted and contemplative life, she begged her parents to allow her to journey to find a spiritual guide. Her parents did not want to deny her pursuit, but they also secretly hoped she would one day take her place beside them as royalty. They agreed to let her continue her quest, but within the confines of the palace.

From that moment on Mandarava immersed herself in every aspect of study that was available. She mastered many languages, read ancient texts, and became a serious scholar and tantric practitioner. With each passing day she became more beautiful and radiant. Tales of her genius, grace, and wisdom resounded throughout the surrounding kingdoms. From every direction suitors laden with gifts of gold came to ask for her hand in marriage.

But Princess Mandarava, wishing only to follow the path of dharma, fled to the forest and cast off her jewels, silken garments, and other symbols of worldly wealth. Naked and without food or drink, Mandarava wandered through the woods until she met a great bodhisattva from whom she gained ordination and took the selfless vows of the bodhisattva path. Her father, seeing her ardent resolve, built his daughter a special palace with a lovely garden where she could live in seclusion with her maids and attendants and continue her practice. But still Mandarava was restless. She longed to meet her true master and guru, the one who would instruct her in the secret practice that brings liberation in one lifetime.

One day while Mandarava was sitting on the grassy hillside with her attendants, in a glittering display of luminosity the great guru Padmasambhava magically appeared before her. Upon seeing this resplendent master, the hearts of the princess and her companions were instantly filled with faith and devotion. They respectfully prostrated themselves before the guru and begged him to come to their palace and turn the wheel of dharma for them.

The guru promised to teach them. In the confines of the palace, preparations were made. Soon Padmasambhava arrived at Mandarava's palace. Doors were sealed, offerings were made. Princess Mandarava and her female retinue began their training under the guidance of the lotus-born guru. He taught them the inner and outer tantras, as well as the secrets of the subtle energy channels, winds, and fluids. But in the midst of this training, a local cowherd happened to catch a glimpse of the women alone with the powerful male yogi. The cowherd began to spread rumors of a secret unsanctioned relationship between Mandarava and her guru. In no time the malicious gossip reached the king's ear. Enraged, he decreed that his daughter be thrown into a pit of thorns and the vajra master burned alive. But Padmasambhava, a fully enlightened master, was beyond cause and effect, form and emptiness. He magically transformed his burning pyre into a huge lake of sesame oil surrounded by flames. In the center of the lake a glistening lotus flower suddenly appeared. Padmasambhava, in the form of an eight-year-old boy, was seated on the flower's calyx. When the king saw this extraordinary manifestation, he fell to the ground and prostrated himself before the living Buddha. First offering Padmasambhava the kingdom itself, the king then decreed that he and his subjects would remain as followers of the great master.

Mandarava was then reunited with her master. Together they journeyed to the sacred cave and place of power known as Maratika. It was here, during the dark age known as the Kali Yuga, that Padmasambhava, as her consort and spiritual teacher, bestowed upon Mandarava countless transmissions and initiations. It was here that they practiced the secret path of total liberation from samsara. And it was here, in the darkness of the cave, as the embodiment of wisdom and skillful means, that they realized the sacred bliss of union. Through the power of their practice they were freed from the chains of birth, sickness, old age, and death and were blessed with the sweet nectar of immortality. Mandarava, as the living embodiment of the dakini, became the keeper of a great treasury of long-life teachings.

From that day on Mandarava journeyed throughout the land healing the sick, teaching both women and men, and selflessly bringing her followers to the path of enlightenment. When her work was completed and she had offered her final teaching, millions of rays of light began to emanate from her heart and into the world. Mandarava's material body slowly dissolved until it became one vast translucent radiant sphere. Like a glistening rainbow fading from the sky, the noble princess vanished from the earth to once again take her place in the luminous realm of the dakinis. In that instant, nine hundred of Mandarava's most dedicated students also dissolved into rainbow light and vanished with her.

The goddesses of fertility, abundance, joy, and eros offer us the possibility of a new relationship with our bodies, senses, and emotions. Through the process of aligning ourselves with their rich nurturing energy, we can walk the path of sacred sensuality—the path of the truly sensuous woman. What does this entail?

A sensuous woman first of all delights in the senses. She lives her life in divine grace, attuned to the rhythms of the universe. Her heart and mind are always constant, ready to react to any situation. Having transformed the negative current of lust into the enlightened wisdom of discernment and spiritual bliss, her creative energy flows naturally and freely, unimpeded by the ignorance of dark passions.

By embracing a mystic alignment with the playful and sensuous Goddess within, the sensuous woman is ready to interact with the powerful currents of the divine Shakti energy that course through her. Transcending the duality of cause and effect, subject and object, she is the luminous essence of her own being rising out of the void, dancing and playing in the ocean of frequencies, shaping them into form. As she dances freely in the joy of this experience her body becomes inundated with the nectar of spiritual light that purifies and transmutes her body into a temple of divine bliss. Filled with a serenity that arises from recognizing her divine nature, the sensuous woman is in tune with the essential spiritual current of her life. Her every act emerges from an extraordinary space of clarity, wisdom, and rapture. Her every feeling, sensation, emotion, expression, movement, and action have been transfigured into sacred gestures through which she assists in the healing, transformation, and liberation of all sentient beings.

The following visualizations and meditations have been created to assist you in walking this glorious path of sacred sensuality. In order to embark on this ancient path, which was fundamental to the training of the priestess, yogini, and soror mystica, it is necessary to become personally acquainted with the rich and revitalizing flow of your Kundalini energy and the playful and passionate sensations of the joyful Goddess. In this way, you can begin to experience the essential sweetness, subtlety, receptivity, and refinement that lie at the heart of true feminine bliss.

Visualization/Meditation:
The Energy Field of the Sensuous Goddess

Stand with your feet slightly apart and your spine straight. Take a deep breath in and turn your thoughts inward. Slowly and gently breathe out, closing your eyes and letting your mind relax into its natural spaciousness. Breathe in. Sense the quiet beauty of this clear, uninterrupted state of mind, as pure and tranquil as a still mountain lake. Breathe out with a soft sigh, releasing all your stress, anxiety, and worries. Allow these disturbing thoughts to melt away like raindrops vanishing into the cool clear waters of that pure mountain lake. Repeat this step a few times.

Breathe in and relax in the great pure empty expanse of the mind. Breathe out with a sigh and let go of all the tension you hold in your body and mind.

Picture yourself standing in the center of a magnificent forest. The fragrance of rose, amber, and sandalwood floats through the air. Sparkling rays of sunlight filter through the trees, bathing the forest in a jewel-like radiance. The soothing sounds of running water fill your ears. Birds chirp joyfully. Breathe in the clear fresh air. Open your senses; let them reach out and expand. Feel the primordial heart of Mother Nature pulsating all around you. Relax for a moment and listen. Feel the sensuous vibration of Mother Nature's primal rhythms running through you. Gently persuade the beat of your heart to come into harmonious resonance with hers, attuning yourself to the strong, unwavering pulse of her divine presence.

At the heart of Mother Earth is a radiant pool of liquid light, a never-ending source of energy and vitality. From the still, quiet center of this magical pool, sinuous streams of liquid light arise and flow through the earth, purifying, nourishing, and cleansing the sacred body of the Mother. In the alchemical and Celtic traditions these flowing currents of feminine energy are known as *telluric* forces. In the Hindu tantric tradition this powerful feminine current is called the Kundalini Shakti, the primordial power of the Goddess visualized as fluid waves of energy and light. According to these traditions, these sacred feminine forces are what animate and sustain us all.

As this Kundalini, or female serpent power, which is latent in all individuals, both female and male, is awakened through periods of deep meditation and visualization, she begins her ascent through the central channel of the body, penetrating, nourishing, and opening each lotus or chakra in turn, leading you to higher and higher levels of cosmic awareness, integration, and divine union.

Take a long, slow, deep breath in. Gently close your eyes and relax as you slowly breathe out. Picture the quiet beauty of the magical pool of life-giving energy at the heart of Mother Earth. Breathe in and imagine that from the depths of the pool uninterrupted streams of luminous liquid light are flowing upward toward your body. Breathe out as you sense this energy of illumination and liberation streaming toward your feet. Breathe in. Open the soles of your feet to receive this radiant feminine current. Breathe out, allowing it to travel up through your ankles, calves, knees and thighs, cleansing and nourishing your entire lower body.

Relax as you feel this sacred energy of the Goddess enter, penetrate, and support the vibrant lotus flower at the base of your spine. Allow the clear energy of the Mother to cleanse and refresh each of its delicate petals, inducing them to spread open and receive her invigorating essence. Picture the blossoming lotus flower floating gently atop Mother Nature's sacred river of light and energy. Rest for a moment, sensing the subtle presence of this energy at the base of your spine.

Inhale softly as you sense the sweet liquid current of feminine energy entering your feet and rising upward until it unites with the Kundalini Shakti, who lies curled around this lotus at the bottom of your spine. Breathe out. Acknowledge the Kundalini Shakti; she is a sacred symbol of your female essence. She is your friend and guide along the path to liberation. Feel her awakening and opening her fiery eyes. Visualize her beginning to uncoil and stretch, her powerful energy blending with the rich telluric current arising from the core of Mother Earth.

Breathe in. Relax and surrender to the Kundalini Shakti's sensuous flow as you feel the supple body of the serpent slowly begin to travel up your spine. Breathe out. Imagine that your coccyx, or tailbone, is absorbing the nourishing light from the conjoined telluric energy of the earth and the kundalini energy within your own body. Sense this revitalizing energy beginning to travel slowly upward into your sacrum.

Breathe in. Gently rock your pelvis forward as you feel the light begin to penetrate the solid bone of the sacrum. Breathe out and gently rock your pelvis backward, encouraging this sinuous energy to rise into your pelvis. Breathe in and rock forward; breathe out and rock back. Again breathe in and rock forward; breathe out and rock back.

Now focus your attention on your pelvis. Feel the sensual light of the Goddess rise up through your sacrum until it contacts the mystic lotus at the base of your womb, which was known in ancient cultures as

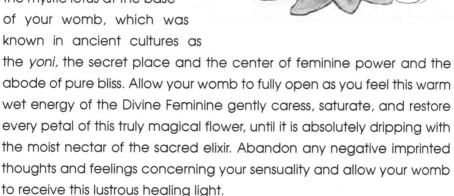

the *yoni,* the secret place and the center of feminine power and the abode of pure bliss. Allow your womb to fully open as you feel this warm wet energy of the Divine Feminine gently caress, saturate, and restore every petal of this truly magical flower, until it is absolutely dripping with the moist nectar of the sacred elixir. Abandon any negative imprinted thoughts and feelings concerning your sensuality and allow your womb to receive this lustrous healing light.

As you continue to breathe in and out, keep up the rocking motion as you feel the soothing sensual nectar of the Goddess slowly encircle each of the five vertebrae of your lumbar spine, bringing them new flexibility and fluidity. Feel this nectar of the Goddess delicately nourish the first, the second, the third, the fourth, and the fifth vertebra. Sense the lotus of your yoni become increasingly flexible and receptive. Feel your womb rise and swell as it becomes pregnant with the fertile energy of the Kundalini Shakti.

Open the soles of your feet. Feel the solidity of the ground beneath them. Breathe in as you visualize the waves of life-enhancing energy rising up from the secret heart of the earth as a fountain of light, again streaming up through your lower body, pelvis, coccyx, sacrum, and lumbar vertebrae. Breathe out and allow the sweet energy of these luminous waters to make contact with the lotus of your navel chakra at the top of your lumbar spine. Relax. Feel the liquid light of the Goddess penetrate this sacred center. Sense the light flowing through each lotus petal, refreshing and revitalizing your entire abdominal cavity.

With each inhale and exhale let the magical healing power of this essential feminine force help you to release any tension you hold in your abdomen as a result of the societal conditioning that says women must possess tight flat stomachs. Totally relax your abdominal muscles and feel how they can naturally support and protect your lower back. Continue to rock your pelvis back and forth as you slowly surrender to this undulating energy of the Kundalini Shakti.

Now picture the pure unpolluted ambrosia of the Goddess rising through your navel center and into the first six of your thoracic vertebrae. Feel the Goddess's warm light caress and pervade each of these vertebrae in turn. Allow your torso to ripple back and forth as your spine receives the pure energy of this throbbing feminine current. Sense it flowing through the first, the second, the third, the fourth, the fifth, and the sixth vertebra until it reaches the mystic lotus at your heart center.

Focus your attention on this sacred heart chakra. Breathe in slowly and deeply. Feel the purifying and nurturing energy of the Kundalini Goddess entering this divine portal to higher dimensions. Breathe out. Feel the gentle yet insistent touch of the Goddess within you; surrender to her your deep-seated fears concerning the vulnerability and sensitivity of your heart. Relax and allow the potent female energy to caress every petal of this delicate lotus of your heart, until it is fully saturated and shining with inner and outer radiance. Picture the Goddess's divine hands effortlessly supporting and sustaining the mystic lotus as it floats quietly upon her sensuous undulating currents of life and light.

Feel your heart begin to beat in time with that of the Divine Mother. Imagine that with each pulsation her sacred energy is flowing through the tender lotus of your heart and pouring outward through its subtle veins and channels to nourish you and all other sentient beings. Rest in the power of this living force of enlightenment.

With each inhalation and exhalation allow your body to sway back and forth as you draw the rich telluric energy from the earth into your spine. Feel it rise toward your throat as it penetrates and revitalizes your next six thoracic vertebrae, bringing them new suppleness and strength. Sense the sacred energy flowing through the seventh, the eighth, the ninth, the tenth, the eleventh, and the twelfth vertebra.

Inhale deeply. Feel the stimulating power of the Kundalini energy as it begins to activate the subtle lotus of your throat. Breathe out. Taste the sweetness of this divine light as it enters and enlivens this sacred flower. Feel the lotus of your throat begin to grow and blossom. Let go of any repressed thoughts or feelings you hold in this region of your body as your throat chakra becomes saturated with the ambrosial nectar of the Goddess. Feel your spirit sing as your voice begins to resonate with the sensuous bliss of the divine Shakti within you.

Relax as you feel her rich liquid energy ripple around each of the seven delicate vertebrae in your neck, or cervical spine. Feel the Kundalini energy nurture, support, and energize the first, the second, the third, the fourth, the fifth, the sixth, and the seventh vertebra. Breathe in, letting the sublime light continue upward into your head until it makes contact with the mysterious lotus of your third eye, the pineal center, or eye of wisdom. This is the chakra known in Hindu tantra as the abode of Shiva, the divine consort of the Great Mother.

Breathe out. As the petals of the radiant lotus of the pineal center slowly and languidly spread open to receive the Goddess's nourishment, picture a luminous ball or seed of white light—symbol of Shiva's male essence—in the core of the beautiful flower. Relax. Feel the Kundalini Shakti penetrate this pure seed essence of his luminosity as she unites with him in the sacred bliss of divine union. Picture the nectar of their union stimulate the root of the glistening thousand-petal lotus at the crown of your head. Feel it quickening and spiraling open like the

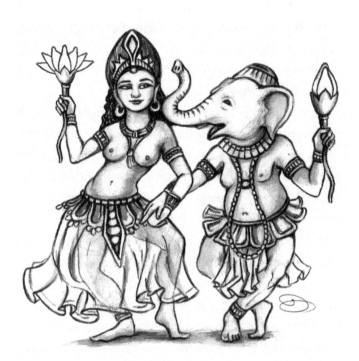

lens of a camera as blissful waves of liquid rainbow light cascade down, around, and through your body. See the light shower you in radiance, suffusing both your physical and luminous energy bodies.

As this vital energy fills you let go of any residual anxiety or confusion about your sexuality and femininity. Allow yourself to surrender body, mind, and spirit to the undulating wavelike rhythm of the feminine.

With each new inhalation and exhalation, feel the sacred light flowing into, through, and around you. Experience the divine dance of goddess and god as the pure distilled essence of their sacred union drips through your body, permeating your every pore. Feel your body become moist and supple. Feel the nipples of your breasts swell.

Open your senses; listen, look, taste, smell, and touch with a newly heightened awareness and sensitivity. Feel your body become a holy chalice filled with the fertile light of union. Let the divine light and energy continue to shower around you and flow from you into the world, magnetizing and inviting others to join you in this joyful display of sacred sensuality.

The Art of Sensuality

Most people today have been conditioned to believe that the range and power of feminine passion is something to be ashamed of. We are told that our erotic feelings should be hidden behind masks of appropriate social behavior. In this cold and colorless scenario we are asked to become as manageable and insensate as the lifeless machines that have increasingly become an integral part of our days. As women born into this patriarchal world, we are conditioned to equate the base feelings of lust, craving, and desire with sexuality. Imprinted by a society that places value only on outer achievements, we too often use our bodies, emotions, and sexuality as tools to seduce and manipulate. From a spiritual perspective, this is completely irresponsible behavior. In doing this we not only hurt ourselves, but those around us as well.

The ancients did not perceive our sensuous, feminine feelings in this manner. They regarded these feelings as fundamental fuel on the path to enlightenment. In the temples and sacred societies of the ancient world transmission of the art of sexual intimacy was one of the most profound aspects of women's mysteries. As documented in Miranda Shaw's eloquent and revealing book, *Passionate Enlightenment: Women in Tantric Buddhism*, tales abound of female tantric adepts who demonstrated magical powers such as clairvoyance, healing, and control of the elements. As experts in ritual gazes these women had the capacity to direct people, animals, and objects merely with the energy they emitted from their eyes.[12] Through years of intensive yogic training these women were taught to awaken and work with the powerful transformative energy of passion.

Fundamental to the development of their extraordinary powers was a thorough knowledge of how to awaken, control, and direct the flow of Kundalini Shakti through their physical and luminous bodies. The sacred ritual of sexual union, often referred to in the Tantric literature as the "worship of women," offers both female and male a directly felt perception of the upward flow of the Kundalini Shakti. When the man's penis fully enters into the woman his action provides her not only with the opportunity to experience intense physical and sensual stimulation, but also to experience a powerful upward surge of her Kundalini energy. If he then one-pointedly focuses his mind on assisting her in opening and purifying her central channel, intense feelings of pleasure and bliss will begin to pervade her body. Naturally receptive, and desirous of their sacred union, she will feel herself open to him like a lotus flower and become the vehicle through which he too can experience divine bliss. In these days of darkness and confusion, of war and devastation, men search the earth to discover, dissect, and manipulate Shakti's secrets. Few of them realize that it is the woman who holds the key to her mysteries.

Expressions of Sensuality

The following exercises have been created to assist you in opening your mind and heart to new possibilities for sensuous expression—ones that arise not from the ignorance, anger, and confusion that has come to motivate much of our actions in this world but from the clarity, wisdom, love, and compassion that arises from real contact with that divine spiritual essence that resides deep within us all.

Through the process of attuning yourself to the fertile transformative energy of the sensuous Goddesses, you will begin to experience a new sense of your own feminine magnetism. You will learn how to refine and direct the flow of your sensuous energy through your eyes in keeping with the enlightened energetic display of the blissful goddesses. Through this process you will begin to release your negative conditioning and discover new levels of feminine pleasure, self-awareness and perception.

❧ Opening Meditation ❧

Begin by breathing in and picturing the calm crystal-clear pool of liquid light at the secret heart of Mother Earth. Breathe out, focusing your mind on its limitless core. Breathe in. Let your senses expand. Rest in the comfort of this pure empty space. As you breathe out notice how the whisper of your breath gently arouses the sacred energy contained in her primordial waters.

Breathe in as you visualize undulating waves rising from this pool through the earth in fertilizing streams of liquid light. Breathe out, bringing your awareness to the soles of your feet. Feel them open as they make contact with the earth below them. Imagine your body to be as firm and supple as a great tree.

Breathe in. Sense the purifying and revitalizing energy of these underground streams and rivulets entering your feet and flowing up through your calves, knees, and thighs. Breathe out. Relax your pelvis as you allow the lotus of your womb to gently open and receive this sacred feminine energy.

Breathe in. Picture the moist serpentine energy rippling up your spine and through your subtle centers until it reaches your third eye, or secret abode of your divine consort. Breathe out. Open your senses to experience the sacred ambrosia of their union in the form of luminous rainbow light. Sense it showering around you at approximately an arm's length from your body.

Breathe in. Feel the sacred energy once again rising up and piercing your pineal center. Allow this divine current of Goddess energy to totally fill your body, spreading through all of the subtle veins and arteries of your luminous body. Feel yourself open even further to welcome this moist soothing elixir as every cell is filled with divine bliss. Relax as you allow the subtle strands of your perception to open and reach beyond your body in delicate weblike patterns, enveloping and embracing the world around you. You are now ready to discover the rich and expressive vocabulary of the sensuous Goddess.

❧ Receptivity ☙

Close your eyes and sense the moist, fertilizing current of the Kundalini Shakti flowing up, around, and through you. Relax the muscles of your pelvis. Feel the muscles and nerves around your womb, your magical abode of bliss, begin to soften and sense the pleasure of this sacred current flowing within you. Slowly breathe in. Keeping your eyes closed and your attention focused inward, simultaneously open your nostrils and softly contract your vaginal muscles as you bring the rich nourishing energy up to your eyes.

Breathe out slowly. Relax your muscles and open your eyes as you feel the energy filling and caressing your eye sockets. Breathe in. Slowly open your eyes wider as you feel them become engorged with this pure radiant light of spirit. Breathe out. Let your senses expand as you gaze outward toward the periphery of your vision.

Relax. Feel your entire body and mind reach out with deep longing for this essential energy of the Goddess. Imagine your body becoming a brilliant crystal-clear vessel eager to receive and merge with the innate light of spirit.

❧ Dreaminess ☙

Close your eyes and relax. Let your breath become soft and fluid. Feel the sacred nectar once again wash over, surround, and pervade your body. Rest even deeper as you imagine yourself floating in a great ocean of spiritual bliss.

Take a long, slow deep breath in. Let your eyes open and roll back in their sockets as the sensuous waves of light flow up through your body. Breathe out. Slowly and gently let your eyelids droop as the soft currents wash downward. Breathe in and out, in and out. Slowly open your eyes and then let your eyelids droop, and open them and allow them to droop. Relax and yield to the subtle caresses of this sweet, warm wetness.

Now feel the current change as the gentle rhythm of the waves rocks you from side to side. With each inhalation and exhalation gently swing your eyes and head from side to side in a half-moon pattern. Let your entire being melt into the warm, dreamy womblike ocean of the Goddess.

❧ Passion ❧

While maintaining this delicate sensation of openness and receptivity, focus your attention on your cervix, the door to your secret place.

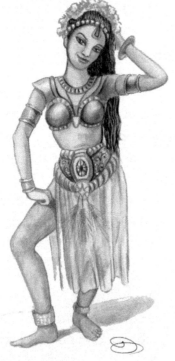

Breathe in as you visualize the warm intoxicating energy of the feminine rising upward, filling the sacred cavern of your womb. Breathe out. Allow its sultry heat to drench your entire lower body with sensuous feelings of pleasure.

Breathe in. Feel your body open further as the revitalizing current of Goddess energy surges upward from your womb, rippling through the central pillar of your body to the secret place of union behind your eyes. Breathe out, letting the rich erotic energy completely suffuse your eyes. Look inward. Let your breath soften and your eyelids relax until your eyes are half shut. Allow a smile of pleasure to form on your lips. Picture yourself as the powerful Kundalini Goddess, ripe with the heat of passion.

Breathe in. Feel the warm wetness of her vital light stream up in delicious waves of sensation from your womb to your eyes Breathe out. Open your eyes and expand your gaze to the periphery, as the distilled energy of passion surges through them in a powerful wave of inner sensation. Breathe in. Slightly contract your eyelids and pupils as you imagine the wave pulling the energy back into the depths of your eyes. Breathe out as you feel the energy stream outward again.

As the intensity of your passion surges and recedes with the flow of your breath, feel your body and eyes begin to pulsate with the pure energy of desire. Allow the powerful waves of this pulsation to be mirrored in your eyes in the form of tiny figure-eight patterns. Revel in the free and spontaneous sensuality of the Goddess.

❧ Demureness ☙

While luxuriating in this fully awakened state of sensuous arousal, picture your treasured consort, your blessed companion on the path of enlightenment, standing before you, as radiant as the sun.

Breathe in as you focus your awareness on your womb, your fertile forest of feminine bliss. Breathe out. Feel its juicy wetness as your whole lower body drips with the divine nectar of the Goddess. Relax and rest for a moment in the pure feeling of this extremely tactile sensation.

Breathe in. Sense the potency of your desire for the sacred bliss of union rush up through your body so powerfully and suddenly that your eyes open wide in astonishment. Breathe out. Wondering if your consort has seen and understood the implications of this intense rush of desire, glance upward quickly with a shy smile.

Relax your breath as you demurely drop your eyelids and lower your gaze toward the ground. Allow your eyelashes to meet and the corners of your mouth to softly curve upward, evoking a sense of modesty.

Repeat. Feel the potent energy of desire surge through your body, startling you with its unabashed power. Peek out of the corner of your eye to see if your devoted consort has noticed. As your eyes humbly meet his, feel a smile of inner contentment form on your face. Relax your gaze and allow your eyelids to languidly meet, evoking a sense of true feminine charm and grace.

❦ Mysteriousness ❧

Breathe in, feeling the sacred ripples of desire subtly stirring in your secret place and evoking an exquisite sense of pleasure. Breathe out, keeping your perception focused on this delicate inner sensation. Breathe in. While staying in touch with the sweet sensation softly stirring in your womb, calmly contract your eyelids and lift your eyebrows almost imperceptibly.

Breathe out. Peek out of the right corners of your eyes. Breathe in, drawing energy first inward and then outward through your eyes as you swing them to the left in a mysterious and beguiling manner.

As you continue to inhale and exhale, swing your eyes from side to side in a half-moon pattern. With your thoughts still lingering in your secret place of delight, let a smile of private pleasure and satisfaction form on your lips, as enigmatic as the smile of the Cheshire cat. In tune with the exquisite bliss of the Goddess, you look as if you possess a great and splendid secret.

❦ Flirtatiousness ❧

Imagine your divine consort, your sovereign lord, seated before you surrounded by a luminous aura of light. Breathe in. Feel the spontaneous, refreshing, and effervescent energy of the Goddess bubble up through your body. Breathe out as you sense the bubbles floating through you, releasing glittering drops of life-enhancing nectar.

Breathe in. Feel a broad smile form on your lips as these exhilarating bubbles tickle your insides. Breathe out. Playfully open your eyes as you imagine that you are glancing upward into your consort's eyes. With each inhalation and exhalation coyly glance downward and inward toward your heart and then send glittering drops of divine energy toward your consort in a figure-eight motion. Allow a playful mischievous smile to appear on your lips.

Maintain the motion and flirtatious expression, while occasionally giving a little wink of your eye. Imagine that you are playfully provoking and arousing your consort's desire by peeking impishly at certain parts of his virile manly body. Let your spirit delight in the divine erotic play of the sensuous Goddess.

Bliss

Picture yourself sitting in a fertile primordial forest. Breathe in, opening your nostrils to inhale the exotic scents of pine, freesia, rose, and amber that waft through the woods. Breathe out. Feel the gentle caress of a soft breeze on your skin. Relax, open your ears, and listen to the refreshing sound of water flowing all around you.

Visualize before you the sacred union of two streams playfully rippling and rushing together. See how naturally they meet and flow together as one. Imagine that from the sacred union of these streams a river of divine nectar is flowing up between your legs, along your inner thighs, and into your womb. Feel this sacred elixir of the Goddess continue to rise through the central pillar of your body, coursing through your inner channels and washing away all impurities and imperfections. Open yourself fully to receive this divine feminine elixir.

Breathe in and in a rush of pleasure let your eyeballs sink into their sockets. Breathe out. Slowly lower your eyelids as you feel the purifying liquid light of the Goddess wash through you. Breathe in and out, in and out. Relax your eyes as your entire being is saturated with warm rapturous feelings. Feel your luminous energy body open, stretch, and grow as your mind, body, and senses become permeated by the sublime energy and bliss of the joyful Goddess.

Joy

Breathe in, picturing the abundant light of the Kundalini Shakti flowing up into your body. Breathe out. Elongate your neck and relax your pelvis as you feel this rich and vibrant energy ripple up the central pillar of your body and into your head, the sacred domain of your senses. Relax. Feel its sparkling incandescence enter into and nourish every sense organ— your ears, mouth, nose, eyes, and skin. Open your eyes, open your ears, open your heart, and open your mind.

Breathe in. Allow the corners of your mouth to turn up in a bright smile of pleasure as you attune yourself to the natural radiance of your essential being. Breathe out. Feel your eyes sparkle with the joy of this inner awareness. Breathe in and out, in and out. With each breath feel these sparks of divine light rise up and ignite behind your eyes. Send spontaneous outbursts of pure glittering light into the world. Experience within yourself the irresistible joy of the sensuous Goddess, as you feel the crystal-clear light of her inherent wisdom shine in a magical display of radiant energy.

❧ Enchantment ☙

From the joyous place of inner awareness of your own essential radiance, again picture your divine consort, your devoted partner on the path, standing before you, resplendent with the light of his own shining spirit.

Take a deep breath in. While keeping your head still and your chin slightly dropped, breathe out and gaze directly into your consort's eyes. Relax as you experience the luminous waves of primordial Shakti energy surging within you like the powerful tide of a moonlit ocean.

Breathe in. Open the gates of your perception. Breathe out. Contract your eyes slightly and look deeper into your consort's eyes, as if you are seeing the beauty of this vast sea reflected in their depths. Relax and expand your vision as you look out of the corners of your eyes, gently attracting your consort's attention. Let the corners of your mouth turn upward in an enticing smile as you imagine the sublime moment of your sacred union.

With each new inhalation and exhalation contract and expand your gaze. Imagine that you are fearlessly riding the waves of pure pleasure that rise, swell, and dissolve within you. Feel the divine elixir of your mystic union saturate your every cell as sparkling drops of nectar shower around your body, exuding the heavenly fragrance of sacred bliss.

❧ Contentment ☙

Relax, letting your breath soften and your muscles loosen. Breathe in with a big yawn and feel your whole being stretch out as it melts into that space of bliss and emptiness that is the secret heart of creation. Stretch your arms, your neck, your fingers; then with a sigh, let them drop. Again, stretch and release.

Breathe in the pure nourishing light of the Goddess. Feel it wash through your body in gentle waves of pleasure. Breathe out, letting your gaze circle down toward your nose, then inward toward the back of your head, and then sideways to the periphery.

Relax. Feel a soft and tranquil smile form on your lips. Let the corners of your eyes turn delicately upward like the soft and tender petals of a lotus flower. Rest peacefully in the sacred heart of the Goddess, the place where the essence of perfect awareness and pure pleasure meet.

❄ Ecstasy ❄

Picture yourself lying at the base of a glistening waterfall. See the water splashing before you. Feel the moistness of its spray as it makes contact with your skin. Open your nostrils and breathe in. Let the desire for pleasure and bliss stir in your secret place as you turn your awareness inward toward this sacred abode of pleasure. Breathe out. Feel your eyelids relax as your womb opens and quivers in anticipation of being suffused with the luscious liquid light of the Goddess.

Breathe in. Open your eyes wide and let your head fall back as the sensuous vibratory energy surges up through your spine in a rush of pleasure and delight. Breathe out as the rich and vibrant light fills your being with an overwhelming sense of joy and vitality.

With each new inhalation and exhalation feel the sacred light of the Goddess rush through every nook and cranny of your body until it radiates from every pore. Let go. Totally immerse yourself in the play of this invigorating energy. Feel it rise up and animate your eyes, making them twinkle with laughter. Allow your head to relax and respond and your eyelids to flutter as waves of delight bubble up and splash outward from you in a brilliant effervescent display. Picture yourself as the joyful Goddess, your body pulsating with light and dancing freely amid the magical display of the phenomenal world.

Love

Begin by closing your eyes and picturing that still, crystal-clear pool of light at the heart of creation. Breathe in as you open your eyes and gaze into the pool's limitless depths—beyond desire or the absence of desire, beyond need or hunger, beyond hope or fear. Breathe out. Look deeply into the mirror of your mind and rest in the serene beauty of your primordial nature.

From this powerful place of self-awareness, breathe in and focus your gaze inward as you sense the pure, essential light of the Goddess who dwells within you. Breathe out slowly as you feel the light saturate the lotus of your heart. Relax. Curve the corners of your mouth upward in a tender smile as you allow the warm feeling of your inner experience to reflect on your face.

Breathe in. Picture before you your precious consort, the radiant being with whom you freely share your most intimate thoughts and feelings. Breathe out. Open your heart, letting waves of light rise from your heart chakra to the center of your eyes. Allow this light to emanate outward from your eyes as you look deeply into your consort's eyes, clearly expressing the innate love and wisdom that resides within the mystical core of your being.

Breathe in. Raise your eyebrows slightly, turning the corners of your eyes upward. Breathe out as you blissfully bathe your consort in this pure healing and invigorating light of the Goddess.

Continue to breathe in and out, fully opening yourself to the warm and nurturing energy of the Goddess within. Feel her fertile nourishing light flowing outward to embrace all of nature. Allow these waves of love and bliss to flow continuously from you, arousing and intermingling with those same energies within the hearts of all sentient beings, awakening within them the knowledge and recognition of their own divine nature.

Now that you have explored the sensuous and joyful domain of the Goddess, let these teachings travel into and through you. Whenever you are feeling low; experiencing PMS or menopausal sensations; having negative thoughts about your body, its inner processes or outward appearance; or even just feeling amorous and eager for intimacy, call on the rich transformative power of the blissful Goddess. Let her inspire you to recognize within yourself the natural beauty and spiritual purity of your female essence, to see the pristine energy of your emotions, heart-felt passions, and delightful erotic sensations rise out of the essence of your being in a magical display of light and vitality.

Open your heart, open your mind, and open your senses. Allow yourself to be impregnated with the fertile light of the Divine Feminine spirit. As the warm, fertile light of the Kundalini Shakti permeates you, you will experience a profound feeling of intimacy with Mother Nature and the world around you. May the sacred bliss, joy, and sensuality of the Goddess flood through you and ceaselessly stream forth from your heart as luminous waves of joy and divine love.

9

Experiencing Love and Compassion

As large as the universe outside, even so large is the universe within the lotus of the heart. Within it are heaven and earth, the sun, the moon, the lightning, and all the stars. What is in the macrocosm is in this microcosm.

—From the Chandyoga Upanishad

The tear drops falling from the eyes, falling on the ground of the heart, are responsible for bringing forth the mysteries of God. Just as merciful rain produces multicolored flowers on the earth, similarly, the eyes that are drenched with tears of remembrance of true Divinity bring forth flowers of spirituality.

—Guru Arjun (1563–1606), spiritual master of
the Sikh tradition

The goddesses of strength and power taught you how to ignite your inner fire, filling you with vitality, inner pride, and security. The sensuous goddesses taught you how to open yourself to the magical world of the senses and how to fill yourself with the fertile, life-enhancing nectar of the Kundalini Shakti and experience the sacred nature of your sexuality. The peaceful goddesses will now lead you on a journey into the recesses of your heart to experience the bliss, serenity, and transformative power of unconditional love.

The goddesses of compassion, healing, and wisdom open our minds and hearts to the vast mystical current of love. They teach us how to reach beyond our imprinted thoughts and feelings and align ourselves with this most delicate of feminine energy

242

currents. But how can one adequately define the profound and exquisitely subtle emotion called love?

Love, which flows through every cell and transcends every boundary, is the life stream of this world. A powerful electrical current that imbues us with vitality and burns away all negativity, love is the sacred alchemical elixir that keeps life in bloom, the richest of all treasures. It is a fluid and peaceful opening of the heart to experience the spark of divinity that is the essence of every living creature.

Love begins with your recognition of this sacred spiritual current within yourself. From this personal experience of the living Goddess, your heart will open like a delicate flower and you will see yourself and the world through the Goddess's loving and infinitely merciful eyes.

Let us journey on the sacred alchemical path of the Divine Feminine as we allow our hearts to overflow with the rich transformative power of love and experience the grace, serenity, rapture, and sovereignty of the peaceful Goddess.

The Goddesses of Love and Compassion

In the sacred texts, paintings, and sculptures of ancient India, Egypt, Tibet, China, and medieval Europe, these radiant and loving female deities—such as Isis, Mary, Kuan Yin, and Tara—are known as the peaceful goddesses. As goddesses of love, healing, and transcendence, they nurture us with the milk of their compassion, purifying us and removing all pain and suffering. Their hearts overflow with the power of unconditional love—the most subtle and refined current of feminine expression. They teach us how to imbue the psychic-energetic landscape with a sense of comfort, warmth, and caring. The realm of these goddesses is a place of subtle beauty and grace in which the pure essence of the feminine spirit radiates as naturally and freely as the morning sun rising from the darkness of night.

As enlightened beings, the loving goddesses shine with the inner light that lies at the heart of darkness. In their all-embracing wisdom they clearly perceive our loneliness, our suffering, our confusion. They remember when we slept peacefully in the dark waters of their wombs, and they experienced the agony of our birth and separation. They feel our pain and longing for release so deeply that waves of compassion spring spontaneously from the depths of their hearts. Committed to the spiritual awakening and sustenance of all sentient beings, these graceful goddesses have vowed to ferry each and every one of their lost and confused children from the material world of ignorance, bondage, and illusion to the heavenly shores of liberation and enlightenment.

The radiant goddesses of healing, mercy, and exaltation offer us the possibility of a truly intimate, honest, and caring relationship with ourselves and with others. They teach us how to look inward and discover that fundamental light of divinity that exists within all sentient beings. As our enlightened role models, these goddesses teach us how to open our eyes and hearts to the perpetual current of truth and beauty that flows throughout our world so that we can fully encounter the most profound and transformative experience that any human being can know: pure, selfless, all-embracing love.

> I am Isis, mistress of the whole land: I am she who rises in the dog star. I am she who separated the heaven from the earth. I have instructed mankind in the mysteries. I have pointed out their paths to the stars. I have ordered the course of the sun and the moon. I am queen of the rivers and winds and sea. I have brought together men and women. I gave mankind their laws, and ordained what no one can alter. I have made justice more powerful than silver and gold. I have caused truth to be considered beautiful.
>
> I am she who is called the Goddess of women. I, Isis, am all that has been, that is or shall be; no mortal man hath ever me unveiled. The fruit which I have brought forth is the sun.
>
> —INSCRIPTION FROM ISIS'S
> TEMPLE AT SAIS

Isis of Egypt is the Universal Goddess, the great healer and keeper of the sacred alchemical mysteries. As the initiator to these mysteries, she oversees the process by which the fecund power of the earth is transmuted and reborn into the spirit. Isis holds the sacred ankh, or the key to the mysteries and the symbol of eternal life. The goddess of transmutation, she is crowned with the risen serpent, the sun, and the horns of the crescent moon. As the personification of wisdom, she waits between the two pillars of opposites that represent the dual nature of our world to enfold us in her golden wings and bring us "face to face with the Divine Reality."[1] Hers is the path of return and renewal, the path in which all opposing forces are reunited in the one supreme source of all becoming.

The sacred hieroglyph or essential symbol of Isis is the throne, which signifies both her earthly power and spiritual authority. She is often pictured standing behind the throne of the pharaoh or her beloved consort Osiris, and is seen as a constant support of those on the path of spiritual awakening. In the ancient myth in which Osiris is murdered and cut into pieces by his evil brother, Set, Isis traverses the land to recover and reunite the pieces of her husband. Her extraordinary magical power gives her the ability to impregnate herself and give birth to Osiris's son, Horus, who later avenges his father's death and restores truth and integrity to the world. Images abound of Isis seated on her throne with her infant son,

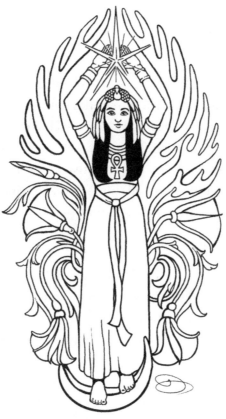

*Isis, the Universal Goddess of Egypt, the great healer and keeper
of the sacred alchemical mysteries. Illustration by DARLENE.*

Horus, suckling at her breast. The ancient Egyptians believed that the pharaohs were
incarnations of Horus, and the goddess Isis ensured their succession to the throne.

In her role as the Universal Mother, healer, and embodiment of wisdom, Isis was
worshipped not only in Egypt but also throughout the entire Greco-Roman world. In
her primal role as caretaker and nurturer, she became the ancient model for the
Blessed Virgin, Mary, the holy mother of divinity. The goddess of magical cures,
visions, dreams, and divine love, Isis is the embodiment of the eternal beauty,
majesty, and healing power of the feminine.

From the primordial space of emptiness and bliss Isis emerged, dancing across the
ocean of existence. She is the first mother. She is the progenitor of all that is to
come. All things manifest in Isis and all things were co-created with her.
Therefore, all of the Goddesses from all of the sacred traditions found on our
planet are essentially Isis. Known in all of the ancient civilizations as the primordial Goddess, she is Shakti, energy divine, the creative force, Goddess of Ten

Thousand Names and Faces. She is the great weaver who ceaselessly weaves the web of space-time, weaves the spiritual into the material, the material into the spiritual.[2]

Isis is the goddess of alchemy whose sacred energy contains a magical healing power. As we feel her transformative current flow within us a subtle reorientation of our luminous bodies begins to take place. The psychic knot that binds the heart is loosened. When this happens great feelings of joy, peace, and love pervade our lives. Fear dissolves and we become warm and receptive to those around us. A heightened sensitivity to the luminous nature of all things develops within us and we are able to gain increasing insight into the fundamental mysteries of universal manifestation.

Hail Mary full of Grace, the Lord is
  with thee.
Blessed art thou amongst women, and
  blessed is the fruit of thy womb Jesus.
Holy Mary, Mother of God, pray for us
  sinners,
Now and at the hour of our death.
—THE "HAIL MARY"

The Blessed Virgin Mary is the living goddess of the West to whom millions of devotees turn in their time of need, or in their fear, suffering, and longing for release. In these dark times, it is Mary's light—the ever-present light of love and compassion—that continues to shine and lead us on the path of spiritual alignment. Like Isis before her, Mary is the radiant mother of divinity, the embodiment of mercy, gentleness, and perfection. Mary assists humanity in lifting its veils of ignorance and delusion to discover the stainless virgin purity of the true spiritual essence that resides within all people. Mary's great devotee Saint Athanasius, bishop of Alexandria, was among the first theologians to christen the goddess Theotokos, or Mother of God. In the following passage, written in A.D. 325, Saint Athanasius demonstrates the similarities between the Blessed Virgin and Isis:

> O dwelling place of the word of God, with whom shall I compare you among all creatures? You are evidently greater than all of them. You are the Ark containing all gold, the receptacle of the true manna that is human and wherein Divinity resides. Shall I not compare you with the fecund earth and its fruits? You surpass them. For it is written, "The earth is the footstool for my feet." Even if I speak of the highest heaven it will not compare to you, for it is written, "Heaven is my throne." (Isaiah 66:1) For you are the dwelling place of God.

In this modern age that is dominated by the masculine, Mary represents for many the feminine ideal, the perfection of woman in her role as mother and spiritual guide.

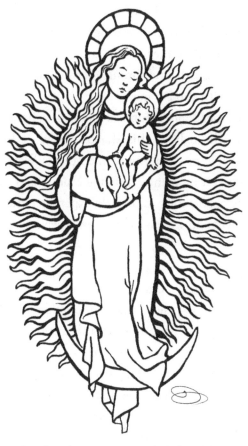

The Blessed Virgin, Mary, the holy mother
of divinity. Illustration by DARLENE.

Appearing in countless visions to her devotees throughout the world, she is the holy mediator between heaven and earth. As the embodiment of the eternal feminine, Mary is always present to listen to our petitions and answer our prayers. From her immaculate heart and overflowing breasts she perpetually pours out the essence of motherly love, shedding tears of mercy for her children, with her graceful hands ever open to lead them on the path to eternal salvation. In the words of the Second Vatican Council:

> Taken up to heaven, she did not lay aside her saving office but by her manifold intercession continues to bring us the gifts of eternal salvation. By her motherly love she cares for her Son's sisters and brothers who still journey on earth surrounded by dangers and difficulties, until they are led into their blessed home. Therefore, the Blessed Virgin is invoked in the church under the titles of Advocate, Helper, benefactress, and Mediatrix.

As the mother of salvation and refuge for all sinners, the Blessed Virgin intercedes at the death of her Catholic practitioners and pleads their cases before the throne of God.[3] The spiritual mother of humanity, Mary waits to take us in her loving arms at the moment of death, and through her sublime mercy she guides our souls to their ultimate union with the Divine.

In every action, Mother Mary exhibits a feminine refinement and beauty that is rare in today's world. Throughout this shadowy Age of Iron it is she who has remained as a steadfast role model for us women of the West, lighting our path and comforting us in our darkest moments. Bringing Mary's light into the holy chalice of our bodies offers us the opportunity to directly experience the power of divine grace. Love illuminates our lives and we see the immense beauty in all things.

The mysterious sound of Kuan Yin's
  name
Is holy like the ocean's thunder—
No other like it in the world!
And therefore we should speak it often.
Call upon it, never doubting,

Kuan Shi Yin—sound pure and holy;
To those who stand in mortal fear
A never-wavering support.
To the perfection of her merits,
To the compassion in her glance,
  To the infinitude of her blessings,
Worshipping, we bow our heads!
—FROM THE LOTUS SUTRA

Kuan Yin of China is the bodhisattva of compassion, the divine savior who hears and responds to the cries of the world. Dressed in robes of white that symbolize her purity, Kuan Yin is often pictured floating effortlessly on the turbulent waves of the ocean of existence, holding a baby in the security and comfort of her loving arms. She is sometimes shown with one hand holding a *mala* (rosary) and the other a vase from which she pours out the pure distilled nectar of compassion. Like Mary and Isis, Kuan Yin is the embodiment of grace, serenity, and generosity—the very essence of selflessness.

Kuan Yin's first appearance in China was as Avalokitisvara, the Buddhist lord of compassion. Around the late eighth century, this male bodhisattva had altered his form and became known as Kuan Shi Yin. Perhaps this was due to the encroaching darkness of the era, with its loss of the power and grace of the feminine current and the longing of the Chinese people for a visible expression of the essence of maternal love.

According to researchers Martin Palmer and Jay Ramsay in their book *Kuan Yin: Myths and Prophecies of the Chinese Goddess of Compassion*, once Kuan Yin took feminine form her worship quickly spread through China and even into Korea and Japan. During this journey many local goddesses were integrated with her.[4] Like her counterpart the Blessed Virgin Mary, Kuan Yin is frequently associated with visionary

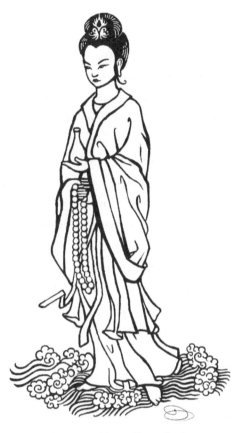

Kuan Yin, a goddess of love, healing,
and transcendence. Illustration by DARLENE.

experiences. Stories abound of her miraculous powers of healing, her undying devotion to her people, and her assistance in their times of fear and anguish. Palmer and Ramsay write, "Kuan Yin's appeal is that she responds to the heartfelt needs of ordinary people. She is accessible to the most ordinary and most lowly. She is the friend that you call upon in times of trouble. She is the hand that guides. She is familiar and she is family."[5] One of the most beautiful meditations for invoking the goddess Kuan Yin comes from an elderly Buddhist nun of Canton who presented her teaching to John Blofeld, Kuan Yin's ardent Western devotee:

> You sit down on a hilltop, or anywhere high enough to see nothing but the sky in front of your eyes. With your eyes you make everything empty. There's nothing there, you say. And you see it like that—nothing, emptiness. Then you say, ah, but there is something. Look, there's the sea and the moon has risen—full, round, white. And you see it like that—sea, silver in the moonlight with little white-topped waves. In the blue-black sky above hangs a great moon—bright, but not

dazzling—a soft brightness you might say. You stare at the moon a long, long time, feeling calm, happy. Then the moon gets smaller, but brighter and brighter till you see it as a pearl or seed so bright that you can only just bear to look at it. The pearl starts to grow and, before you know what's happened, it is Kuan Yin Herself standing up against the sky, all dressed in gleaming white and with Her feet resting on a lotus that floats on the waves. You see her, once you know how to do it, as clearly as I see you sitting there, clearer, because Her face is not in shadow, also Her robes are shining, and there's a halo round her head, besides the bigger oval-shaped halo cast by her body. She smiles at you—such a lovely smile. She's so glad to see you that tears of happiness sparkle in Her eyes. If you keep your mind calm by just whispering Her name and not trying too hard, She will stay a long, long time. When she does go, it's by getting smaller. She doesn't go back to being a pearl, but just gets so small that you can't see Her. Then you notice that the sky and sea have vanished, too. Just space is left—lovely, lovely space going on forever. That space stays long if you can do without you. Not you and space, you see, just space, no you.[6]

No matter what difficulty you may find yourself in, as the "bodhisattva who hears and responds to the cries of the world," Kuan Yin always makes her generosity, warmth, and love available to you. Whenever you are in need of healing, assistance, or spiritual sustenance, you need only recite her sacred mantra *Om Mani Padme Hung* (I pay homage to the jewel in the lotus) and she will quickly come to your aid. As you bring the divine light of Kuan Yin into your life, pain and suffering begins to dissolve and you are filled with renewed faith in your spiritual practice.

OM TARE TUTARE TURE SOHA
OM, I Praise the Venerable Exalted Tara
I Praise You Tare Liberator Swift And
    Courageous
Through Tutare Remover Of All Fear
Through Ture Bestower Of Good
    Fortune
Through Soha I Bow At Your Lotus Feet
—OPENING MANTRA FROM *THE TWENTY ONE PRAISES OF TARA*[7]

Tara is the supreme source of sustenance and the refuge, mother, protector, guide, and healer of the Tibetan people. Enlightened dakini of the three realms—the underground realm of the *nagas*, of the earthly realm of humans, and the divine realm of the gods—Tara is the harbinger of freedom and symbolizes the visible manifestation of the enlightened energy, radiance, and wisdom of our own primordial being. Blissful and smiling, having transcended the realms of suffering, Tara sits serenely on an open lotus flower patiently waiting to assist us in crossing the ocean of samsara, or suffering. Her powerful story is a great inspiration to all female seekers on the path of enlightenment.

The Story of Tara

Based on *The Golden Rosary of Tara* by Taranatha (circa 1575), and other Tibetan Buddhist teachings[8]

Many mahayugas ago, in a time and place before our planet even existed, there lived a lovely and graceful princess named Jnanachandra, or "Wisdom Moon." In this world known as Various Lights, the Buddha dharma flourished and sentient beings had the capacity to live long and fruitful lives. Knowing how rare it was to have the opportunity to take birth in a physical body in a place where the dharma was openly taught, the pious and noble Jnanachandra spent hundreds of years immersed in the ritual practices of purification, meditation, and offering. She wholeheartedly dedicated every moment of her life—both awake and in the dream state—to these practices. This heartfelt devotion to the path of dharma—of righteousness, wisdom, and compassion—made her ripe to receive the fruit of enlightenment.

And so Jnanachandra was brought before the great buddha of this realm named Turya, or "Sound of Drums." The monks who sat at the buddha's feet perceived Jnanachandra's abiding faith and perseverance in the practice and instructed her, "Due to your unwavering devotion to the path of dharma, you now have the opportunity to receive the ultimate liberation. Therefore, you must make a heartfelt wish to be reborn in the body of a man, for only in this way can you receive the true nectar of enlightenment."

But the clear-hearted and perceptive princess replied, "There is no wisdom in this offer, for in reality, there is no duality, no birth and rebirth, no self and other, no male and female. There is only the shining light of the primordial state itself, beyond cause and effect, samsara and nirvana. To think otherwise is only delusion. Many are those who work to achieve enlightenment in the body of a man. And so until the vast ocean of samsara is emptied, I shall remain in the precious body of a woman, working ceaselessly for the benefit of all beings." For countless ages she manifested throughout the universe in this feminine form, assisting all beings on the pristine path of self-liberation.

Through the great love of Avalokitisvara, the Lord of Compassion, Jnanachandra appeared to those of us in this earthly realm. Avalokitisvara was devoted to the awakening and liberation of all sentient beings, and at one point in time he had succeeded in emptying all of samsara. But as soon as this arduous task was complete, to his dismay

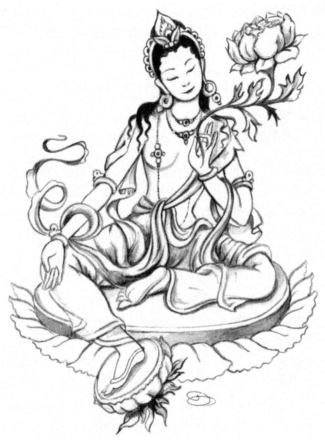

*Tara, the refuge, mother, protector, guide, and healer
of the Tibetan people. Illustration by* DARLENE.

it was immediately filled up again. Overwhelmed by the immensity of this task, a single teardrop fell from his shining eye and immediately transformed into Green Tara, who then spontaneously manifested in twenty-one forms, each offering refuge and spiritual sustenance to those of us who dwell upon the earth. The following description of her five main forms will provide you with insight into the great healing and transformative power she brings into the lives of those who pay homage to her.

Tara's most familiar image is in the color green—the color of Mother Nature. As Green Tara, she embodies the energy and power of the karma, or action, family; Green Tara's presence symbolizes the compassionate activity of all the buddhas. Like the air, she is swift moving, and she is always eager to assist all beings. As mother, liberator, remover of fear, and provider of sustenance and refuge she transmits her love, compassion, and blessing to all sentient beings. Green Tara teaches us how to transform jealously into wisdom.

White Tara is of the buddha, or mind, family. Bringer of truth, virtue, and serenity, she sits on the pure white lotus, symbolizing the stainless essence of our being. The luminous white light emanating from the depths of her heart purifies, removes pain, and bestows long life to her devotees. The goddess of grace, tranquility, and longevity, White Tara rides on the waves of samsara, holding out her hand to us, always ready to transmute our false ignorance and disease into the radiant light of health and vitality. The embodiment of the emptiness of space, White Tara teaches us how to transform sloth, lethargy, and ignorance into omnipotence.

Yellow Tara is of the *ratna*, or wealth, family; she bestows prosperity and good fortune. Glowing brightly like the sun, Yellow Tara's golden radiance pervades all realms and all times. From her heart center she emanates rays of golden light, and she gives to her disciples the blessings of penetrating intellect and material and spiritual abundance. As the gracious goddess and the embodiment of the riches of the earth, she teaches us how to transform pride and arrogance into the wisdom of equanimity.

Blue Tara is of the *vajra*, or skillful means, family; she is the strong and wrathful protector. With keen eyes that flash like lightning, Blue Tara is the remover of obstacles. She subdues evil spirits and destroys negative thoughts and misconceptions. The goddess of power and active compassion, Blue Tara is the embodiment of water, who teaches us to transform the distorted energy of wrath and anger into the wisdom of clarity.

Red Tara is of the *padma*, or lotus, family; she is the joyful transmitter of the divine ecstasy that comes with true spiritual ripening. Filled with the sacred fire of divine and uncontaminated sensuality, Red Tara dances joyfully amid the three worlds. She is the embodiment of inexhaustible bliss and the giver of magical attainments such as healing powers and clairvoyance. The vital energy of Red Tara's playful laughter magnetizes and enchants all beings. She teaches us how to transform the dark poison of lust into the wisdom of discernment.

Divine healer and protectress, embodiment of all that is pure and beautiful, the radiant light of Tara provides a constant source of refuge for we who are lost in the delusions of samsara. May the three worlds ceaselessly resound with the divine liberating power of her sacred mantra: *Om Tare Tutare Ture Soha.*

Human love as we have come to perceive and experience it in this age of materialism is greedy, selfish, and manipulative in nature. Unable to see beyond the infantile cravings of our own egos, many of us fall in what we imagine as love not with a person, but with what we think that person can give us or do for us to advance our position. However, as soon as that person is unable to live up to or fulfill these egotistical cravings, the energy of what we thought was love dissolves. At this point we hunger to meet another, someone who perhaps this time will assist us in accomplishing our egoistic goals.

Another type of supposed love in this society stems from the need to fill one's sexual cravings. In this scenario, one may imagine that she "falls in love" with someone who can satiate her lust or for a few moments offer a strong sensation, a temporary feeling of security, or fill a secret desire for dark and nefarious pleasures. Since this relationship is again based upon possession and ego fulfillment, as soon as it becomes easy to have the desires quenched the person will move on to make another conquest.

Another type of love that is prevalent in our media-dominated society is based on the outer qualities or superficial appearance of another. One may imagine that he is in love with another for her slim, healthy body, or her boundless energy, or her material wealth. However, once this external attractiveness dissipates or vanishes due to illness, age, or difficult circumstances, the love suddenly vanishes along with it.

Isis, Mary, Kuan Yin, and Tara offer us the means to move beyond these imprinted versions of love and create a truly intimate, honest, and caring relationship with those around us. As we bring their divine healing current into the holy chalice of our bodies, we begin to realize the fundamentally selfless nature of love. This direct perception of love takes us far beyond the self-centered, needy feelings so many of us have been conditioned to mistake for love. There is no greed, possessiveness, or excessive self-indulgence associated with a genuine expression of love. It is not produced by or dependent on outward appearances, material circumstances, or another person's actions. It arises as naturally and effortlessly as the radiant light of the sun, ceaselessly shining for the benefit of all beings in a generous and unrestricted way.

Now that you have gained insight into the extraordinary spiritual power and healing energy of these loving and compassionate goddesses, it is time to travel deeper, to dive into their mystical realm of feeling and emotion. The following meditation has been designed to assist you in opening your heart to the rich transformative power of love, release your tensions and fears, and fill your luminous energy body with radiance so that you can fully experience the divine grace and blessings of the peaceful goddesses.

Visualization/Meditation: The Energy Field of the Peaceful Goddess

Begin by sitting in a comfortable position with your spine straight. Close your eyes and turn your thoughts inward. Take a deep breath and allow your inner awareness to concentrate in your heart, the seat of the indestructible essence of your being. Breathe out, letting your mind and senses expand into the world. Breathe into your heart, and breathe out to the world. Gaze into your heart and out at the world.

As you continue to breathe in and out, notice any pain or anxiety in your being. If you observe yourself carefully, you will begin to notice that any discomfort, stress, or tension that you feel may be coming not from a disturbance of your physical body, but

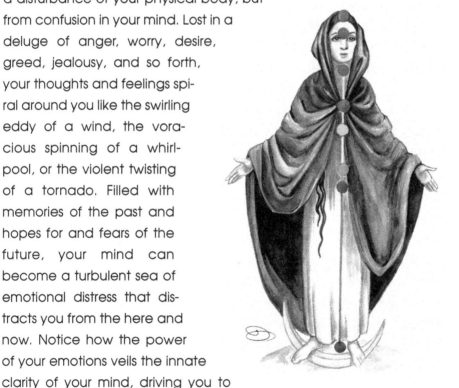

from confusion in your mind. Lost in a deluge of anger, worry, desire, greed, jealousy, and so forth, your thoughts and feelings spiral around you like the swirling eddy of a wind, the voracious spinning of a whirlpool, or the violent twisting of a tornado. Filled with memories of the past and hopes for and fears of the future, your mind can become a turbulent sea of emotional distress that distracts you from the here and now. Notice how the power of your emotions veils the innate clarity of your mind, driving you to lose track of the beauty and spaciousness of the present moment.

Let your breathing soften as you focus again on that clear empty ground of being at the center of your heart. Journey deep into the inner realm of the feminine, into the womb of creation, into the bindu, or source, the still point at the heart of manifestation. Feel yourself floating into the emptiness. Feel your worries and tensions fall away as you descend into the vortex, into the heart of the Divine Mother.

Breathe in. Let the goddess's soothing darkness envelop you. Breathe out. Feel your entire being yield to her spaciousness. Allow your mind—your watcher, the voice that incessantly chatters inside your head—to relax and dissolve into the Goddess's all-embracing emptiness. Release the last remnants of your anger, fear, and frustration as you imagine yourself sitting on a pure and delicate lotus flower that is gently floating in the clear endless ocean of the Goddess's heart. No longer are you in the world of darkness and pain; you have transcended that world and awakened to the realm of the wise, merciful, and loving Goddess. This is the realm known to seers and mystics from the world's sacred traditions, a realm of refinement, beauty, and grace.

Picture that at your base chakra you have roots that extend deep into the peaceful waters of the Goddess. Feel the soft nurturing energy of her divine energetic current begin to rouse and stir and flow upward through these roots in purifying waves of liquid light. Visualize your base chakra, the subtle lotus that supports and grounds you, awakening and responding to her gentle touch. See the lotus spiral open like the lens of a camera to receive this powerful cleansing energy.

Breathe in the liquid light of the Goddess. Breathe out. Feel its pure healing energy radiating through the petals of the lotus, imbuing them with life. Sense this divine energy of the Goddess pouring into your thighs, knees, calves, and feet, washing away any tension or pain you hold there. Breathe in, letting the warm nurturing energy flow upward through your central channel to your second chakra, or the lotus of your yoni. Breathe out. Feel how the warmth of this sacred energy stimulates its petals to gently turn and spread.

Breathe in. Feel your womb drink in this purifying essence. Breathe out. Let your entire pelvis be impregnated by the radiant moisture of this blessed liquid light. Relax. Accept that all of your mental impurities, all of those dark, imprinted thoughts that veil the true purity and guilessness of your femininity and sexuality are being washed away through their contact with these distilled primordial waters.

Breathe in. Sense the healing light of the Goddess flowing up through the central pillar of your body in rippling waves of love and kindness. Breathe out. See the light rise, pouring its purifying nectar into the lotus of your solar plexus, the seat of your will, and place where so many of us women retain our fears and anxieties. Rest for a moment and really let yourself feel the amount of tension you have in this area. Picture the tension as a weakly flickering wheel of light, its spokes covered with mud. Become aware of how deeply it longs to recover its flexibility and radiance.

Allow the gentle flow of your breath to bring the pure healing light of the Goddess into this subtle center. Feel it sweep through every spoke of the wheel, clearing away the psychic dirt and dissolving your distrust and tension. See the wheel start to turn and sparkle, sending currents of life-enhancing energy through every fiber of your nervous system and luminous energy body. Let yourself relax and be renewed as you are filled with the warm soothing light of the goddess.

Bring your attention to your heart center. Breathe in. Sense the distilled light of the Goddess soaring into your heart chakra. Breathe out. Feel the silken touch of her hand as she plants the precious seed of enlightenment into its mystic core. Relax. See the clear sparkling water of her divine tears falling on the fertile ground of your heart. Feel the sacred seed start to germinate and take root deep within your heart center.

Breathe in. See the seed grow and open into an exquisite flower, shining with the pure light of divinity. Breathe out. Feel the nectar of the Goddess's compassion streaming into each one of the flower's glistening petals. Rest for a moment as you let the mystic light and energy flow through these petals like a healing balm. Feel the light continue outward through all the subtle channels of your luminous energy body, washing away all sadness, loneliness, and pain like a cleansing summer rain.

Breathe in as you feel the sweet nectar of the Goddess's divine love ascend to your throat chakra. Breathe out. Taste the nourishing essence of the nectar as it fills this sacred abode of sound. Breathe in. Drink in the rich restorative milk of the Goddess. Breathe out. Sense the lotus of your throat center spiral open as it is saturated by the warmth of the blessed liquid light. Breathe in and feel the subtle vibration of the Goddess's healing current purifying your every thought and word. Breathe out the full, clear, sacred breath of compassion. As the breath continues to flow gently into and out of your lungs, imagine that glittering rays of light are emanating from your mouth and your speech is becoming resonant with the sweet melodic tones of your feminine voice.

Inhale deeply, letting the luminous light of the Goddess rise up into your head. Breathe out. Feel the distilled essence of her love permeate your pineal center—your wisdom eye, the eye of gnosis and center of inner vision. Breathe in. Sense the powerful energy of her divine love awakening the clear natural radiance of your mind. Breathe out. Feel the purifying light of her infinite compassion wash through all your sense organs like crystalline waves breaking on the ocean of your awareness.

Breathe in, feeling the innate rapture of the experience incite the holy waters to rise and swell upward through your central channel like a fountain. Breathe out. Feel the energy stimulate the thousand-petaled lotus at the crown of your head. Relax as you see the flower begin to open and spin with joy, sending streams of luminous rainbow light around your body in a spherical, toroidal shape. Breathe in the powerful current of divine love. Breathe out. Feel the energy flowing up, around, and through you.

With each inhalation and exhalation feel the potency of this cleansing light spiraling up your central channel and washing through every cell of your body. Open yourself to the transformative power of the pure healing light. Drown yourself in this ocean of love and be born anew. Picture yourself as the Great Goddess herself, sailing lightly upon the vast sparkling ocean on a glowing white moon, sending sparkling waves of love, compassion, and exaltation to all sentient beings.

The Art of Love and Compassion

The path of the priestess is a path of attunement to the subtle light and energy of Shakti, the Divine Feminine current that resides within us all. In the temples and sacred societies of the ancient world, an essential part of the training of the priestess, yogini, and soror mystica was education in the art of healing. Through specialized exercises, they were provided with the knowledge of how to open their hearts to the Goddess's powerful current of love and grace and skillfully channel it through their hearts, hands, and eyes. These women would sit together in silent contemplation and open their awareness to the ebb and flow of the psychic-energetic-emotional land-scape.

By transforming into the goddesses of love and compassion or just aligning them-selves to the essential light of their divine nature, the women would gain insight into the correct means for balancing and harmonizing the energies of those who came to them for healing and nurturing. They would spend periods of time in seclusion searching within their own hearts and luminous energy bodies for any distortions or disturbances that needed to be healed and consequently released. For these percep-tive women knew that in order to become true healers they must first heal them-selves. Leaving their earthly ambitions behind, they would dedicate their lives to the service of humanity.

Fully actualizing the power of restraint they spoke only when they felt it was nec-essary. When they did so it was with great clarity of perception, their words designed to strike a responsive chord in the heart of the listener. For these sensitive women knew how to see beyond the physical eyes directly into the eyes of the soul. As they spoke, their eyes shone with an inner light, for their words came directly from the depths of their hearts.

They were so filled with the radiant current of divine love that to those around them they appeared to be in this world but not of it. Wherever they went, the atmos-phere was suffused with light and grace. For these loving and compassionate women, these priestesses of the great temple of healing were so in touch with their own divine natures that they could transmit the essence of this grace to others with a look, a ges-ture, or a touch.

Expressions of Love and Compassion

The following exercises have been created to teach you how to bring your heart into resonance with the Divine Mother and feel the immense power of her healing power within you. As you practice the exercises, simple gifts of faith, charity, patience, gentleness, and kindness will fill your life. A new understanding of the needs and concerns of others will develop and your heart will be filled with spontaneous feelings of generosity, love, and compassion.

✺ Opening Meditation ✺

Breathe in, picturing the clear empty ocean of divinity at the still point or womb of manifestation. Breathe out. Witness how the whisper of your breath begins to stir those dark waters, creating a silently spinning vortex from which streams of life-giving energy spontaneously spring. Relax and imagine that from the center of this vortex, from the very heart of the Goddess, a radiant lotus flower is rising, with you seated tranquilly on its soft petals.

As you rest peacefully on this lotus notice how the sparkling waters seem to move and twirl and dance around you. See how they rise and swell and reach out to support you, as if the Great Mother is gently rocking you in the sweet cradle of her arms. Breathe in and out, in and out. Let all your cares and worries melt away, purified by the powerful tide of the Goddess's deep and selfless love. See your problems dissolve like tears or raindrops into the shining sea of feminine bliss.

As you rest quietly atop the glorious fountain of love, feel the rich cleansing current begin to caress your spine. Sense the energy flowing up your central channel through the lotuses of your womb, solar plexus, heart, throat, pineal, and crown centers. Experience the luminous waters gently nourishing each of these chakras, stimulating them to stir and spin open like beautiful blossoming flowers.

Breathe in the sacred baptismal water of the Goddess. Feel it swell up and around your luminous energy body, washing through every subtle channel until you are totally immersed in its radiance. Breathe out. Allow the secret gates of your perception to swing open and your hidden passageways to be filled to overflowing with this holy essence. Feel the life-enhancing energy stream out of your body and envelop the world in a magnificent shower of sparkling crystalline dew.

The following exercises are designed to attune you to the purifying and transformative energy of the goddesses of love and compassion and teach you how to refine and direct the flow of this sacred healing energy from your heart through your eyes. Through the process of attuning yourself to the serene, harmonious, and merciful energy of these goddesses, your heart will be strengthened and a great sense of inner peace will fill you. From this clear tranquil place you will begin to trust your own insight and intuition so that you can more deeply explore the subtle passageways between your heart, the world around you, and the multidimensional universe we inhabit.

❧ Humility ❧

Take a few slow deep breaths in and out while gently dropping your chin toward your chest. Lower your eyes and look inward toward the lotus of your heart, the sacred abode of the Divine Mother. Close your eyes and allow your eyelids to softly tremble as you see her standing there, her body blazing with the clear light of truth, sincerity, and compassion.

Breathe in. Gently lift your eyelids as you look deeply into the Goddess's warm and loving eyes. Breathe out. Let your eyes become soft and passive as they gaze into hers. Slowly lower your gaze in deference to her extraordinary healing power. Bow your head as you stand humbly before her, surrendering your small egotistical self to the vast healing current of her love.

As you continue to breathe softly in and out, relinquish your fear, lust, arrogance, jealousy, and pride. Drown yourself in the ocean of her wisdom, allowing the corners of your mouth and the corners of your eyes to turn upward in a soft smile of inner peace and serenity.

❧ Inspiration ❧

Inhale sharply, lifting your head and eyes up toward the right diagonal as you feel the sacred energy of the Goddess surge through your body.

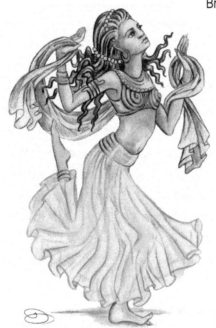

Breathe out. Open your eyes wide as you imagine that your mind is soaring upward like a bird, spreading its wings and flying effortlessly on the powerful currents of the wind.

Breathe in, reaching out with your vision as you picture your mind rising even farther, beyond the clouds, toward the sun, and into the heavenly realms of light. Breathe out. As a sparkling ray of sunlight extends down and strikes your third eye, it illuminates your mind and stimulates your imagination, providing you with insight into the sacred mysteries of life. Rest in this powerful feeling of inner clarity, awakening, and gnosis.

❊ Gratitude ❊

Close your eyes and relax. Inhale slowly and deeply and allow your spine to lengthen, your head to fall back, and your eyes to turn toward the sky as you feel a rejuvenating wave of divine energy wash up through your central channel, infusing your body with new life and light. Breathe out, letting your gaze expand out to the periphery as you feel the sacred nectar of the Goddess shower your body in gentle waves of love and kindness.

Breathe in. Follow the upward motion of the light with your eyes as the energy swells up into your heart and fills it with the distilled essence of the Goddess's love. Breathe out. Allow your eyes to fill with moisture as you open your heart to the extraordinary healing power of this love. Relax and with each breath feel the generous warmth of her divine love spreading out from your heart to permeate every cell of your body.

As you sense each fresh wave of love swell into your heart, gently lower and blink your eyes in acknowledgment of and appreciation for the boundless generosity of the loving Goddess and the sacred gifts and blessings she is continuously bestowing upon you.

❧ Devotion ❧

Breathe in and close your eyes. Focus your awareness inward toward the glistening lotus of your heart. Picture the magnificent Goddess standing serenely in its center. Breathe out with a whisper. See the loving Goddess emerge from your heart on a glistening wave of light as you slowly open your eyes and gently sweep your gaze outward.

Relax. Let your gaze rest on the Goddess's translucent image, which is now floating in the air before you. Recognize her; feast your eyes upon her, for she is the glittering reflection of your own divine essence—pure, fresh, and vital. She is the shining one who opens the door to your heart and guides you on the path to ultimate liberation.

As you slowly breathe in widen your gaze; allow it to be clear, open, and unobstructed as you sense vibrant beams of light flowing directly from the Goddess's heart to yours. Slowly breathe out. Contract your eyes slightly, projecting the pure untainted energy of your faith and trust in this powerful transformative process deep into the Goddess's loving heart. Look deeply into her wise and shining eyes as you take refuge in her glorious path of love, wisdom, and compassion.

❧ Divine Love ❧

Breathe in and out, in and out. As you breathe rock your chin forward and back and turn your gaze inward and out from your heart. Feel the attraction of the strong magnetic current that flows between you and the glistening Goddess, who is the shining reflection of your own divinity.

On the next inhale allow your eyelids to relax as you picture the Goddess riding on a shimmering moonbeam, streaming into the pure lotus of your heart. Breathe out. Let the corners of your eyes and mouth turn up as you feel the light of her divine being dissolve into your heart and flow through all the subtle channels of your body, like a snowflake melts into a clear mountain lake.

With each gentle inhalation and exhalation feel the divine energy of the Goddess permeate your being until your body and mind become inseparable from hers. Feel your face and eyes begin to glow with the innate knowledge and wisdom of the Goddess within. Let the sparkling light of your essential spirit shine out, as clear and radiant as the morning sun. As you do so, recognize and nourish the spark of divinity that exists deep within the heart of all human beings.

❧ Empathy ❧

Inhale slowly and deeply. Close your eyes and focus your attention on your heart. Hold your breath for a moment and feel the vital power of its pulsation. Breathe out. Sense your eyeballs gently pulsating in synchronicity with your heart's primal rhythm. Breathe in. Gently open your eyes and let a soft smile form on your lips as you feel the rich, healing light of the Goddess flowing into the mystic lotus of your heart. Breathe out. With every beat sense the Goddess's warm cleansing energy swirling around and washing through every inch of your heart.

Breathe in. Look inward and picture your heart as a bridge between the Goddess's sacred realm of light and love and the material world we inhabit. Breathe out. Reach out with the subtle antennas of your awareness and visualize before you the people of this world.

As you continue to breathe in and out, feel your heart becoming warm, soft, and receptive to these people. Notice that as you open yourself to these feelings your heart begins to beat in gentle harmony with their hearts. Soften your eyes and see the ripples of light and energy flowing out of the luminous energy bodies of these people; this light and energy is a subtle energetic display of their every thought, feeling, and action. Let your eyes fill with the tenderness of the merciful Goddess, as your heart becomes a clear and direct channel for her warm and loving energy.

❧ Nobility ❧

Breathe in, recalling the calm translucent sea of the Goddess. Breathe out. Rest your mind in the beauty and serenity of its mirrorlike clarity. Breathe in and out, in and out.

With each breath feel the sparkling light that resides in the depths of the shining sea begin to course through and around you, showering your body with waves of vital energy. Allow the divine nectar of the Goddess to revive and replenish you, elongating your spine, lifting your chest, and filling your eyes with light.

Feel your senses expand and gaze serenely out toward the horizon. Feel the restorative energy fill you with a sense of spaciousness, freedom, and possibility, as if you are the Universal Mother standing on a mountain overlooking the whole of your creation.

Slowly inhale and exhale. With a feeling of dignity and love for your children, turn your head from right to left, your eyes scanning the horizon. As you continue to gaze from side to side, open your eyes even wider to take in the wondrous beauty of your world.

Bring your head and your gaze back to the center. Let your breath become soft and fluid as you lift your chin slightly. Feel your eyes glow with a sense of motherly pride, respect, and reverence as you look upon your vast shining kingdom.

✢ Compassion ✣

Breathe in. Feel the purifying stream of celestial grace arise from the empty essence of divinity. Sense it flowing up through your body and into the sweet, sensitive ocean of your heart. Breathe out. Let your eyes be soft and full as you picture the sparkling liquid light gently flooding into the depths of your heart, filling it with love and mercy as naturally as a river flows into the sea.

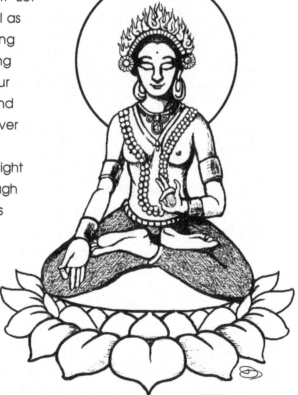

Relax. As this nurturing light of the Goddess pours through you, picture your eyes as deep caverns overflowing with the distilled essence of her love. Imagine that you are the Great Mother riding on a cloud in your pure land of light and wisdom.

Softly and slowly breathe in and out, in and out. Lower your head and tilt it to the right as you cast your eyes down toward your nose. As the Great Mother, regard the pain and suffering of your lost children. Sense their loneliness and isolation, their deep longing for release. With each gentle breath, feel great currents of love and kindness swell in you. Slowly blink your eyes as they become wet with the glistening jewel-like teardrops of your compassion. Do not hold back the tears; let them flow freely like a warm healing rain falling on a parched field.

Visualize the distilled essential light of your compassion piercing the hearts and permeating the bodies of these sad and lonely beings, dissolving all negativity, obscuration, pain, and sorrow. Fill the luminous energy bodies of your children with radiance and their minds with a new sense of clarity, freedom, and possibility.

❧ Meditative Bliss ❧

Delicately close your eyes as you picture the clear light of divinity rising through your central channel like a star rising over the sea—a light so bright it dispels all darkness. Breathe in. Raise your eyelids slightly as you feel your pupils drift slowly to the outer corners of your eyes. Breathe out. Let your gaze expand to the periphery as you sense the sacred light showering around you like a fine mist.

Take a long, slow deep breath in. Allow the corners of your eyes and mouth to turn upward in a soft smile as the warm healing light of the Goddess pervades your luminous energy body and seeps into the very marrow of your bones. Breathe out. Feel your heart chakra open like a blossoming flower. Having fully surrendered your small self to the clear light of your divine essence, a feeling of total relaxation and release sweeps over you. Your eyelids relax and your eyes shine as glittering rays of light stream from your every pore. The entire atmosphere is charged with joy. Rest in this lucid state of pure immediate presence that is the essential nature of mind.

❧ Soothingness ❧

Breathe in, and with a soft smile of serenity recall the primal beauty of the deep and calm sea—the sacred dwelling place of the living Goddess. Breathe out. Rest in the pure liquid essence of her divine healing waters. Breathe in. Focus your gaze inward as you feel the radiant energy of her life-giving waters stream up and fill your luminous energy body. Breathe out, letting your smile expand and your eyes shine with the splendor of this sweet inner sensation. Allow your breath to soften as you open yourself to the Goddess's cleansing light. Let it wash through and dissolve into you, until your body and mind are completely mixed with the Goddess's.

Notice that your feet are gently resting on a crescent moon, peacefully riding on the luminous waves of the sacred ocean. Let your eyelids droop slowly and your gaze expand to the outward corners of your eyes until you sense the same boatlike shape as this crescent moon. With each gentle breath rock your eyes back and forth in a fluid swinging motion. Allow them to open and close in time with the gentle, relaxing rhythm of the waves. Picture yourself as the Great Mother floating serenely on a boat of light. Send soothing vibrations of love and harmony into the hearts of your children as you ferry them across the ocean of suffering to the shining shore of freedom and enlightenment.

✢ Radiance ✣

Breathe in, letting the pure crystalline light of the Goddess rise into the center of your eyeballs like the full moon rising in the night sky. Breathe out. Imagine that from this central point eight pathways reach out like the spokes of a wheel. As you breathe softly, allow the light to flow out through the pathways until your eyes are shining like two stars.

Breathe in. Feel your spine elongate. Lift your head and chin up high. Breathe out. Visualize yourself as the grand and virtuous Goddess, your head encircled with a bright halo of stars. Breathe in. Open your eyes wide, curving the corners of your eyes gently upward. Breathe out. Feel your eyes fill with the shimmering light of the Goddess until they become as radiant as two glowing orbs.

With each new breath feel the energy of the divine light simultaneously burst through each of the eight channels with the blazing intensity of shooting stars searing through the darkness of the night sky. See the light permeate all spiritual and material regions like showers of crystalline dew edged with colors of the rainbow. Immerse yourself in the splendor, majesty, and illustriousness that is the natural domain of the loving Goddess.

❧ Rapture ❧

Softly close your eyes, drop your chin to your chest, and look inward. Breathe in slowly, letting your head lift and fall back as you feel a moist intoxicating wave of divine energy swell up through your body. Feel it flow up through your womb and solar plexus, filling your heart with joy. Feel it rise even farther until, as you breathe out, the wave curls and breaks over the top your head, delightfully splashing around your body.

Relax. Focus your awareness on your heart as you lower your chin to your chest in preparation for the next pure rush of light and energy. As the next wave swells and breaks, breathe in, lift your chest, and raise your head and eyes to the sky. Gently lower you gaze toward your heart as you surrender your body, mind, and spirit to the pure healing power of the Goddess's loving current.

As the next wave rushes through you, breathe in. Let your gaze expand, your heart open, and your face shine with a radiant smile. All suffering dissolves and you feel as if your heart is taking wing and flying into the pure realms of heavenly bliss. Breathe out. Let your eyes shine with celestial glory and your eyelids softly tremble. Feel your heart soar on the wings of the Goddess's divine love.

With each breath feel your heart fully open to welcome and embrace the vast healing energy of the Divine Mother. Let your heart overflow with the sacred nectar of her love as you blissfully ride on this sacred current of joy and exaltation.

Now that you have explored the pure, compassionate, and contemplative realm of the peaceful Goddess, let these teachings travel with you. Whenever you feel frightened, anxious, lonely, or sad, do not hesitate to call upon the vast healing power and grace of the merciful Goddess. Let the pure cleansing energy of her boundless compassion fill your heart and permeate your being. Feel it radiate through your body and mind, transforming your fears, anxieties, and negative emotions until you become a shining vessel of divinity, fully awake, aware, and responsive to all that surrounds you.

Like the Great Goddess herself, dedicate your life to the sustenance, protection, and education of all sentient beings. Every day, in every moment, with every breath, feel the power of your inherent wisdom shining from your heart in a magnificent display of sparkling rainbow light as you invite others to take your hand and travel with you on the sacred path of love, liberation, and enlightenment.

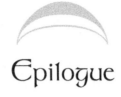

Epilogue

I am always within light, O Mother,
Always returning home to light,
When these physical eyes close for the last time,
Darkness will dissolve into light
And light into you.

RAMPRASAD SEN (TRANSLATED BY LEX HIXON)

ach and every one of us has the potential to perceive, regulate, and transmit the sacred current of the Divine Feminine that illuminates our reality. Providing you with an understanding of women's primary role as Keepers of the Light has been at the heart of the teachings I have presented in this book. But this book is only an introduction.

As you have seen, over the centuries the sacred women's mysteries were transmitted through the oral tradition without the use of the written word. I wish I could sit or stand before you like my teachers sat or stood before me and using this ancient means of education directly demonstrate to you the energy and power of these teachings. So many levels of information are communicated through expression, movement, gesture, sound, and feeling. These are subtle levels of knowledge that are beyond the power of the written word. In the writing of this book, I have done my best to offer you an experience of the beauty, value, and subtle energy of these ancient teachings and provide you with the knowledge of where you may go to seek out the teachings and transmissions that will lead you to deeper levels of the mysteries.

Over the years women have asked me, " What can I do in my everyday life to stay in touch with the Path of the Priestess, the ancient ways of the goddess?" This is my answer:

Remember the power of silence, stillness, and truth. Whenever possible, allow yourself to let go and relax into the silence. Simply sit down, close your eyes, take a deep breath, and feel the immense light and healing power of the goddess flowing through you. Never forget that her divine love and energy is always available to you.

Recognize that every lie, even the smallest falsehood you utter distorts not only your own luminous energy body but that of the larger world as well. So be honest with others, but most of all, be honest with yourself.

Be aware. Open your senses and become cognizant of the signs, symbols, and messages offered to you as they manifest throughout the psychic-energetic-emotional landscape. Allow them to inform and illuminate your actions.

Remember that all aspects of human life are sacred. All bodily motion, be it walking, standing, sitting, stretching, or gesticulating should be performed with total focus, in total presence with one pointed concentration upon the here and now, the present moment, and directly perceived experience.

Spend time in communion with Mother Nature. Open your eyes to the beauty of the manifest world. With every step you take, sense your feet making contact with the earth, the sacred body of the mother. Feel her blissful and rejuvenating current of light flowing through you. With every glass of water you drink, close your eyes and visualize that the goddess is filling your physical and luminous energy bodies with her divine nectar. With every breath you take feel yourself becoming saturated and rejuvenated by her life-enhancing radiance.

When you go to sleep, visualize the goddess abiding in the sacred lotus of your heart. When you wake up, see that she is still there offering the riches of her divine strength, love, and wisdom. As you go through your day-to-day activities continue to hold her in your heart, allowing her divine presence to fill you with clarity, insight, and inspiration.

I pray that the teachings you have encountered during the course of this book have been of benefit to you, bringing you new insight into the essential nature of the feminine experience and encouraging you to cast aside your worn out imprints and realize how powerful, sensuous, and loving we women really are.

I pay homage to the goddesses and dakinis who have allowed me to be a conduit for their sacred teachings and been my constant companions throughout the writing of this book. May they bestow their blessings upon you and fill your life with bliss, strength, serenity and love.

Continue the journey on the path of the priestess with the Sacred Mysteries videos *Awakening the Feminine: Exercises from the Path of the Priestess* and *Isis and the Black Madonna: The Alchemical Goddesses* featuring Sharron Rose. For more information go to www.sacredmysteries.com or write to Sacred Mysteries, PO Box 1853, Buellton, CA, 93427.

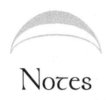

Notes

Chapter 1: The Call of the Goddess

1. For greater insight into the history and development of Kathak dance see Reginald and Jamilla Massey, *The Dances of India* (London: Tricolor Books, 1989), pp. 73–83.

2. Enakshi Bhavani, *The Dance in India* (Bombay: D. B. Taraporevala Sons and Co., 1965), p. 36. This book is an excellent resource on the many forms of classical folk and tribal dance in India.

3. Bhavani, 37. The *Natya Shastra*, or ancient text on the science of dramaturgy known as the fifth Veda, states that the classical dance in India was first performed in the Himalayas.

4. For more on the origins of the *Natya Shastra* see Tara Michael, *The Symbolic Gestures of the Hands* (Paris: Editions Semaphore, 1985), pp. vii–xxv. Or for an extensive explanation of the mudras employed in Indian dance, their multifaceted meanings, and their usage see Bhavani or Bharatmuni, *The Natya Shastra* (New Delhi: Sri Satguru, n.d.), chapter 9.

5. Richard Thompson, *Mysteries of the Sacred Universe* (San Diego: Govardhan Hill, 2000), p. 188.

6. Dr. Pushpendra Kumar, Ph.D., *Shakti Cult in Ancient India* (Varanasi: Bhartiya Publishing, 1974), p. 25.

7. Bharatmuni, pp. 4, 45–47.

8. Throughout India there are numerous statues and paintings depicting the Goddess or God standing or sitting on a lotus flower. These images have been created to inspire the devotees in their process of transformation. The images reveal that these deities, born from and rising above the lotus flower, have not only emerged from but have also transcended the human condition. This is why the lotus is considered a most sacred plant in the East, for it symbolizes the struggle of humanity to rise up from its dark and harmful thoughts and actions and liberate itself into the clear light of wisdom and compassion.

9. For more information on the life and poetry of Mirabai, see Louise Landes-Levi, *Sweet on My Lips: The Love Poems of Mirabai* (New York: Cool Grove Publishing, 1997). In the appendix of this exquisite translation (pp. 63–65), Landes-Levi relates how Mirabai wandered barefoot throughout the countryside, teaching the village women dance and even singing for the great Moghul emperor Akbar. She also speaks of Mirabai's attainment of the ultimate body of light.

10. In the depth of Mirabai's devotion, the manner in which she directs her inner passions toward her Lord, and the poetic depiction of her states of longing, rapture, and spiritual ecstasy, I am reminded of the writings of female mystics of medieval Christianity, such as Hildegard of Bingen, Mechthild of Magdeburg, and Beatrice of Nazareth. For more information on the writings of these remarkable female visionaries of the Western tradition, see Emilie Zum Brunn and Georgette Epiney-Burgard, *Women Mystics in Medieval Europe* (New York: Paragon House, 1989).

Chapter 2: The Dance of the Dakini

1. For a more detailed description of Chögyal Namkhai Norbu Rinpoche's early life and training see Namkhai Norbu, *The Crystal and the Way of Light* (New York: Routledge and Keegan Paul, 1986), pp. 1–10.

2. Ibid., pp. 129–131.

3. For a detailed description of the many facets and manifestations of the dakini see Tsultrim Allione, *Women of Wisdom* (Ithaca, N.Y.: Snow Lion, 2000), pp. 103–109.

4. In his book *The Crystal and the Way of Light* (pp. 126–128) Norbu relates the story of his uncle Dogdan's realization of the rainbow body in Tibet during the time of the Cultural Revolution. During this extraordinary process of transmutation Dogdan's body first shrank to the size of a small child's and then later disappeared altogether, leaving only the hair and fingernails, which are considered impurities. Evidence of this level of transmutation by masters, yogis, yoginis, and practitioners exists throughout Tibetan lore.

5. For more information on the terma tradition and its relationship to the dakinis see Allione, pp. 119–121.

6. For a more detailed explanation of the energetic aspects of these Tantric practices see Norbu and Clemente, pp. 77–81. Norbu and Clemente, *The Supreme Source* (Ithaca, N.Y.: Snow Lion, 1999), pp. 77–81.

7. Allione, p. 92. Allione is a teacher and yogini who has been empowered to transmit the teachings. Because she is an American woman who was raised with our modern Western imprints, she has great insight into working with and releasing the obstacles we female seekers may encounter on the path.

8. Norbu, *The Cycle of Day and Night* (Oakland: Zhang Zhung Editions, 1984), 27.

9. For the biography of this excellent female practitioner and yogini see Allione, pp. 137–164. Modern scientific research has discovered that when we are in the dark, melatonin, a hormone secreted by the pineal gland, regenerates the body, induces dream states, and causes sleep. From a scientific perspective, this could account for Ayu Kandro's youthful appearance.

10. For further insight into the practice of the dark see Norbu, *The Crystal and the Way of Light*, pp. 113–114. For a fascinating look into some of the visionary experiences that can unfold in dark retreat, see Tenzin Wangyal, *Wonders of the Natural Mind* (Barrytown, N.Y.: Station Hill Press, 1993), pp. 10–19. Wangyal is a Lama in the ancient Bon tradition of Tibet, a tradition that also carries the Dzogchen lineage.

11. For more information on the practice of chod see Norbu, *The Crystal and the Way of Light*, pp. 47–49, and Allione, pp. 168–171.

12. See Namkhai Norbu *Dream Yoga and the Practice of Natural Light* (Ithaca, N.Y.: Snow Lion, 1992). This book offers a powerful perspective on dream yoga.

13. For teachings on the power of karma and the process of reincarnation or transmigration see Norbu, *The Crystal and the Way of Light*, pp. 57–58.

14. Ibid., p. 72.

15. For further insight into the channels and chakras see Norbu, *The Crystal and the Way of Light*, pp. 88–93.

16. The work of visionary artist Alex Grey and the teachings of Dr. Alberto Villoldo present a powerful vision of the beauty of the luminous body and the effects of negative emotions on it. See Alex Grey, *Transfigurations* (Rochester, Vt.: Inner Traditions International, 2001), and Alberto Villoldo, *Shaman, Healer, Sage* (New York: Harmony Books, 2000). Also see the videos *ArtMind: The Healing Power of Sacred Art* with Alex Grey (Los Olivos, Calif.: Sacred Mysteries Productions, 2002) and *Healing the Luminous Body: The Way of the Shaman* (Los Olivos, Calif.: Sacred Mysteries Productions, 2002).

Chapter 3: Opening the Mystic Eye

1. For a full exposition on the healing art of craniosacral therapy see John E. Upledger and Jon Vredevoogd, *Craniosacral Therapy* (Seattle: Eastland Press, 1983).

2. Robert Masters, *The Goddess Sekhmet: Psychospiritual Exercises of the Fifth Way* (St. Paul: Llewellyn, 1991), pp. 73–74.

3. See R. A. Schwaller de Lubicz, *The Temple of Man* (Rochester, Vt.: Inner Traditions International, 1998), p. 390. In this text, which reports on a gaping head wound that penetrates to the bones, fracturing and tearing open the viscera of the patient's skull, the pulse is described as "something that throbs and flutters under your fingers like the weak place on an infant's crown before it becomes knit together."

4. Exercises such as these can be found in Dr. Masters's books *Psychophysical Method Exercises*, volumes I–VI, (Pomona, N.Y.: Kontrakundabuffer, 1983) and *Listening to the Body: The Psychophysical Way to Health and Awareness* (New York: Dell, 1978), which was coauthored with Dr. Houston, as well as the audiotape series *Masters Psychophysical Method* (Pomona, N.Y.: Kontrakundabuffer, 1983).

Chapter 4: The Keepers of the Light

1. For an in-depth view of the history and the impact of the modern Puritanical mind-set on this once sacred feminine art form, see Wendy Buonaventura, *Serpent of the Nile* (Brooklyn: Interlink Books, 1994).

2. Michael S. Schneider, *A Beginner's Guide to Constructing the Universe* (New York: HarperPerennial, 1995), p. 268. This book is an excellent introduction to the sacred geometry inherent in the patterns of nature, art, architecture, and science.

3. The translation that Jay used of the *Isis the Prophetess* text was from the book *Alchemy* by Marie-Louise von Franz (Toronto: Inner City Books, 1980). In this book, Ms. von Franz provides an excellent analysis of the text as well as a look at Greek and Arabic alchemy from a Jungian perspective.

4. This translation of *The Book of Comarios* is from the book *Alchemy: The Golden Art* (Rome: Gremese, 1995). In *The Book of Comarios* Kleopatra states, "The soul now summons the body filled with light and says, 'Awaken now from the depths of Hades, come forth from the darkness, awaken and leave the darkness behind. Because you have regained a spiritual and divine nature, the voice of resurrection has spoken and the pharmakon [medicine] of life has penetrated within you.'"

5. Ibid., pp. 23–40, for the analysis that inspired this teaching.

6. Fulcanelli, *Les Mysteres des Cathedrales* (Suffolk, England: Neville Spearman, 1977), p. 45.

7. For a fascinating look at the relationship between Isis, the Black Madonna, and the alchemical arts see the video *Isis and the Black Madonna: The Alchemical Goddesses*, by Jay Weidner and Sharron Rose (Los Olivos, Calif.: Sacred Mysteries Productions, 2003).

8. Ean Begg, *The Cult of the Black Virgin* (London: Penguin Books, 1996), pp. 64, 73.

9. Fulcanelli, *Les Mysteres des Cathedrales*, p. 58.

10. See Jansen. Based on thorough research, Jansen presents both historical sources and legendary material about the rise and development of the cult of Mary Magdalene in Europe, especially in France, during the Middle Ages. Jansen, Katherine Ludwig, *The Making of the Magdalene* (Princeton, N.J.: Princeton University Press, 2000).

11. Jansen, p. 40.

12. From a conversation between the author and Laura Lea Cannon, coauthor of the play *My Magdalene* (written with her husband, David Tresemer), for which I created the choreography. In her travels through France, Cannon discovered a tradition of using the healing oils of Mary Magdalene that was said to have been passed down to living healers in the south of France.

13. Begg, p. 99.

14. From the forward by Leslie Shepard to G. R. S. Meade, *Pistis Sophia* (Secaucus, N.J.: University Books, 1974), p. xvii.

15. Meade, p. 20, chapter 17, chapter 18.

16. Jean-Yves Leloup, *The Gospel of Mary Magdalene* (Rochester, Vt.: Inner Traditions International, 2002), p. 37.

17. James M. Robinson, ed. *The Nag Hammadi Library* (San Francisco: HarperSan Francisco, 1978), p. 148.

18. Michael Baigent, Richard Lee, and Henry Lincoln, *Holy Blood Holy Grail* (New York: Dell, 1982). This best-selling book opened the door for many others to the relationship between Jesus, Mary Magdalene, and the bloodline of the French royalty.

19. For further speculation on these themes see David Tresemer and Laura Lea Cannon's introduction to Leloup's *The Gospel of Mary Magdalene*.

20. Gershom Scholem, *On the Mystical Shape of Godhead: Basic Concepts in the Kabbalah* (New York: Schoken Books, 1991), p. 167. This book contains an entire chapter on the Shekhina.

21. Scholem, *On the Mystical Shape of Godhead*, p. 147.

22. Raphael Patai, *The Hebrew Goddess* (Detroit: Wayne University State Press, 1990), p. 99.

23. Gershom Scholem, *On the Kabbalah and Its Symbolism* (New York: Schocken Books, 1969), p. 107. This metaphorical perspective on the exile of the soul is also delineated in the gnostic text titled *The Exegesis on the Soul*, which was discovered in 1945 in Nag Hammadi. This treatise describes the process by which the feminine soul descends into the darkness of matter to grow, learn, and be reunited with her divine husband. It begins, "Wise men of old gave the soul a feminine name. Indeed she is female in her nature as well. She even has a womb. As long as she was alone with the Father she was virgin and in form androgynous. But when she fell down into a body, she then fell into the hands of many robbers. And the wanton creatures passed her from one to another. Some made use of her by force, while others did so by seducing her with a gift. In short, they defiled her. And in her body she prostituted herself and gave herself to one and all considering each one she was about to embrace as her husband."

24. Scholem, *On the Kabbalah and Its Symbolism*, p. 108. It is fascinating to note that with the *Bahir* the ancient concept of reincarnation enters the Hebrew mythos. Through the medium of parable, the *Bahir* tells us that as punishment for their sins, souls must "circulate from generation to generation," until "from [the realm of the Shekhina,] which is both the terrestrial world and a mystical region, all the souls are gathered anew, 'when the days have passed'—that is . . . at the end of time." See also Gershom Scholem, *Origins of the Kabbalah* (Princeton: Princeton University Press, 1987), pp. 176–177. Here we discover that at the end of time the Divine Feminine gathers her children and brings them home.

25. In *On the Kabbalah and Its Symbolism* Scholem tells us, "To the Kabbalists, the union between man and woman within its holy limits was a venerable mystery, as one may judge from the fact that the most classical and widely circulated Kabbalistic definition of mystical meditation is to be found in a treatise [Joseph Gikatila's *Iggereth ha Kodesh*, c. 1300] about the meaning of sexual union in marriage."

26. Patai, p. 162.

27. Ibid., p. 275.

28. Ibid.

29. Zoe Oldenbourg, *Massacre at Montsegur* (New York: Pantheon Books, 1961), p. 41.

30. For a more thorough view of the perception of the Divine Feminine in the gnostic teachings see Elaine Pagels, *The Gnostic Gospels* (New York: Vintage Books, 1989), pp. 48–69.

31. Oldenbourg, p. 44.

Chapter 5: History and the Feminine Mysteries

1. For a better understanding of the symbolic representations of the ages according to the Western tradition see Fulcanelli, *Les Mysteres des Cathedrales*, p. 169. Fulcanelli states, "In Medieval times, these four phases of the great cyclic period, whose continuous rotation was expressed in antiquity by means of a circle divided by perpendicular diameters, were generally represented by the four

evangelists, or by their symbolic letter, which was the Greek *alpha*, or more often still, by the four evangelical beasts surrounding Christ, the living human representation of the cross." He equates this symbolism with images from the great Gothic cathedrals of France, the visionary writings of Saint John and Ezekiel, and the ancient Hindu teachings. For the alchemical perspective see Fulcanelli, *The Dwellings of the Philosophers* (Boulder: Archive Press, 1999), pp. 520–522.

2. In Arthur Avalon's introduction to his translation of *The Tantra of the Great Liberation* (New York: Dover Books, 1972), pp. xivi–l, he describes from the ancient Hindu tantric perspective the yugic cycle and the resulting consequences to humanity's longevity, spiritual strength, and stature. He also describes the primary scriptures and teachings of each age and the places of pilgrimage and the avatars.

3. For further information on the end times of the current cosmic cycle and the time of transition from the Kali Yuga to the Golden Age, see Weidner and Bridges, *A Monument to the End of Time* (Mt. Gilead, N.C.: Athyrea Books, 1999); John Major Jenkins, *Maya Cosmogenesis 2012* (Santa Fe: Bear and Co., 1998); Villoldo; and the teachings of the Brahma Kumaris, a spiritual group in the Hindu Vedanta tradition.

4. Fulcanelli, *Les Mysteres des Cathedrales*, pp. 170–171.

5. For a description of manifestation from the ancient Tibetan Bon perspective see Norbu, *The Crystal and the Way of Light*, p. 59. For the ancient Hindu perspective see Manley P. Hall, *Lectures on Ancient Philosophy* (Los Angeles: The Philosophical Research Society, 1984), pp. 228–229.

6. From a personal conversation between the author and a member of the Brahma Kumaris about Brahma Kumaris spiritual knowledge at Zaca Lake Retreat (Los Olivos, Calif.: August, 2001).

7. Réné Guénon, *The Reign of Quantity and the Signs of the Times* (New Delhi: Munshiram Manoharlal, 2000), pp. 10–12.

8. Ibid., pp. 175–176. The alchemical tradition contains references to this view. In his introduction to Fulcanelli's book *Les Mysteres des Cathedrales*, Walter Lang writes, "One of the most arcane of human traditions suggests that the humanity of our Adam was not the earth's first human race. Some very advanced alchemists have hinted at a range of previous humanities in excess of thirty."

9. Avalon, pp. xivi–xivii.

10. Heinrich Zimmer, *Artistic Form in Yoga in the Sacred Images of India* (Princeton: Princeton University Press, 1984), pp. 24–25. Zimmer presents the cosmic vision of the unfolding of creation from the Hindu tantric perspective.

11. Teachings of the Brahma Kumaris.

12. Johanna Lambert, ed., *Wise Women of the Dreamtime: Aboriginal Tales of the Ancestral Powers* (Rochester, Vt.: Inner Traditions International, 1993), p. 7. For an analysis and comparison of the Aboriginal view with that of the tantric see also Robert Lawlor, *Voices of the First Day: Awakening in the Aboriginal Dreamtime* (Rochester, Vt.: Inner Traditions International, 1991), pp. 68–77.

13. Norbu, *The Crystal and the Way of Light*, p. 130. It is interesting to turn to the Tibetan Buddhist description of the Sambhogakaya realms—or realms of light inhabited by the realized beings such as spiritual masters, dakas, and dakinis—for their perspective on who we once were.

14. Lawlor, *Voices of the First Day: Awakening in the Aboriginal Dreamtime*, p. 106.

15. Ibid., p. 104

16. For a better understanding of the inner fire practice that has been handed down through the Tibetan tantric lineage see Geshe Kelsang Gyatso, *Clear Light of Bliss* (London: Wisdom Publications, 1982), chapter 2.

17. From a teaching given to the author at Zaca Lake Retreat (Los Olivos, Calif.) prior to the sacred ceremony of the Bear Dance in July 2001. In many of the traditional cultures, such as the Zulu of South Africa and Native American tribes, a woman is considered the spiritual leader and elder of the tribe, and she chooses the chief or worldly leader.

18. For an in-depth view of women during the hunter-gatherer epoch see Marija Gimbutas, *The Language of the Goddess* (San Francisco: Harper and Row, 1989) and Rianne Eisler, *The Chalice and the Blade: Our History, Our Future* (San Francisco: HarperSanFrancisco, 1988).

19. Nancy Qualls-Corbett, *The Sacred Prostitute* (Toronto: Inner City Books, 1988), p. 30.

20. Teachings of the Brahma Kumaris.

21. For a more complete picture of the results of this shift in perspective see William Irwin Thompson, *The Time Falling Bodies Take to Light* (New York: St. Martin's Press, 1981), pp. 118–159.

22. Teachings of the Brahma Kumaris.

23. R. A. Schwaller de Lubicz, *The Temple of Man*. This two-volume set describes the sacred teaching of ancient Egypt as evidenced in the architecture of the Temple of Luxor.

24. In *The Dance of India*, Bhavani states, "Art was meant for all and through it Hindu religious thought and philosophy were conveyed to all classes of society. To make these abstract theological teachings understood by the average person, symbols were created which clarified the inner meaning of the highly philosophical precepts of the Vedas, etc. A great culture developed where the highly abstruse, ethical philosophies were put into concrete, explicit form."

25. For more on the origins of the *Natya Shastra* see Michael, pp. vii–ix.

26. Vatsyayana, *Kama Sutra* (New York: Castle Books, 1963), pp. 13–15.

27. For information on the priestesses in the temples of the ancient Middle Eastern, Greek, Roman, and Celtic traditions see Norma Lorre Goodrich, *Priestesses* (New York: Harper Perennial, 1989). In this extensive book Goodrich explores the lives of the priestesses.

28. For a compelling view of the moment in the Middle Ages when the sacred view of sound shifted in the European mindset, see Naydler, pp. 139–140. Jeremy Naydler, *The Temple of the Cosmos* (Rochester, Vt.: Inner Traditions International, 1996) (first revision).

29. See Robert Lawlor's introduction to R. A. Schwaller de Lubicz, *Symbol and Symbolique* (Rochester, Vt.: Inner Traditions International, 1978), pp. 10–11.

30. For an extensive exposition on the effect of the written word on humanity, with emphasis on its impact on women, see Leonard Shlain, *The Alphabet Versus the Goddess* (New York: Penguin Putnam, Inc., 1998).

31. Guénon, *The Reign of Quantity and the Signs of the Times*, pp. 66–77.

32. Elaine Pagels, *Adam, Eve and the Serpent* (New York: Vintage Books, 1988), p. 133.

33. There have even been tales of women who were found guilty merely because their male inquisitors became sexually aroused during torture.

34. Guénon, *The Reign of Quantity and the Signs of the Times*, pp. 65–67.

35. In a conversation with a swami of the Hare Krishnas at Zaca Lake Retreat, I learned that they believe that the Kali Yuga began 5,000 years ago and that we still have 432,000 years left before the end of the cycle and the beginning of the new Golden Age.

36. Villoldo, pp. 233–234.

37. Isha Schwaller de Lubicz, *The Opening of the Way* (Rochester, Vt.: Inner Traditions International, 1981), p. 11. Writes de Lubicz, "Behind all religions there is only one 'Truth,' and the revelation of this truth through their different myths and symbols brings harmony instead of discord. Every sincere seeker has in his heart this 'will toward the Light' and if he listens to it, he will not seek in vain."

38. See John Reynolds, trans., *Self-Liberation Through Seeing with Naked Awareness* (Barrytown, N.Y.: Station Hill Press, 1989), p. 38

39. Namkhai Norbu and Adriano Clemente, *The Supreme Source* (Ithaca, N.Y.: Snow Lion, 1999), p. 22. In this Tantra the location of these worlds and the nature of the beings that dwell in them are described.

Chapter 6: Lifting the Veil from the Face of Modernity

1. For more information on the history, practices, and biographies of priestesses, yoginis, and temple dancers see Miranda Shaw, *Passionate Enlightenment: Women in Tantric Buddhism* (Princeton, N.J.: Princeton University Press, 1994); Allione; and Frederique Apffel Marglin, *Wives of the God-King: The Rituals of the Devadasis of Puri* (Delhi: Oxford Press, 1985); and Goodrich.

2. According to Jansen, p. 27, in early Christianity the feminine principle was associated with "vision, prophesy and spiritual understanding as embodied by Mary Magdalene" and the masculine principle was associated with "apostolic tradition, hierarchy and acquired knowledge as represented by Peter." For information on the Tibetan Buddhist view of the natural roles and inclinations of the female and the male see Keith Dowman, *Sky Dancer: The Secret Life and Songs of the Lady Yeshe Tsogyel* (London: Routledge and Kegan Paul, 1984), pp. 253–255.

3. Kumar, p.100. This belief is particularly evident in Hindu tantra.

4. For more insight into this metaphor see Scholem, *On the Kabbalah and Its Symbolism*, pp. 106–107, and Maddalena Scopello's introduction in *The Nag Hammadi Library*, pp. 190–192.

5. From the Tibetan tantric viewpoint women's innate wisdom, sensitivity, and insight into the magical display of forms that arise from the empty nature of reality made them ripe for this significant task.

6. Based on a conversation between the author and the scholar Robert Lawlor in Nederland, Colorado, in July 1997.

7. Lambert, p. 78.

8. See Lynn Picknett and Clive Prince, *The Stargate Conspiracy* (London: Little, Brown and Company, 1999), pp. 350–351.

9. See Patai, pp. 273–276.

10. See Matityahu Glazerson, *Building Blocks of the Soul: Studies on the Letters and Words of the Hebrew Language* (Northvale, N.J.: Jason Aronson, Inc., 1997), pp. 115, 122. This excellent book on *gematria*, or interpretive Jewish numerology, brings new insight into the significance of and reverence for the woman in the Jewish tradition in her role as protector and "Keeper of the Light."

11. Judith Simmer-Brown, *Dakini's Warm Breath* (Boston: Shambhala, 2001), p. 35.

12. Namkhai Ningpo, *Mother of Knowledge: The Enlightenment of Yeshe Tsogyel* (Berkeley, Calif.: Dharma Publishing, 1983), p. 102.

13. Elaine Pagels, *The Gnostic Gospels* (New York: Vintage Books, 1989), pp. 54–59.

14. Leloup, p. 31.

15. For an in-depth look at these issues see Betty Friedan, *The Feminine Mystique* (New York: W. W. Norton and Company, 1997), pp. 182–183.

16. Friedan, p. 186.

17. For insight into the impact of the theories and methods of Freud and his fellow psychotherapists on modern society and on women see Friedan, chapter 5.

18. "Obit: Edward L. Bernays: Father of PR," *PR Watch* (March 9, 1995), p. 103.

19. Tim O'Shea, *The Doors of Perception: Why Americans Will Believe Almost Anything* (Rense.com, August 18, 2001).

20. Sheldon Rampton and John Stauber, *Trust Us, We're Experts* (Los Angeles: Tarcher/Putnam, 2001), pp. 22, 45, 92.

21. Evidence of this mystic alignment comes to us through the teachings and practices of Indo-Tibetan tantra and temple dance, in which students are presented with specific deity practices for attuning their energies and emotions to a more enlightened level of awareness.

22. Naomi Wolf, *The Beauty Myth* (New York: Anchor Books, 1991), p. 10.

23. Lambert, p. 7.

24. Kelly Patricia O'Meara, *Doping Kids* (*Insight in the News Magazine*, June 28, 1999). According to investigative reporter O'Meara, there are nearly six million children in America between the ages of six and eighteen taking mind-altering pharmaceuticals. In addition, I recently heard a news report that stated that more prescriptions for Ritalin are written for toddlers than any other pharmaceutical, including antibiotics.

25. Confirmations took place in the Roman Catholic faith and bar mitzvahs still existed in the Jewish tradition, but in the immigrant communities rushing to assimilate the secular value of materialism

these time-honored rites of passage almost became parodies of the ancient rites. From my perspective as a child growing up in the Jewish tradition, I felt that both parents and their children appeared to be more concerned with how lavishly they could throw a party and how many gifts would be received than with the spiritual nature of the rite. Many Western esoteric scholars believe that the lineage of transmission was broken in the West at the end of the Middle Ages. Julius Evola, in his excellent book *The Hermetic Tradition, Symbols and Teachings of the Royal Art* (Rochester, Vt.: Inner Traditions International, 1971), states, "Modern civilization stands on one side and on the other the entirety of all the civilizations that have preceded it. (For the West, we can put the dividing line at the Middle Ages). There are two worlds, one which has separated itself by cutting off nearly every contact with the past. For the great majority of moderns, that means any possibility of understanding the traditional world has been completely lost."

26. For a scathing commentary on the rise of neospiritualism in the West and the machinations of the counterfeit initiation see Réné Guénon, *The Reign of Quantity and the Signs of the Times*.

27. Réné Guénon, *Perspectives on Initiation* (Ghent: Sophia Perennis, 2001). Chapter 22 of this book contains an excellent description of the traditional problems for the initiate that are inherent in the acquisition and development of "psychic powers." For deeper insight into the Tibetan Buddhist perspective on "magic" see Chogyam Trungpa, *Journey Without a Goal* (Boston: Shambhala, Inc, 1981), pp. 109–115.

28. Goodrich, pp. 201–202.

29. Guénon, *Perspectives on Initiation*, pp. 48–55.

30. In his training program for Western shamans, Dr. Alberto Villoldo often speaks about these issues. In the video *Healing the Luminous Body: The Way of the Shaman* (Los Olivos, Calif.: Sacred Mysteries Productions, 2002) he states, "There are dangers associated with energy medicine. These are dangers seldom pointed out by practitioners. I've had many people come to my office after they have seen an energy healer who has applied energy to their cancer only to have their cancer metastasize throughout their body. We have to be very careful, for these are extraordinarily powerful practices that can disinhibit the immune response or accelerate the growth of a cancer in the body."

31. In *The Crystal and the Way of Light*, p. 139, Namkhai Norbu Rinpoche states, "Our mind is the basis of everything, and from our mind everything arises, Samsara and Nirvana, ordinary sentient beings and Enlightened Ones . . . Even though the Essence of the Mind, the true nature of our mind, is totally pure right from the beginning, nevertheless, because pure mind is temporarily obscured by the impurity of ignorance, there is no recognition of our own State. Through this lack of self-recognition arise illusory thoughts and actions created by the passions."

Chapter 7: Discovering Strength and Power

1. For a better understanding of the essence and manifestations of Kali, see Lex Hixon, *Mother of the Universe: Visions of the Goddess and Tantric Hymns of Enlightenment* (Wheaton, Ill.: Quest Books, 1994). This book is an exploration and recreation of the mystic poetry of Ramprasad Sen. These hymns to and revelations of the activities and attributes of the Great Goddess provide insight into one man's hunger for completion and union with the Divine Feminine.

2. Masters, *The Goddess Sekhmet*, p. 48.

3. Alison Roberts, *Hathor Rising* (Rochester, Vt.: Inner Traditions International, 1995), pp. 10–11. She is the "confused one in the night," totally out of control and "wading in their blood as far as Heracleopolis." All this, says the goddess, "is balm for my heart."

4. Weidner and Bridges, pp. 194, 233.

5. The Hindu scripture the *Devi Mahatmyam* dates back to the twelfth century A.D., and first appears in the *Markandeya Purana* composed by the sage Markandeya. However, it is clear from the statuary that dates back to the fourth century, as well as from tales of her connection with the indigenous

Dravidian or pre-Aryan culture of India, that she is a much older goddess whose worship dates to before the advent of the written word.

6. See Nik Douglas and Penny Slinger, *Sexual Secrets* (Rochester, Vt.: Destiny Books, 1979), pp. 108, 109, and John Myrdhin Reynolds, *The Golden Letters* (Ithaca, N.Y.: Snow Lion, 1996), p. 157 for more in-depth information concerning these subtle channels.

Chapter 8: Exploring Sensuality

1. Heinrich Zimmer, *Myths and Symbols in Indian Art and Civilization* (New York: Harper and Row, 1962), pp. 91–93.
2. David Kinsley, *Hindu Goddesses* (New Delhi: Motilal Banarsidass, 1986), p. 31.
3. Ibid., p. 29.
4. Murray Hope, *Practical Egyptian Magic* (New York: St. Martin's Press, 1984), p. 106.
5. E. A. Wallis Budge, *The Gods of the Ancient Egyptians* (1904; reprint, New York: Dover, 1969), p. 429.
6. Ibid., p. 435.
7. This translation is taken from James Wasserman and Dr. Raymond O. Falkner, *The Egyptian Book of the Dead* (San Francisco: Chronicle Books, 1994), plate 37.
8. Diane Wolkstein and Samuel Noah Kramer, *Inanna, Queen of Heaven and Earth* (New York: Harper and Row, 1983), pp. 16–18.
9. For a thorough analysis of this tale see Wolkstein and Kramer, pp. 146–150.
10. Ibid., p. 37.
11. Lama Chonam and Sangye Khandro, *The Lives and Liberation of Princess Mandarava* (Boston: Wisdom Publications, 1998). This retelling of Mandarava's story is based on a translation of the terma, or wisdom text, of the yogi Samten Lingpa, who was born circa 1871.
12. Shaw, p. 79. This work presents extensive evidence of the fundamental role women played in the transmission of the tantric arts, particularly in the domain of sexuality.

Chapter 9: Experiencing Love and Compassion

1. Manley P. Hall, *The Secret Teachings of All Ages* (Los Angeles: The Philosophical Research Society, Inc., 1988), p. xiv. For an evocative account of Isis and her symbolism and insight into her mysteries as performed throughout the ancient world, see the chapter "Isis, the Virgin of the World."
2. Weidner and Rose, *Isis and the Black Madonna; The Alchemical Goddesses* (video), (Los Olivos, Calif.: Sacred Mysteries Productions, 2003).
3. Maria Warner, *Alone of All Her Sex: The Myth and the Cult of the Virgin Mary* (New York: Alfred A. Knopf, 1976), pp. 315–316.
4. Martin Palmer and Jay Ramsay with Man-Ho Kwok, *Kuan Yin: Myths and Prophecies of the Chinese Goddess of Compassion* (London: Thorsons, 1995), p. 25.
5. Ibid., p. 26.
6. John Blofeld, *Bodhisattva of Compassion: The Mystical Tradition of Kuan Yin* (Boston: Shambhala, 1988). A personal account of Blofeld's search for the history, legends, rituals, and worship of Kuan Yin.
7. This prayer was taught to me by Prema Dasara, a talented sacred dancer and spiritual teacher, at a retreat she held in Woodstock, New York, in the summer of 1994. During this retreat she gave instruction in the Dance of the Twenty-One Taras.
8. See John Reynolds, trans., *The Golden Rosary of Tara* (Arcidosso, Italy: Shang-Shung Edizioni, 1985) for deeper insight into her history and manifestations.

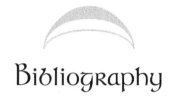

Bibliography

Allione, Tsultrim. *Women of Wisdom*. Ithaca, N.Y.: Snow Lion, 2000.

Avalon, Arthur. *The Serpent Power*. New York: Dover, 1974.

_____. *The Tantra of the Great Liberation*. New York: Dover, 1972.

Bach, Hilde. *Indian Love Paintings*. New Delhi: Lustre Press, 1985.

Baigent, Michael, Richard Lee, and Henry Lincoln. *Holy Blood, Holy Grail*. New York: Dell, 1982.

Balyoz, Harold. *Three Remarkable Women*. Flagstaff, Ariz.: Altai, 1986.

Bamford, Christopher, ed. *Rediscovering Sacred Science*. Edinburg: Floris, 1994.

Banerji, Projesh. *Dance of India*. Allahabad, India: Allahabad Law Journal Press, 1947.

Begg, Ean. *The Cult of the Black Virgin*. London: Penguin, 1996.

Beyer, Stephen. *The Cult of Tara*. Berkeley, Calif.: University of California Press, 1978.

Bharatmuni. *The Natya Shastra*. New Delhi: Sri Satguru, n.d.

Bhattacharya, Shiva. *Principles of Tantra*. Madras: Ganesh and Company, 1978.

Bhavani, Enakshi. *The Dance in India*. Bombay: D. B. Taraporevala Sons and Co., 1965.

Birks, Walter, and R.A. Gilbert. *The Treasure of Montsegur*. Great Britain: Crucible, 1987.

Blofeld, John. *Bodhisattva of Compassion: The Mystical Tradition of Kuan Yin*. Boston: Shambhala, 1988.

Bolen, Jean Shinoda. *Goddesses in Everywoman*. New York: Harper and Row, 1984.

Brunn, Emilie Zum and Georgette Epiney-Burgard. *Women Mystics in Medieval Europe*. New York: Paragon House, 1989.

Budge, E. A. Wallis. *Egyptian Magic*. New York: Dover, 1971.

_____. *The Gods of the Ancient Egyptians*. New York: Dover, 1969.

Bumiller, Elisabeth. *May You Be the Mother of a Hundred Sons: A Journey among the Women in India*. New York: Random House, 1990.

Buonaventura, Wendy. *Serpent of the Nile*. Brooklyn: Interlink, 1994.

Capel, Anne K., and Glenn E. Markoe, eds. *Mistress of the House, Mistress of Heaven: Women in Ancient Egypt*. New York: Hudson Hills, 1996.

Chailley, Jacques. *The Magic Flute Unveiled*. Rochester, Vt.: Inner Traditions International, 1992.

Charpentier, Louis. *The Mysteries of Chartres Cathedral*. Haverhill: Rilko, 1972.

Chonam, Lama, and Sangye Khandro. *The Lives and Liberation of Princess Mandarava*. Boston: Wisdom Publications, 1998.

Compton, Madonna. *Archetypes on the Tree of Life*. St. Paul: Llewellyn, 1991.

Coomarswamy, Ananda K. *The Dance of Shiva: Essays on Indian Art and Culture.* New York: Harper and Row, 1984.

Coomarswamy, Ananda K., and Gopala Kristnayya Duggirala. *The Mirror of Gesture.* New Delhi: Munshiram Manoharlal, 1977.

Dagyab, Loden Sherab Rinpoche. *Buddhist Symbols in Tibetan Culture.* Boston: Wisdom Publications, 1995.

Das, H. C. *Tantricism: A Study of the Yogini Cult.* New Delhi: Sterling Publishers, 1981.

De Boer, Esther. *Mary Magdalene: Beyond the Myth.* Harrisburg: Trinity Press, 1997.

Deneck, Margarite-Marie. *Indian Art.* London: Paul Hamlyn, 1967.

DePascalis, Andrea. *Alchemy: The Golden Art.* Rome: Gremese International, 1995.

Doresse, Jean. *The Secret Books of the Egyptian Gnostics.* New York: MJF Books, 1986.

De Rola, Stanislas Klossowski. *The Golden Game.* London: Thames and Hudson, 1988.

Douglas, Kenneth, and Gwendolyn Bays, trans. *The Life and Liberation of Padmasambhava.* Berkeley, Calif.: Dharma Publications, 1978.

Douglas, Nik, and Penny Slinger. *Sexual Secrets.* Rochester, Vt.: Destiny Books, 1979.

Dowman, Keith, trans. *The Flight of the Garuda.* Boston: Wisdom Publications, 1994.

————. *Sky Dancer: The Secret Life and Songs of the Lady Yeshe Tsogyel.* London: Routledge and Kegan Paul, 1984.

Eisler, Rianne. *The Chalice and the Blade.* San Francisco: HarperSanFrancisco, 1988.

Eliade, Mircea. *The Sacred and the Profane.* New York: Harcourt, Brace and World, 1959.

Evola, Julius. *The Hermetic Tradition: Symbols and Teachings of the Royal Art.* Rochester, Vt.: Inner Traditions International, 1971.

Evans-Wentz, W. Y. *Tibetan Yoga.* London: Oxford University Press, 1958.

Filoramo, Giovanni. *A History of Gnosticism.* Oxford: Blackwell Publishers, 1990.

Fortune, Dion. *The Mystical Qabalah.* York Beach, Me.: Samuel Weiser, 1984.

Fredrikksson, Marianne. *According to Mary Magdalene.* Charlottesville, Va.: Hampton Roads, 1999.

Friedan, Betty. *The Feminine Mystique.* New York: W. W. Norton, 1997.

Fulcanelli. *Les Mysteres des Cathedrales.* Suffolk, England: Neville Spearman Limited, 1977.

————. *The Dwellings of the Philosophers.* Boulder: Archive Press, 1999.

Gimbutas, Marija. *The Language of the Goddess.* San Francisco: Harper and Row, 1989.

Glazerson, Matityahu. *Building Blocks of the Soul: Studies on the Letters and Words of the Hebrew Language.* Northvale: Jason Aronson, 1997.

Godwin, Joscelyn, Christian Chanel, and John P. Deveny. *The Hermetic Brotherhood of Luxor.* York Beach, Me.: Samuel Weiser, 1995.

Goodrich, Norma Lorre. *Priestesses.* New York: Harper Perennial, 1989.

Gordon, Antoinette. *The Iconography of Tibetan Lamaism.* Rutland, Vt.: Charles E. Tuttle, 1939.

Graves, Robert. *The White Goddess.* New York: Farrar, Straus and Giroux, 1948.

Gray, William G. *The Office of the Holy Tree of Life.* Dallas: Sounds of Light, 1970.

Green, Miranda. *Celtic Goddesses.* London: British Museum Press, 1995.

Greer, Germaine. *The Female Eunich.* New York: McGraw-Hill, 1970.

Grey, Alex. *Art Mind: The Healing Power of Sacred Art* (video). Los Olivos, Calif.: Sacred Mysteries Productions, 2002.

Grey, Alex. *Transfigurations.* Rochester, Vt.: Inner Traditions International, 2001.

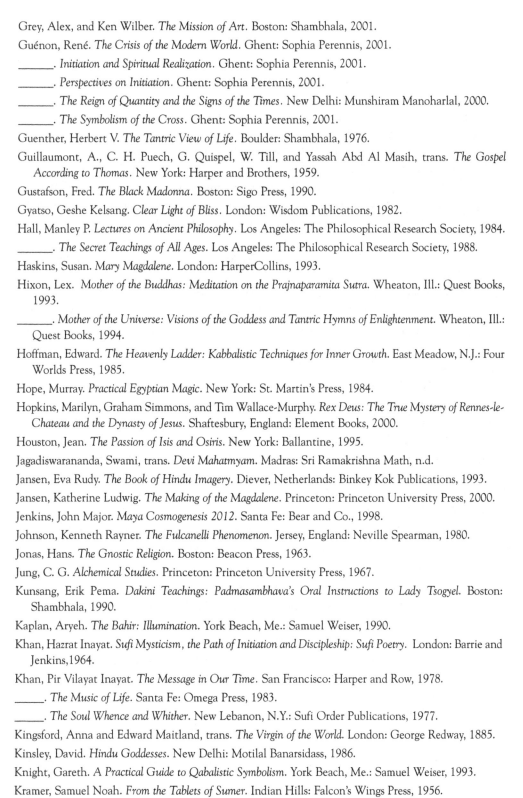

Grey, Alex, and Ken Wilber. *The Mission of Art*. Boston: Shambhala, 2001.

Guénon, René. *The Crisis of the Modern World*. Ghent: Sophia Perennis, 2001.

_____. *Initiation and Spiritual Realization*. Ghent: Sophia Perennis, 2001.

_____. *Perspectives on Initiation*. Ghent: Sophia Perennis, 2001.

_____. *The Reign of Quantity and the Signs of the Times*. New Delhi: Munshiram Manoharlal, 2000.

_____. *The Symbolism of the Cross*. Ghent: Sophia Perennis, 2001.

Guenther, Herbert V. *The Tantric View of Life*. Boulder: Shambhala, 1976.

Guillaumont, A., C. H. Puech, G. Quispel, W. Till, and Yassah Abd Al Masih, trans. *The Gospel According to Thomas*. New York: Harper and Brothers, 1959.

Gustafson, Fred. *The Black Madonna*. Boston: Sigo Press, 1990.

Gyatso, Geshe Kelsang. *Clear Light of Bliss*. London: Wisdom Publications, 1982.

Hall, Manley P. *Lectures on Ancient Philosophy*. Los Angeles: The Philosophical Research Society, 1984.

_____. *The Secret Teachings of All Ages*. Los Angeles: The Philosophical Research Society, 1988.

Haskins, Susan. *Mary Magdalene*. London: HarperCollins, 1993.

Hixon, Lex. *Mother of the Buddhas: Meditation on the Prajnaparamita Sutra*. Wheaton, Ill.: Quest Books, 1993.

_____. *Mother of the Universe: Visions of the Goddess and Tantric Hymns of Enlightenment*. Wheaton, Ill.: Quest Books, 1994.

Hoffman, Edward. *The Heavenly Ladder: Kabbalistic Techniques for Inner Growth*. East Meadow, N.J.: Four Worlds Press, 1985.

Hope, Murray. *Practical Egyptian Magic*. New York: St. Martin's Press, 1984.

Hopkins, Marilyn, Graham Simmons, and Tim Wallace-Murphy. *Rex Deus: The True Mystery of Rennes-le-Chateau and the Dynasty of Jesus*. Shaftesbury, England: Element Books, 2000.

Houston, Jean. *The Passion of Isis and Osiris*. New York: Ballantine, 1995.

Jagadiswarananda, Swami, trans. *Devi Mahatmyam*. Madras: Sri Ramakrishna Math, n.d.

Jansen, Eva Rudy. *The Book of Hindu Imagery*. Diever, Netherlands: Binkey Kok Publications, 1993.

Jansen, Katherine Ludwig. *The Making of the Magdalene*. Princeton: Princeton University Press, 2000.

Jenkins, John Major. *Maya Cosmogenesis 2012*. Santa Fe: Bear and Co., 1998.

Johnson, Kenneth Rayner. *The Fulcanelli Phenomenon*. Jersey, England: Neville Spearman, 1980.

Jonas, Hans. *The Gnostic Religion*. Boston: Beacon Press, 1963.

Jung, C. G. *Alchemical Studies*. Princeton: Princeton University Press, 1967.

Kunsang, Erik Pema. *Dakini Teachings: Padmasambhava's Oral Instructions to Lady Tsogyel*. Boston: Shambhala, 1990.

Kaplan, Aryeh. *The Bahir: Illumination*. York Beach, Me.: Samuel Weiser, 1990.

Khan, Hazrat Inayat. *Sufi Mysticism, the Path of Initiation and Discipleship: Sufi Poetry*. London: Barrie and Jenkins, 1964.

Khan, Pir Vilayat Inayat. *The Message in Our Time*. San Francisco: Harper and Row, 1978.

_____. *The Music of Life*. Santa Fe: Omega Press, 1983.

_____. *The Soul Whence and Whither*. New Lebanon, N.Y.: Sufi Order Publications, 1977.

Kingsford, Anna and Edward Maitland, trans. *The Virgin of the World*. London: George Redway, 1885.

Kinsley, David. *Hindu Goddesses*. New Delhi: Motilal Banarsidass, 1986.

Knight, Gareth. *A Practical Guide to Qabalistic Symbolism*. York Beach, Me.: Samuel Weiser, 1993.

Kramer, Samuel Noah. *From the Tablets of Sumer*. Indian Hills: Falcon's Wings Press, 1956.

Kramrisch, Stella. *The Presence of Shiva*. Princeton: Princeton University Press, 1981.

Kumar, Dr. Pushpendra, Ph.D. *Shakti Cult in Ancient India*. Varanasi, India: Bhartiya Publishing, 1974.

Lacarrier, Jacques. *The Gnostics*. San Francisco: City Lights, 1989.

Lambert, Johanna, ed. *Wise Women of the Dreamtime: Aboriginal Tales of the Ancestral Powers*. Rochester, Vt.: Inner Traditions International, 1993.

Lawlor, Robert. *Voices of the First Day: Awakening in the Aboriginal Dreamtime*. Rochester, Vt.: Inner Traditions International, 1991.

Leet, Leonora. *Renewing the Covenant: A Kabbalistic Guide to Jewish Spirituality*. Rochester, Vt.: Inner Traditions International, 1999.

_____. *The Secret Doctrine of the Kabbalah*. Rochester, Vt.: Inner Traditions International, 1999.

Leloup, Jean-Yves. *The Gospel of Mary Magdalene*. Rochester, Vt.: Inner Traditions International, 2002.

Levi, Louise Landes. *Sweet on My Lips: The Love Poems of Mirabai*. New York: Cool Grove Publishing, 1997.

Marglin, Frederique Apffel. *Wives of the God-King: The Rituals of the Devadasis of Puri*. Delhi: Oxford Press, 1985.

Massey, Reginald, and Jamilla Massey. *The Dances of India*. London: Tricolor Books, 1989.

Masters, Robert. *The Goddess Sekhmet: Psychospiritual Exercises of the Fifth Way*. St. Paul: Llewellyn, 1991.

Masters, Robert, and Jean Houston. *Listening to the Body: The Psychophysical Way to Health and Awareness*. New York: Dell, 1978.

_____. *Mind Games*. New York: Dorset Press, 1972.

_____. *Neurospeak*. Wheaton, Ill.: Quest Books, 1994.

_____. *Psychophysical Method Exercises*, vol. 1–6. Pomona, N.Y.: Kontrakundabuffer, 1983.

Matthews, Caitlin. *Sophia, Goddess of Wisdom*. London: Thorsons, 1992.

Meade, G. R. S. *Pistis Sophia*. Secaucus, N.J.: University Books, 1974.

Meltzer, David, ed. *The Secret Garden: An Anthology of the Kabbalah*. Barrytown, N.Y.: Station Hill Press, 1999.

Meyer, Marvin W., ed. *The Ancient Mysteries*. San Francisco: Harper and Row, 1987.

Michael, Tara. *The Symbolic Gestures of the Hands*. Paris: Editions Semaphore, 1985.

Mookerjee, Ajit. *Kundalini: The Arousal of the Inner Energy*. Rochester, Vt.: Destiny Books, 1986.

_____. *Tantra Asana: A Way to Self-Realization*. Basel: Basilius Press, 1971.

Moor, Edward. *The Hindu Pantheon*. Los Angeles: The Philosophical Research Society, 1976.

Naydler, Jeremy. *The Temple of the Cosmos*. Rochester, Vt.: Inner Traditions International, 1996.

Ningpo, Namkhai. *Mother of Knowledge: The Enlightenment of Yeshe Tsogyel*. Berkeley, Calif.: Dharma Publishing, 1983.

Norbu, Namkhai. *The Crystal and the Way of Light*. New York: Routledge and Keegan Paul, 1986.

_____. *The Cycle of Day and Night: An Essential Tibetan Text on the Practice of Contemplation*. Oakland, Calif.: Zhang Zhung Editions, 1984.

_____. *The Cycle of Day and Night: An Essential Tibetan Text on the Practice of Contemplation*. Barrytown, N.Y.: Station Hill Press, 1987.

Norbu, Namkhai, and Adriano Clemente. *The Supreme Source*, Ithaca, N.Y.: Snow Lion Publications, 1999.

Norbu, Namkhai, and Michael Katz, ed. *Dream Yoga and the Practice of Natural Light*, Ithaca, N.Y.: Snow Lion, 1992.

Norbu, Namkhai, and Kennard Lippman, trans. *Primordial Experience: An Introduction to Dzogs-Chen Meditation*. Boston: Shambhala, 1978.

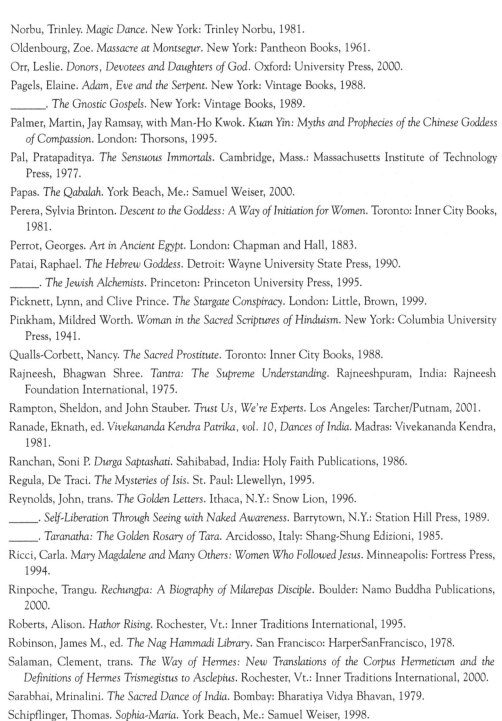

Norbu, Trinley. *Magic Dance*. New York: Trinley Norbu, 1981.

Oldenbourg, Zoe. *Massacre at Montsegur*. New York: Pantheon Books, 1961.

Orr, Leslie. *Donors, Devotees and Daughters of God*. Oxford: University Press, 2000.

Pagels, Elaine. *Adam, Eve and the Serpent*. New York: Vintage Books, 1988.

_____. *The Gnostic Gospels*. New York: Vintage Books, 1989.

Palmer, Martin, Jay Ramsay, with Man-Ho Kwok. *Kuan Yin: Myths and Prophecies of the Chinese Goddess of Compassion*. London: Thorsons, 1995.

Pal, Pratapaditya. *The Sensuous Immortals*. Cambridge, Mass.: Massachusetts Institute of Technology Press, 1977.

Papas. *The Qabalah*. York Beach, Me.: Samuel Weiser, 2000.

Perera, Sylvia Brinton. *Descent to the Goddess: A Way of Initiation for Women*. Toronto: Inner City Books, 1981.

Perrot, Georges. *Art in Ancient Egypt*. London: Chapman and Hall, 1883.

Patai, Raphael. *The Hebrew Goddess*. Detroit: Wayne University State Press, 1990.

_____. *The Jewish Alchemists*. Princeton: Princeton University Press, 1995.

Picknett, Lynn, and Clive Prince. *The Stargate Conspiracy*. London: Little, Brown, 1999.

Pinkham, Mildred Worth. *Woman in the Sacred Scriptures of Hinduism*. New York: Columbia University Press, 1941.

Qualls-Corbett, Nancy. *The Sacred Prostitute*. Toronto: Inner City Books, 1988.

Rajneesh, Bhagwan Shree. *Tantra: The Supreme Understanding*. Rajneeshpuram, India: Rajneesh Foundation International, 1975.

Rampton, Sheldon, and John Stauber. *Trust Us, We're Experts*. Los Angeles: Tarcher/Putnam, 2001.

Ranade, Eknath, ed. *Vivekananda Kendra Patrika, vol. 10, Dances of India*. Madras: Vivekananda Kendra, 1981.

Ranchan, Soni P. *Durga Saptashati*. Sahibabad, India: Holy Faith Publications, 1986.

Regula, De Traci. *The Mysteries of Isis*. St. Paul: Llewellyn, 1995.

Reynolds, John, trans. *The Golden Letters*. Ithaca, N.Y.: Snow Lion, 1996.

_____. *Self-Liberation Through Seeing with Naked Awareness*. Barrytown, N.Y.: Station Hill Press, 1989.

_____. *Taranatha: The Golden Rosary of Tara*. Arcidosso, Italy: Shang-Shung Edizioni, 1985.

Ricci, Carla. *Mary Magdalene and Many Others: Women Who Followed Jesus*. Minneapolis: Fortress Press, 1994.

Rinpoche, Trangu. *Rechungpa: A Biography of Milarepas Disciple*. Boulder: Namo Buddha Publications, 2000.

Roberts, Alison. *Hathor Rising*. Rochester, Vt.: Inner Traditions International, 1995.

Robinson, James M., ed. *The Nag Hammadi Library*. San Francisco: HarperSanFrancisco, 1978.

Salaman, Clement, trans. *The Way of Hermes: New Translations of the Corpus Hermeticum and the Definitions of Hermes Trismegistus to Asclepius*. Rochester, Vt.: Inner Traditions International, 2000.

Sarabhai, Mrinalini. *The Sacred Dance of India*. Bombay: Bharatiya Vidya Bhavan, 1979.

Schipflinger, Thomas. *Sophia-Maria*. York Beach, Me.: Samuel Weiser, 1998.

Scholem, Gershon. *On the Kabbalah and Its Symbolism*. New York: Schocken Books, 1969.

_____. *On the Mystical Shape of Godhead: Basic Concepts in the Kabbalah*, New York: Schocken Books, 1991.

_____. *Origins of the Kabbalah*. Princeton: Princeton University Press, 1987.

Schneider, Michael S. *A Beginner's Guide to Constructing the Universe*. New York: HarperPerennial, 1995.

Schwaller de Lubicz, Isha. *The Opening of the Way*. Rochester, Vt.: Inner Traditions International, 1981.

Schwaller de Lubicz, R. A. *Esotericism and Symbol*. Rochester, Vt.: Inner Traditions International, 1985.

_____. *Nature Word*. Rochester, Vt.: Inner Traditions International, 1990.

_____. *Symbol and Symbolique*. Rochester, Vt.: Inner Traditions International, 1978.

_____. *The Temple of Man*. Rochester, Vt.: Inner Traditions International, 1998.

Shaw, Miranda. *Passionate Enlightenment: Women in Tantric Buddhism*. Princeton: Princeton University Press, 1994.

Shlain, Leonard. *The Alphabet Versus the Goddess*. New York: Penguin Putnam, 1998.

Simmer-Brown, Judith. *Dakini's Warm Breath*. Boston: Shambhala, 2001.

Singh, Hazur Maharaj Sawan. *Philosophy of the Masters*. Punjab, India: Radha Soami Satsang, 1964.

Singh, Jaideva. *Vijnanabhairava or Divine Consciousness*. New Delhi, India: Motilal Banarsidass, 1981.

Starbird, Margaret. *The Woman with the Alabaster Jar*. Santa Fe: Bear and Co., 1993.

Stevens, John. *Lust for Enlightenment*. Boston: Shambhala, 1990.

Svoboda, Robert E. *Aghora: At the Left Hand of God*. Albuquerque: Brotherhood of Life, 1986.

_____. *Aghora II*. Albuquerque: Brotherhood of Life, 1993.

Thompson, Richard. *Mysteries of the Sacred Universe*. San Diego: Govardhan Hill, 2000.

Thompson, William Irwin. *Darkness and Scattered Light*. Garden City, N.Y.: Anchor Press, 1978.

_____. *The Time Falling Bodies Take to Light*. New York: St. Martin's Press, 1981.

Trungpa, Chogyam. *Cutting Through Spiritual Materialism*. Boston: Shambhala, 1973.

_____. *Journey Without a Goal*. Boston: Shambhala, 1981.

_____. *The Myth of Freedom*. Berkeley: Shambhala, 1976.

Tyldesley, Joyce. *Daughters of Isis: Women of Ancient Egypt*. London: Viking, 1994.

Upledger, John E. *Craniosacral Therapy II*. Seattle: Eastland, 1987.

Upledger, John E. and Jon Vredevoogd. *Craniosacral Therapy*. Seattle: Eastland, 1983.

Vatsyayana. *Kama Sutra*. New York: Castle Books, 1963.

Vatsyayan, Dr. Kapila. *Classical Indian Dance in Literature and the Arts*. New Delhi: Sangeet Nayak Akademi, 1968.

Villoldo, Alberto. *Healing the Luminous Body: The Way of the Shaman* (video). Los Olivos, Calif.: Sacred Mysteries Productions, 2002.

———. *Shaman, Healer, Sage*. New York: Harmony Books, 2000.

Von Franz, Marie-Louise. *Alchemy*. Toronto: Inner City Books, 1980.

Von Simson, Otto. *The Gothic Cathedral*. New York: Harper and Row, 1956.

Wangyal, Tenzin. *Wonders of the Natural Mind*. Barrytown, N.Y.: Station Hill Press, 1993.

Warner, Maria. *Alone of All Her Sex: The Myth and the Cult of the Virgin Mary*. New York: Alfred A. Knopf, 1976.

Wasserman, James, and Dr. Raymond O. Falkner. *The Egyptian Book of the Dead*. San Francisco: Chronicle Books, 1994.

Weidner, Jay, and Sharron Rose. *Isis and the Black Madonna: The Alchemical Goddesses* (video). Los Olivos, Calif.: Sacred Mysteries Productions, 2003.

Weidner, Jay, and Vincent Bridges. *A Monument to the End of Time: Alchemy, Fulcanelli and the Great Cross*. Mount Gilead, N.C.: Aethyrea Books, 1999.

Wilkinson, Richard H. *Reading Egyptian Art: A Hieroglyphic Guide to Ancient Egyptian Painting and Sculpture*. London: Thames and Hudson, 1994.

_____. *Symbol and Magic in Egyptian Art*. London: Thames and Hudson, 1999.

Wilder, Alexander, trans. *Theurgia or the Egyptian Mysteries: 1911*. Kila, Mont.: Kessinger Publications, 1998.

Winston, Richard, and Clara Winston. *Notre-Dame De Paris*. New York: Newsweek Books, 1971.

Witt, R. E. *Isis in the Ancient World*. Baltimore: Johns Hopkins University Press, 1997.

Wolf, Naomi. *The Beauty Myth*. New York: Anchor Books, 1991.

Wolkstein, Diane, and Samuel Noah Kramer. *Inanna, Queen of Heaven and Earth*. New York: Harper and Row, 1983.

Woods, David. *Genesis: The First Book of Revelations*. London: Baton Press, 1985.

Zimmer, Heinrich. *Artistic Form in Yoga in the Sacred Images of India*. Princeton: Princeton University Press, 1984.

_____. *Myths and Symbols in Indian Art and Civilization*. New York: Harper and Row, 1962.

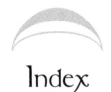

Index

adornment, 171, 172
agrarian civilizations, 136
alchemy, 96, 97, 100–105, 112
   See also Fulcanelli; telluric
     energy
Allione, Tsultrim, 54
altered states of consciousness,
   86
amusement, 204
ancestors, reverence for, 15–16
ankh, 78, 108, *109*, 110, 244
art, sacred, 137–39, 142
astral body, 82
Athena, 83
Aufu, 82
Australian aborigines, 129–30,
   133, 155, 172, 179
Avalokitisvara, 248, 251–52

bardo, 62
base chakra, 256
beauty, 171, 172, 173
Begg, Ean, 111
Bernays, Edward, 161–62
bhakti, 30
Bhavani, Enakshi, 8
bindu, 194
Black Madonna, 111–14
Black Virgin, 101–2, 111–12
   See also prima materia
Blessed Virgin Mary, 85, 181,
   245, 246–48
bliss, 171, 237, 266
Blofeld, John, 249–50

Book of the Dead, 115, 217
Brahma Kumaris, 146
breath, 194
Bronze Age, 135–40
Budge, Wallis, 216–17

Cathari, 106, 120–23
Catholic Church, 105, 120, 122
Celts, 98, 111, 225
central channel, 195
cervix, 195
chakras, 28
   See also specific chakras
Chartres Cathedral, 111,
   112–13
children, 173
chod, 59–61
Christ, 46, 104–5, 114–16, 117,
   121
civilization, 141–42
clothing, 17–18, 171
Communism, 144
compassion. *See* love and compassion
conditioning, negative, 87–88
consumerism, 160–61
   See also materialism
contentment, 238–39
cow, 126–27
craniosacral therapy, 69–71, 82
creation, 127
cross, 110
crown chakra, 198, 229–30, 258
crucible, 100, 108

culture, 137–38

dakinis
   described, 44, 45, 47, 49
   as enlightened energy,
     50–51
   as essence of Divine
     Feminine, 52
   transforming into, 47, 48
   See also Mandarava;
     Simhamukha; Tara
dark retreat, 59, 63–66
deliberation, 206
demureness, 235–36
determination, 208
devotion, 25, 263
Diamond Age, 146
divine love, 263–64
Divine Mother. *See* Goddess
dreaminess, 233–34
dreaming, 9, 164
Dreamtime, 128–30, 155, 179,
   181
dream yoga, 61, 62–63
Durga
   dance of, 32–34
   described, 188–89
   myth of, 189–92
   Sitara Devi as, 10, 12–13
Dzogchen, 41, 43, 54, 59,
   63–66
   See also Norbu, Namkhai

ecstasy, 239–40

Edlibi, Ramzi El, 92, 93, 96
elders, 172–73
elements, five, 132
elixir of life, 100
emotions
    expressing, 199–200
    physical body and, 87
    purification of, 53–54
    transmuting, 192–93
    true nature of, 58
empathy, 264
enchantment, 238
end of the world, 146
energy body, 65, 83–84, 165,
    177, 271
enlightenment, 44, 62, 145,
    212, 231
entropy, 127
extrasensory perception, 136,
    176, 178
eyes, 199, 200, 203, 259

female body, 21, 212
femininity
    clothing and, 17–18
    distortion of, 30, 37
    in modern times, 151–52,
    159
    sensuality and, 26, 29–30,
    34
feminism, 4, 151–52, 159,
    162–63, 171–72
fierceness, 205–6
fiery Goddess. See strength and
    power
Filoramo, Giovanni, 104
Finney, Jean, 38–39
flirtatiousness, 236–37
Friedan, Betty, 159, 160
Fulcanelli, 90, 99, 100, 101,
    106, 111–12, 129

Ganges river, 19–21
Garden of Eden, 128–29
gesture
    sacred, 17, 18
    See also mudra
glance of penetration, 203

See also eyes
gnostics, 104–5, 114–16,
    120–23, 156–57
Goddess
    healing power of, 259,
    260–61
    manifestations of, 164
    as role model, 153, 164
    Sitara Devi as, 12–13
    statues of, 81
    Triple Goddess, 164–65, 182
    women and, 153, 154,
    164–71, 183–84
    See also goddesses; Shakti
goddesses
    of love and compassion,
    164, 168, 243–53, 254
    peaceful goddess, 255–58
    as personifications, 137
    of sensuality, 164, 171,
    212–24
    of strength and power, 164,
    166, 184–93
Golden Age, 13, 126, 128–30,
    146
Gothic cathedrals, 105–11
gratitude, 262–63
Great Mother, 17, 24
Grey, Alex, 165, 177
Gunga, 19, 21

Haidit, 82
Hathor, 215–17
healing
    craniosacral therapy as,
    69–71
    dieties of, 85
    in Egypt, 83
    Goddess and, 259, 260–61
    modalities, 69, 88
    Sekhmet and, 81–82, 88
heart center, 196, 228, 257
hieroglyphs, 94
history of humanity. See yugas
Homo luminous, 146
honesty, 271
Hope, Murray, 215
Horus, 108, 244–45

Houston, Jean, 71–72, 80–81,
    87, 94
humility, 261
hunter-gatherers, 133, 134, 136

iaret, 76
Inanna, 180, 217–19
Incan shamans, 146
Indian classical dance. See
    Kathak classical dance
industrialization, 144
initiation, 36, 54–55
inner eye. See mystic eye
Inquisition, 143–44
inspiration, 261–62
intoxication, 207–8
Iron Age, 13, 105, 106, 126,
    140–45, 220
Isis
    alchemical secrets of,
    100–101
    ankh and, 108
    as Black Virgin, 112
    dance of, 94–96
    described, 181, 244–45
    embodying, 92, 93, 94, 95,
    110–11

joy, 237–38
Judaism. See Kabbalah
Jung, Carl, 60

Ka, 82
Kabbalah, 106, 117–18, 119,
    120, 156
Kali, 13, 126, 180–81, 184–85
Kali Yuga. See Iron Age
Kama Sutra, 28
Kandro, Ayu, 59
karma, 43, 61–62
Kathak classical dance, 6–8,
    14–15, 21, 25, 26
Katha Nritya, 14–15
Khan, Ustad Imrat, 8
Khu, 82
Kleopatra, 103
Krishna, 29, 31
Kuan Yin, 85, 248–50

Kundalini Shakti. *See* Shakti

Lakshmi, 13, 213–15
Lambert, Johanna, 130, 155, 172
Lapdron, Machig, 59–60
Lawlor, Robert, 67, 130, 133
Leake, Paul, 41, 42
light, 46, 146–47
   See also rainbow body
light body practice, 103
love and compassion
   divine, 263–64
   goddesses of, 164, 168, 243–53, 254
   spiritual awakening and, 25, 147
   visualizations, 240, 255–68
   See also Isis; Kuan Yin; Tara
luminosity, 44
luminous ball of light, 43, 64
luminous energy body, 65, 83–84, *165*, *177*, 271

magical body, 82
majesty, 204–5
mandalas, 52
Mandarava, 47, 117, 180, 219–23
mantras
   creation of, 131
   dakinis and, 51–52
   Om Mani Padme Hung, 250
   Om Tare Tutare Ture Svaha, 65, 250, 253
   Sa Sekham Sâhu, 73–74, 85
Markert, Margaret Ann, 69–71
Mary Magdalene, 114–16, 117, 156–57
masculinity, 131
Masters, Robert, 71–89
materialism, 37, 136, 145, 161, 162, 174–79
   See also consumerism
matriarchy, 135
men, 135, 137, 142, 153–54
   See also patriarchy
menopause, 172

Middle Eastern dance, 91–92
mind, 55–56, 179–80
Mirabai, 30–32
Montsegur, *112*, 120, 122
Mother Earth, 225, 226, 232
Mother Nature, 136, 142, 143, 225, 241, 271
mudras, 18, 70, 131
mysteries, 135, 143–44, 153, 157, 270
mysteriousness, 236
mystical marriage, 94, 103
mystic eye, 28, 85
myths/legends, 125, 129, 131, 137

namaste, 17
Narby, Jeremy, 155
navel chakra, 228
Naydler, Jeremy, 215–16
neters, 80, 130
New Age, 175–79
nobility, 264–65
Norbu, Namkhai
   about, 39–41, 42
   chod practice of, 59
   on dakinis, 44, 48, 50–51
   teachings of, 43, 54, 55–56, 57–58, 62–63
Notre Dame Cathedral, 106–11

oracles, 178
Osiris, 92, 94, 244

pacification, 206–7
Padilla, Adelina Avla, 134
Padmasambhava, 38, 43–44, 50, 116–17, 156, 220, 222–23
Palmer, Martin, 248, 249
passion, 54, 209, 212, 234–35
Patai, Raphael, 119
patriarchy, 143
peaceful goddess, 255–58
philosopher's stone, 102
playfulness, 208–9
pleasure, 87
power. *See* strength and power
prayer, 164

pregnancy/birth, 134
pride, divine, 202–3
priestesses
   hierarchy of, 137
   sacred role of, 18, 24–25
   as sexual initiators, 26
   temple priestesses, 139
prima materia, 100, 101–2, 107, 108, 111–12
primordial state, 42–43, 54–55, 58
protection techniques, 83–84, 85
psychedelics, 5–6, 175
psychics, 154, 176
psychophysical work, 86
pujas, 25
purification, 182

Radha, *27*, 29
radiance, 267–68
rainbow body, 46, 82, 103
Ramsay, Jay, 248, 249
Rangdrol, Jatang Tsokdruk, 180
rapture, 268
receptivity, 233
reincarnation, 46
religion, 133
resurrection, 46, 103, 104–5
Reynolds, John Myrdhin, 187–88
rigpa, 54
rites of passage, 153–54
ritual, 131, 138, 140–41
role models, 153, 157, 164, 180

sacred dance, 2, 16, 164
   See also transformation
Sâhu. *See* rainbow body
Saint Athanasius, 246
Sambhogakaya, 130
Saraswati, 13, 21–24
Scholem, Gershom, 118, 119
second chakra, 195–96, 256
sekhem, 75
Sekhmet, 72–85, 88, 186–87
self-confidence, 202
self-observation, 57–58
sensuality
   art of, 231–41

goddesses of, 164, 171,
    212–24
visualizations, 225–30
See also Hathor; Inanna;
    Lakshmi; Mandarava
sexual union, 26, 30, 97–98,
    119, 143, 231
shadow body, 82
Shakti
    attunement to, 199, 259
    awakening of, 26, 28,
        225–27, 231, 241
    cerebrospinal fluid and, 70
    conduits for, 132
    described, 12
    as luminosity, 44
    protection and, 83
    Sekhmet and, 73
    strength from, 147
    women as incarnation of, 13
shamans, 133–34, 146, 155
Shaw, Miranda, 231
Shekhina, 117–18, 119, 127,
    147
Shiva, 12, 19, 20, 21, 127, 190,
    191
Silver Age, 130–35
Simhamukha, 47, 79, 166,
    187–88
Sitara Devi, 8–35
Skinner, B.F., 160
sky-dancers. See dakinis
solar plexus chakra, 257
soothingness, 266–67
soul retrieval, 67–68
sound, sacred, 15
statues, 81
strength and power
    emotional expression as,
        199–200
    goddesses of, 164, 166,
        184–93
    visualizations, 194–209
    See also Durga; Kali;
        Sekhmet; Simhamukha

Talukdar, Dulal, 6–7
tantra
    alchemy and, 102
    beginning stages of, 19
    described, 51–52
    goddess worship of, 13
    protection techniques,
        83–84, 85
    women and, 156
    See also Durga; Kali; Shakti;
        Tibetan Tantric
        Buddhism
Tara, 47, 48, 64–65, 85,
    169–70, 250–53
teachings, hidden, 10, 50, 101
telluric energy, 225, 229
temple dance, 164
temples, 67, 80–81, 84, 138
termas, 10, 50, 101
theater, 18, 139
third eye, 197, 229, 258
throat chakra, 197, 229, 258
Tibetan Tantric Buddhism
    development of, 38–39,
        43–44
    Dzogchen and, 54
    Golden Age and, 130
    lineage of, 41–42
    path of, 43
    See also dakinis; Dzogchen;
        Simhamukha
Tolkien, J.R.R., 140
Tower of Babel, 136
transfiguration, 103
transformation
    healing and, 259
    into a goddess/dakini,
        84–85, 153
    Kali and, 126
    purification from, 53–54
    sacred art of, 14–15, 16, 50,
        52
transmission, 42, 54–55
tree of life, 106–8
Triple Goddess, 164–65, 182
twilight language, 50

Universal Mother, 110, 213

Villoldo, Alberto, 146
Virgin Mary. See Blessed Virgin
    Mary
Vishnu, 213, 214

Way of the Five Bodies of
    Sekhmet, 81–82, 88
Weidner, Jay, 96–123
wildness, 209
Withers, Maida, 4
Wolf, Naomi, 171, 172
Wolkstein, Diane, 217
women
    emotional nature of, 54
    extrasensory perception and,
        178
    feminine expression dis-
        torted in, 30, 37
    Great Goddess and, 153,
        154, 164–71, 183–84
    as incarnation of Shakti, 13
    as inferior, 142–43
    men and, 153–54
    mysteries of, 135, 143–44,
        153, 157, 270
    role of, 134–35, 136–37,
        153, 154–58, 179, 180
    See also femininity
wrathful Goddess. See strength
    and power
written language, 141, 142

Yeshe Tsogyel, 44, 50, 116–17,
    156
yoni, 227–28
yugas
    Bronze Age, 135–40
    Diamond Age, 146
    Golden Age, 13, 126,
        128–30, 146
    Iron Age, 13, 105, 106, 126,
        140–45, 220
    Silver Age, 130–35
    transition time, 145–47

BOOKS OF RELATED INTEREST

THE TRIPLE GODDESS TAROT
The Power of the Major Arcana, Chakra Healing,
and the Divine Feminine
by Isha Lerner
Illustrated by Mara Friedman

THE WOMAN WITH THE ALABASTER JAR
Mary Magdalen and the Holy Grail
by Margaret Starbird

SACRED WOMAN, SACRED DANCE
Awakening Spirituality Through Movement and Ritual
by Iris J. Stewart

THE GODDESS IN EVERY GIRL
Develop Your Teen Feminine Power
by M. J. Abadie

THE GREAT GODDESS
Reverence of the Divine Feminine from the Paleolithic to the Present
by Jean Markale

THE GODDESS IN INDIA
The Five Faces of the Eternal Feminine
by Devdutt Pattanaik

A YOGA OF INDIAN CLASSICAL DANCE
The Yogini's Mirror
by Roxanne Kamayani Gupta, Ph.D.

HATHOR RISING
The Power of the Goddess in Ancient Egypt
by Alison Roberts, Ph.D.

Inner Traditions • Bear & Company
P.O. Box 388
Rochester, VT 05767
1-800-246-8648
www.InnerTraditions.com

Or contact your local bookseller